Epidemic of Cardiovascular Disease and Diabetes

Epidemic of Cardiovascular Disease and Diabetes

Explaining the Phenomenon in South Asians Worldwide

Raj S. Bhopal, **CBE, DSc(hon), BSc, MBchB, MPH, MD, FRCP, FFPH**

Bruce and John Usher Chair of Public Health
and Honorary Consultant in Public Health Medicine
The University of Edinburgh
and
NHS Lothian Health Board

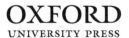

OXFORD
UNIVERSITY PRESS

OXFORD
UNIVERSITY PRESS

Great Clarendon Street, Oxford, OX2 6DP,
United Kingdom

Oxford University Press is a department of the University of Oxford.
It furthers the University's objective of excellence in research, scholarship,
and education by publishing worldwide. Oxford is a registered trade mark of
Oxford University Press in the UK and in certain other countries

Published in the United States of America by Oxford University Press
198 Madison Avenue, New York, NY 10016, United States of America

British Library Cataloguing in Publication Data

Data available

Library of Congress Control Number: 2019930898

ISBN 978–0–19–883324–6

Printed and bound by
CPI Group (UK) Ltd, Croydon, CR0 4YY

I dedicate this book to my sons Sunil, Vijay, Anand, and Rajan; my daughters-in-law Hannah and Manu; and my grandchildren Leo and Ethan. It is their love and inspiration, and the quest for their health and well-being and especially the hope that they will avoid cardiovascular diseases and type 2 diabetes that have been the scourge of my extended family, which has provided me with the energy and motivation to complete this work.

Forewords

I met Dr Raj Bhopal in New Delhi about 10 years back for the first time. I was immediately struck by his forthrightness and boyish effervescence. We talked about India, food, and his life in UK. But in between such mundane discussion, he would ask me incisive academic questions to pick on my brains. I already knew he was trying to gauge my present and future research expanse. It is as if I already knew him closely by reading his papers, especially several hypotheses. I always refer to and project a slide of his brilliant 'adipose tissue compartment overflow' hypothesis. It was like knowing Stephen King's brain and personality by reading his books, not having met him or visited Castle Rock, Main (USA).

I did not believe he could put together so many papers, hypotheses and views so elegantly in one place. This book is an all encompassing compendium of knowledge on cardiovascular and diabetes in south Asians. Clarity in Dr Raj Bhopal's approach is visible throughout. For example, people (many researchers) do not know what 'south Asians' means or what is their historical background.

Mastery of biostatistics and public health is also evident. Among the unique features of this book (including summaries of interview with key researchers worldwide), I found filling the jigsaw puzzle of determinants and risk factors brilliant. I liked the way Dr Bhopal has built up the puzzle in much of a 'Hitchcock' style and completed it at the end of the book. A discussion on 'non-traditional risk factors' is often overdone my many writers, but Dr Raj Bhopal has put it cleverly and concisely. His masterful insight into diet and culture of south Asians stems from his own ethnic background and constantly keeping his keen eye on the ground.

People may ask; is this book too intellectually angled? I think it is the opposite as the analysis is simple and helpful; hypotheses are clearly explained; and the text reads like solving a mystery and a jigsaw puzzle; and clues for future research are hidden throughout yet in plain sight. Numerous researchers and physicians interested in this area are going to love this book. For me, the most important outcome may be that this book may launch a thousand research studies!

Anoop Misra
New Delhi, India
August 2018

There are two indisputable facts which underpin the quest to interpret and explain the epidemic of cardiovascular disease in south Asian populations. First of all, the world is now a much smaller place with the advent of globalisation. As a consequence, we are veering away from the dogma that populations are indigenous, to the ancient aboriginal wisdom that people belong to the land, not land to the people. South Asians are therefore not restricted to south Asia and migration to European pastures and beyond has generated patterns of cardiovascular disease which are fertile ground for academic inquisition. Secondly we are all more similar than we are different. So why then do south Asians have different patterns of cardiovascular disease despite sharing similar genotypes and risk factors? High income countries not only have much to contribute but much to learn from the study of a diaspora. If ever there was one academic mind which has the rigour and discipline to seek answers to the question of why we are so similar yet so different, it is Raj Bhopal. Here we have an exemplary approach to exploring the questions, hypotheses and answers which have emerged in an organised manner as Raj has opened up Pandora's box.

Dr Kiran Patel
Medical Director, NHS England (West Midlands)

Preface

In 1984 when I was in my early training in public health I was confronted by this question—a googly—by Professor William Littler, professor of cardiovascular medicine at Birmingham University who I met at a conference: What do you think of South Asians' risk of coronary heart disease? (I paraphrase.) I replied that I would expect them to have less risk because of their lower prevalence of smoking and higher prevalence of vegetarianism. At the same conference, shortly thereafter, Professor Michael Marmot presented the first UK data showing that men in England and Wales who were born in the Indian Subcontinent had an age-standardized mortality ratio about 15% higher than in those predominantly White European origin people born in England and Wales. Professor Littler surely knew South Asians had a relatively high risk of coronary heart disease (CHD) but he had the good grace not to refute my youthful ignorance based on first principles. In 1985 the Southall Diabetes Survey in London showed an extraordinarily high prevalence of diabetes mellitus in the predominantly Indian, Punjabi-origin population there. I had a premonition that what was happening to South Asians in the UK was a forewarning of what would happen in South Asia as it 'modernized'.

My research and scholarship has taken many directions since 1984 but the question of why South Asians are prone to CHD, stroke, and type 2 DM_2 diabetes has never left my mind since that conversation with Professor Littler. It has been a challenge and a privilege to synthesize international research and scholarship on his question, but broadening it to stroke and DM_2.

Science works best when it is either based on an explicit theory or, in the absence of one, is undertaking empirical work that leads to one. Unfortunately, the state of the art on South Asians' tendency to cardiovascular diseases and DM_2 does not yet lead to a theory that is widely accepted. Nonetheless, to progress towards one I have purposively integrated work on three different kinds of scientific endeavour:

a) Expositions of causal hypotheses or general causal ideas

b) Reviews of the topic providing contextual background and information on the burden of disease and socio-economic circumstances and relationships between them

c) Studies of specific risk factors and their relationship to the outcomes of interest

With one exception (the thrifty phenotype), given its centrality in current thinking, and the lack of an alternative quantitative review, I have not delved into the details of the methods and results of a set of specific studies but relied on others' reviews, and what struck me as being important individual studies. I think readers will recognize that as a practical and appropriate approach.

I have done something unusual—perhaps even unique—in that after drafting my book, I then discussed with twenty-two internationally recognized researchers/scholars about their favoured explanations for South Asians' susceptibility to CHD, stroke, or DM_2. Their accounts are given as an appendix and summarized in the text in Chapter 9.

I hope I have accomplished my aim of producing an easy to read, up-to-date synthesis of the state of knowledge on the chosen topic. I have set out new directions and ideas and been able to de-emphasize those that do not look to me as if they will stand the test of time. Of course, I have inevitably reached some wrong conclusions. As this book will be published after my retirement, I now hand over the baton to the up-and-coming generation to build on my work just as I have done with that of others. Surely, they will correct my errors and misjudgements for the benefit of hundreds of millions of people like me and my family who are affected unnecessarily by these almost wholly preventable chronic diseases.

Raj Bhopal
30 May 2018

Acknowledgements

The opportunity to think long and hard, and to read extensively, is rare in modern academic and professional life. I am, therefore, deeply grateful to my employers, The University of Edinburgh and NHS Lothian Board for nine months of sabbatical leave to lay the foundation for this project. My colleagues David Weller, Sarah Cunningham-Burley, Harry Campbell, and Alison McCallum were instrumental in paving the way for me, and I thank them and many colleagues at the Usher Institute of Population Health Sciences and Informatics for this opportunity.

Many colleagues have helped me think about the questions raised in this book but twenty-two of them shared their innermost thoughts on the topic. They are listed in the appendix together with a digest of their ideas.

I was invited by the Cardiological Society of India to give a plenary lecture in Kolkata, India, at their 69th conference in November/December 2017 and to summarize the ideas here in twelve minutes. The focusing of the mind in meeting this challenge, and the discussions with colleagues there, helped with the concluding chapters of the book.

Sometimes, given the complexity and difficulty of this project, I have felt foolish in attempting it. Encouraging and supportive words from my colleagues, especially in the Edinburgh Migration and Ethnicity Health Research Group, have given me courage and especially by providing me feedback when presenting my arguments. One member—Dr Danijela Gasivec—even read the whole manuscript and gave me immensely useful feedback, which was both critically constructive and energizing because of its positivity. I cannot fully express my gratitude especially as she has a young child to look after and relocated to Australia during this period.

Expert and enthusiastic help was provided by my secretary, Anne Houghton until she retired in December 2017, and subsequently by my personal assistant, Jayne Richards, and by Dawn Cattanach who prepared some of the figures.

I first mentioned the idea of this book to OUP's then commissioning editor, Helen Liepman, in the mid-1990s. It is testimony to my lasting relationship with OUP that this plan has come to fruition under the guiding hand of Nicola Wilson, Senior Commissioning Editor of OUP and her team.

My wife Roma was, as ever, patient and understanding when I converted the spare bedroom into a study during my nine-month sabbatical. After my previous books I have offered her a Caribbean Cruise but she has never taken up this invitation. I need to increase my offer. Might the Galapagos Islands tempt her as more adequate thanks?

Contents

Abbreviations

AGE	advanced glycation end product	ICD	International Classification of Diseases
Apo (A, B)	apolipoprotein A or B	ICMR-INDIAB	Indian council for Medical Research-India diabetes study
ATP	adenosine triphosphate		
BMI	body mass index		
BP	blood pressure	IHD	ischaemic heart disease
CAD	coronary artery disease (see CHD, synonym)	IMT	intima media thickness
		LDL-C	low density lipoprotein cholesterol
CARRS	Centre for Cardiometabolic Risk Reduction in South Asia Surveillance Study	Lp(a)	lipoprotein (a)
		MI	myocardial infarction
CHD	coronary heart disease	NFC(s)	neo-formed contaminant(s) (see TFAs and AGEs)
CRP/hs-CRP	high sensivity C-reactive protein		
CT	computed tomography	OXPHOS	oxidative phosphorylation
CVD	cardiovascular disease (sometimes used to mean cerebro-vascular disease but not so here)	PURE	Prospective Urban Rural Epidemiology Study
DAG	directed acyclic graph	PWV	pulse wave velocity
DARTS	Diabetes Audit and Research in Tayside Scotland	RNA	ribonucleic acid
		SHELS	Scottish Health and Ethnicity Linkage Study
DM/DM$_2$	type 2 diabetes mellitus	SNP	single nucleotide polymorphism
DNA	deoxyribonucleic acid		
DOHAD	developmental origins of health and adult disease	TFA(s)	trans fatty acid(s)
		UK	United Kingdom
		UN	United Nations
FFA(s)	free fatty acid(s)	US(A)	United States of America
GWAS	genome-wide association study		
		VLDL-c	very low density lipoprotein cholesterol
HDL-c	high density lipoprotein cholesterol	WHO	World Health Organization
HOMA (IR or B)	homeostatic model assessment (insulin resistance or beta-cell function)		

Glossary

I want this book to be accessible and easy for all readers and not just medical professionals. I have minimized medical, epidemiological, and other jargon but technical words are unavoidable. I have explained technical words at first mention but, nonetheless, readers may not be reading sequentially or may need reminding of the meanings of unfamiliar words. Of course, it is easy to check meanings in dictionaries and especially with internet access. Yet, I don't want my readers to go to such trouble especially as such resources can be complex. My glossary is simple and expressed in my words, although, sensibly, I have cross-checked my entries using various sources. I have drawn upon my glossaries in *Concepts of Epidemiology* and *Migration, Ethnicity, Race and Health*.

Word/phrase Definition

Adiponectin A hormone produced in adipose tissue that has several functions including in glucose metabolism, which is statistically associated with protection from cardiovascular disease.

Adiposity/adipose tissue The connective tissue that is predominately fat cells and part of the vital body organ that is fat. Adiposity is the amount of such tissue.

Adrenaline See catecholamines.

Adipocyte The main cell in fat tissue that stores fat.

Advanced glycation end products Glycated proteins and lipids formed naturally but accelerated by various processes including heating of food.

Allostasis The capacity to alter the value of a variable and maintain homeostasis around that new value, e.g. raised or lowered blood pressure or body weight.

Apolipoproteins Proteins that bind lipids for transport around the body as lipoproteins, e.g. low density lipoprotein cholesterol.

Angina (pectoris) This is a discomfort or pain, traditionally in the chest (hence pectoris; Latin for chest is pectus). However, angina can be elsewhere, e.g. the jaw or back, and such atypical presentations are especially important in South Asians, and again especially in South Asian women.

Arrhythmias A variety of disturbances characterized by irregularity or abnormally slow or fast beating of the heart. Some are not generally harmful, e.g. ectopic beats, and some often fatal, e.g. ventricular fibrillation.

Arterial stiffness The result of reduced elasticity of the arterial wall (see also arteriosclerosis) with adverse effects on cardiovascular function. The pulse wave when the heart beats then travels faster.

Arteriosclerosis The loss of elasticity of the wall of the artery usually a result of thickening and hardening. It is usually thought of as a feature of aging.

Arteriole A small, narrow, and thin-walled artery that precedes the capillary. The arteriole is part of the microcirculation.

Artery The blood vessels that leave the heart either to conduct blood to the lungs (pulmonary circulation) or the rest of the body. These blood vessels have thick muscular walls and need their own blood supply (vasa vasorum—see below).

Asystole There is no detectable pulse indicating the left ventricle of the heart is not functioning properly. Death is imminent without cardiac resuscitation (or has already occurred).

Atherosclerosis A complex pathological process whereby a fibrous and fatty material, together with inflammatory cells and calcium, is deposited inside the arterial wall, often as quite discrete plaques. This process is the core pathology in the modern epidemic of ischaemic heart disease and stroke. The plaques narrow the artery, and may rupture or be the focus of thrombosis.

ATP (adenosine triphosphate) This is the molecule that stores and supplies energy for molecular functions at the level of the individual cell. ATP production in humans is mainly in mitochondria.

Autonomic nervous system The nervous system that regulates bodily functions, e.g. heart rate, but is not under conscious control, consisting primarily of the hypothalamus in the brain and the sympathetic and parasympathetic nervous systems.

Bangladeshi A person whose ancestry lies in the Indian subcontinent who self-identifies, or is identified, as Bangladeshi. (See also South Asian.) Between 1947 and 1971 the land known as Bangladesh was East Pakistan and before that India.

Bidis (or beedis) A form of cigarette where instead of paper a leaf is used to roll the tobacco. They are cheap and popular in South Asia.

Beta cells The cells in the Islets of Langerhans in the pancreas that produce insulin.

Biraderi/beraderi This is a subgrouping akin to a clan or tribe, the word being derived from one meaning brotherhood. It is often closely related to sub-groups within castes.

Blood pressure (BP) Usually refers to the pressure in the arteries supplying the body except for the lungs (i.e. not veins and pulmonary arteries) as measured by a sphygmomanometer (see below).

Body mass index (BMI) This is a simple way of assessing weight while adjusting for height. The formula is weight in kilogrammes divided by height in metres squared. The WHO defines a BMI of more than 25 kg/m² overweight and 30kg/m² or more as obese. These cut-offs are considered by many as too high for South Asians.

Cardiometabolic A term to encapsulate the connection between the cardiovascular and metabolic diseases, particularly but not solely, diabetes mellitus.

Cardiovascular disease A phrase that includes a range of disorders of the heart and blood vessels.

Caste A form of social hierarchy created around broad kinds of occupations that are associated with certain groups of people across many generations, with movement inhibited in or out of the group. The group is the caste. The caste determines a multiplicity of social factors, e.g. who you marry so it fosters a degree of inbreeding as well as wealth-related inequality. Caste is ingrained in the Indian subcontinent even though it is now outlawed.

Catecholamines The term for adrenaline (**epinephrine**) and noradrenaline (**norepinephrine**), and dopamine hormonal products .

Cause/causation Something which has an effect, in the case of epidemiology this effect being (primarily) a change in the frequency of risk factors or adverse health outcomes.

Cerebral arteries The main arteries in the front of the neck going to the brain are the cerebral arteries and the blood supply is called the cerebral circulation.

Cerebrovascular disease A general term for a range of diseases of the circulation of the brain, but most commonly called stroke, so the two are often synonymous.

Chinese A person with ancestral origins in China, who self-identifies, or is identified, as Chinese.

Cholesterol A lipid (fatty substance) that is essential to many bodily functions that is transported in the blood via lipoproteins. Cholesterol and other lipids carried by low/very low-density lipoproteins (LDL/VLDL) are a risk factor for cardiovascular diseases.

Chromosome See gene.

Clot (blood) Congealed blood, the change from liquid to semi-solid being a result of the clotting mechanism. The medical term is thrombosis and hence the phrase coronary thrombosis which is sometimes used for an acute myocardial infarction.

Collateral circulation Blood vessels that provide a back-up for the main blood supply, opening up when needed.

Consanguinity Inbreeding.

Coronary artery disease A group of diseases resulting from reduced blood supply to the heart, most often caused by narrowing or blockage of the coronary arteries that provide the blood supply to the heart. More commonly this is known as coronary heart disease.

Coronary heart disease (CHD) See coronary artery disease.

Cortisol A steroid hormone produced by the adrenal gland and essential for many functions. It is considered a good masker of psychosocial stress and is involved in glucose production and hence is of special interest in cardiovascular disease and diabetes mellitus type 2 research.

C-reactive protein/hs-CRP C-reactive protein (CRP)/high sensitivity-CRP (hs-CRP) molecule is increased in the course of inflammation. It is one of the most important clinical markers of inflammation, including that associated with atherosclerosis (when hs-CRP is used).

Creole An uncommon word used to describe people of mixed European and African ancestry living or originating from the West Indies and parts of South America. The main use of this term in ethnicity and health research is in Dutch studies of the Surinamese, who are divided mainly into Creole and Hindu (see also Hindu). Creole is also a language.

Demographic transition The change in the age structure of the population after death rates and fertility rates decline, with a comparatively older population being the result.

Diabetes mellitus type 1 A disease characterized by high levels of glucose in the blood caused by lack of the hormone insulin.

Diabetes mellitus type 2 A disease characterized by high levels of glucose in the blood caused by either lack or ineffectiveness of the hormone insulin.

Diaspora A scattering of people, as in migration of South Asians far and wide. In this context it refers to those outside the country of origin.

Diastolic (blood pressure) The blood pressure when the heart is not beating.

DNA See gene.

DOHAD (hypothesis) The complex of ideas that fetal and early life determines susceptibility to adult health and disease. The hypothesis is discussed in detail in the book. See also thrifty phenotype.

Ectopic fat The word ectopic implies the fat is out of place, which is a misnomer. It is actually used, in practice, to refer to adipose tissue depots or deposition in higher than usual amount around and in the organs, e.g. pericardial fat and intrahepatic fat. There is much interest in ectopic fat in South Asian populations.

Effect modification The phenomenon whereby the relative risk associated with a factor is altered by the presence of another characteristic. The classic example is that the risk of lung cancer is much greater in smokers who were also exposed to asbestos. In our context, the question is whether the effects of risk factors such as smoking vary by migrant status, race, or ethnic group.

Embolus An object moving through the circulation of blood sometimes causing a harmful blockage downstream usually in the smaller arteries or arterioles. In this book's context the emboli that matter are fragments of atheromatous plaque or of blood clots.

Endothelial dysfunction This refers to the state where the arterial wall is not functioning optimally, e.g. dilating, because the lining of the artery, the endothelium, is not releasing chemicals such as the dilator nitric oxide in the required amount or time.

Endothelium The single layer of interconnected cells that lines the entire vascular system including the heart and the venous and arterial circulations. Impairment of this layer is thought to be central to atherosclerosis.

Environment A broad conception, sometimes to mean everything except genetic and biological factors, and sometimes qualified and narrowed, e.g. physical environment.

Epidemic Traditionally this was the occurrence of large numbers of cases of infectious diseases but is now applied to all health outcomes where the number substantially exceeds that expected given past experience as in the epidemic of CHD.

Epidemiological transition The change in disease patterns that accompanies the demographic transition, with both transitions usually following economic, educational, or social improvements.

Epidemiology The science and craft that studies the pattern of diseases (and health, though usually indirectly) in populations to help understand both their causes and the burden they impose. This information is applied to prevent, control, or manage the problems under study.

Epigenetics The study of the process whereby the function (expression) of the genes is altered as a result of the non-genetic (environmental) influences. One of the important processes is through methylation.

Epinephrine See catecholamines.

Ethnicity The social group a person belongs to, and either identifies with or is identified with by others, as a result of a mix of cultural and other factors including one or more of language, diet, religion, ancestry, and physical features traditionally associated with race. Increasingly, the concept is being used synonymously with race but the trend is pragmatic rather than scientific.

European/White European See White European.

Fat oxidation/lipid oxidation The breakdown of fatty acids, mainly in the mitochondria, to generate energy. The process is important for atherosclerosis too as lipids such as low density lipo protein-c can be oxidized and have complex effects including uptake by macrophages. Oxidized fats/lipids have been associated with atherosclerosis.

Fatty acids See free fatty acids.

Fatty liver A build-up of fat in the liver, often a result of being overweight to a greater extent than normal. A common resulting problem relevant to this book is impairment of glucose metabolism as a result of hepatic insulin resistance.

Fetal origins hypothesis See DOHAD (Developmental origins of health and adult disease).

Fibrinogen An important molecule in the blood clotting pathway which is a commonly used clinical marker.

Fibrosis The process whereby connective tissues are laid down to cause hardening and scarring of tissues, often as part of repair or ageing process. Fibrosis is part of the process of atherosclerosis and repair of the heart and other organs after myocardial infraction.

Fitness (cardio-respiratory) The ability of the heart, lungs, and muscle to function during prolonged and vigorous physical activity. It is usually measured by maximal oxygen use during such physical activity: fit people use more oxygen.

Free fatty acids Lipids (fats) are mostly held in storage, e.g. in subcutaneous or intraabdominal depots as triglycerides. However, as they are transported in the bloodstream they are bound to proteins. In this form they are called fatty acids; when there is no ester bond they are called free fatty acids. In this form they are an alternative fuel to glucose and increase insulin resistance.

Gene The discrete basic unit (made of DNA or deoxyribonucleic acid) of the chromosome, which itself consists of numerous genes and other DNA material. Genes carry information coding for specific functions, e.g. making proteins. This information is carried to the cell by a chemical very similar to DNA, i.e. RNA (ribonucleic acid) There are two genes (one from the father, the other from the mother) at a particular location on a chromosome—both for the same function. Variants of the same gene on a particular location are called alleles. There are 23 pairs of chromosomes in each cell in human beings (46 in total), and the number of genes is estimated at about 20,000.

Genetics The study of heredity, nowadays the structure and function of the chromosomes and their components such as genes including their interaction with the environment through epigenetics.

Genotype The genetic makeup of a cell, and hence the individual (as all normal cells except sperm and ova contain the same genes).

Ghee Butter is heated and the non-fat components separated. The fat components become ghee, a product greatly coveted in much of South Asia as a food with health and religious properties. As ghee is high in saturated and trans fats, there have been concerns about its health effects. It is easily confused with Vanaspati hydrogenated oil formulated to be like ghee, which is very high in trans fats.

Glycaemic food index This refers to the estimate of how a food or drink will be digested and release glucose (from the intestine) into the bloodstream. It is based on the carbohydrate content of the food and ranks foods on how they change blood glucose.

Glomerulus A cluster of blood vessels, nerve ending, and other tissues in a globular shape at the top of the nephron which is key functioning unit of the kidney, reabsorbing necessary fluids and electrolytes, and excreting the remainder as urine.

Glycosylation The binding of carbohydrates to proteins, lipids, and other molecules. It is an important normal process. In the context of this book the binding of glucose and other simple sugars is of particular interest (glycation or non-enzymatic glycosylation). This is potentially damaging. See also glycosylated haemoglobin (HbA1c).

Genome-wide association study (GWAS) A large number of SNPs (see below) are identified across the genome and in a large population associations are sought between the variants and outcomes of interest. If an association is found it locates a chromosome and a section of the chromosome to the outcome. Further studies are needed to pinpoint the genes and gene functions that are potentially causally related.

Haemoglobin The molecule in the red blood cell that carries oxygen from the lungs to the tissues.

Haemorrhage A bleed; in our context one that occurs in the brain or in an atherosclerotic plaque.

HbA1c/glycosylated haemoglobin This is the glycation (glycosylation) of haemoglobin the oxygen-carrying molecule in red blood cells. A high number reflects high levels of glucose over the previous two/three months. It is a key measure of well controlled diabetes mellitus and is also used for diagnosis.

Heart attack See myocardial infarction.

High density lipoprotein (HDL) See lipoprotein.

Hindu Anyone who practices the religion of Hinduism. In some countries, including the Netherlands, it is commonly used to describe South Asian populations, particularly those coming from Surinam.

Homeostasis This is the capacity to maintain equilibrium (stability) in an organism in the face of external forces for change. Homeostasis is maintained by complex regulatory mechanisms.

Hyperglycaemic High levels of glucose in the blood variably defined using cut-offs for impaired fasting glucose, impaired glucose tolerance, and diabetes mellitus type 2.

Hypertriglyceridemia High levels of the lipid triglyceride in the blood (the cut-off will vary by laboratory but is about 150mg/dl).

Hypertension A condition of having blood pressure above an arbitrarily defined level (presently 140/90). Hypertension is associated with many adverse outcomes, particularly atherosclerotic diseases.

Hypothesis A proposition that is amenable to test by scientific methods.

Impaired fasting glucose (IFG) A higher than recommended blood glucose after an overnight fast.

Impaired glucose tolerance (IGT) An abnormality of glucose metabolism detected after glucose measurements following a fast and the ingestion of a standard glucose load. It predicts a higher risk of CHD and of diabetes.

Imprinting A psychological or physical process whereby a permanent change occurs in an organism as a result of an early life experience. This is relevant to the concept of programming in the fetal/developmental origins of adult disease hypothesis (see DOHAD).

Incidence The number of new cases of an outcome, usually calculated as an incidence rate (or risk or incidence proportion) which allows easy comparison between populations taking population size and structure into account.

Indian A person whose ancestry lies in the Indian subcontinent who identifies, or is identified, as Indian (see South Asian). (There were major changes to India's geographical boundaries in 1947 when Pakistan was created.) The term may also be used to refer to Native Americans (North American Indians).

Indian Asian Synonymous for Indian (used to distinguish from Native American).

Inflammation A complex, multifaceted process essential for repairing damage, maintaining immunity against the threat of infection and fighting against foreign bodies including but, not solely, microbes. Inflammation is central in the causation and consequences of atherosclerosis. It is also enhanced with increasing adiposity.

Islets of Langerhans Clusters of cells in the pancreas including beta cells that produce insulin and alpha cells that produce glucagon, a hormone that opposes the actions of glucose.

Interaction A statistical term used in the measurement of effect modification. See also Effect modification.

Intima-media thickness The thickness of the intima and media layers of the artery, usually measured by ultrasound in the carotid artery, as a marker for atherosclerosis.

Insulin A hormone produced in the beta cell of the Islets of Langerhans in the pancreas. Insufficient functional insulin leads to diabetes mellitus as one of its many functions is to permit glucose to enter cells. With few exceptions (brain, placenta) insulin is essential for glucose entry.

Insulin resistance The action of insulin in permitting the entry of glucose into cells, especially muscle cells, is impaired. Hepatic (liver) insulin resistance is when insulin's capacity to switch off the production of glucose in the liver is impaired. The result is raised blood glucose. Fat in the liver and in muscles (the latter in Europeans but not in Indians) increases insulin resistance.

Lipids A range of chemicals of which triglycerides and fatty acids are a subclass. In the context of cardiovascular disease the focus is on blood lipids such as cholesterol.

Lipoproteins Molecules that can transport lipids, in our context, in the blood. LDL-c, for instance, consists mostly of apolipoprotein B in a membrane with the lipid inside. The membrane is lipophilic (attracted to lipid) on the inside and hydrophilic (attracted to water) on the outside.

Low density protein (LDL) As triglyceride is removed from very low density lipoprotein, the lipoprotein remaining becomes cholesterol rich and lower in density. LDL-c is the lipid most agreed as being causally related to atherosclerosis.

Lp(a) (Lipoprotein (a)) An important lipoprotein generally agreed as one of the causes of CHD and one some scholars consider is especially important in South Asians.

Menarche The age of occurrence of first menstruation (periods).

Mendelian inheritance A relatively simple form of genetic inheritance obeying Gregor Mendel's laws of inheritance.

Mendelian randomization The genes from the pair of chromosomes in the germ cells (from mother and father) are fairly randomly exchanged, in the process known as meiosis, to form a sperm cell or ovum that contain 23 chromosomes each. When the sperm and ovum unite there are, again, 46 chromosomes, the correct number. The random process is used to study the effects of gene variants on disease outcomes as an experiment of nature.

Metabolic syndrome A complex clinical concept whereby certain characteristics cluster together, e.g. high blood pressure, insulin resistance, central obesity, blood lipid abnormalities, and hyperglycaemia. The clinical definition varies. There are several sets of criteria.

Microcirculation The small vessels of the circulation, i.e. the arterioles, capillaries, and venules. In addition, the small vessels of the lymphatic system are part of the microcirculation.

Mitochondria Subcellular structures that perform the crucial task of energy and heat production.

mm Mercury (mmHg) By convention, given the widespread historical use of mercury in the sphygmomanometer, the apparatus used for measuring blood pressure, the pressure is described as the height of the column of mercury sustained by the pressure (Hg being the chemical abbreviation for mercury). BP of 120mmHg means the BP has the pressure exerted by a column of mercury 120mm high.

Mortality Death.

Morbidity Health problems excepting death (mortality), usually referring to disease.

Mutagen A substance such as radiation that damages the structure of DNA (or RNA) through mutations (i.e. permanent alterations) in the chemical structure of DNA. A single nucleotide polymorphism (SNP) is an example of the outcome of mutation at the gene level, where the nucleotide structure is altered.

Myocardial infarction The death of heart muscle from insufficient blood supply to the heart, usually caused by blockage of the coronary arteries (see also arteriosclerosis and coronary heart disease).

Neurons The cells responsible for the nervous system, i.e. brain and spinal cord and autonomic nervous system function. (There are other types of supportive cells in the nervous system).

Noradrenaline See catecholamines.

Normoglycemic The glucose levels in the blood are normal, a presumption usually made for people who do not have demonstrated IFG, IGT, diabetes mellitus type 2 or high levels of Hba1c.

Norepinephrine See catecholamines.

Nucleotides The chemicals, nucleic acids, that hold the genetic code in the genes (DNA and RNA), i.e. adenine, guanine, cytosine, and thymine (uracil in RNA).

Oxidative phosphorylation The chemical process whereby ATP is formed from ADP in the mitochondria.

Pancreas The organ in the abdomen that has several functions including digestion and the production of insulin and glucagon.

Pandemic When an epidemic has spread across all geographical regions it is a pandemic. Cardiovascular disease and diabetes mellitus type 2 are accepted as near pandemic now.

Pakistani A person whose ancestry lies in the Indian subcontinent who identifies, or is identified, as Pakistani (see South Asian). Some Pakistanis may have birth or ancestral roots in the current territory of India but identify with Pakistan, a country created in 1947.

Parasympathetic nervous system See autonomic nervous system.

Peritoneal/peritoneum Within the abdomen, and encapsulating the abdominal organs, is a membrane—the peritoneal membrane. Peritoneal refers to the membrane (peritoneum) and the space it encapsulates.

Phenotype The characteristics of an organism, in our case, a human being that result from the combined effects of the genotype and the environment (in the sense of non-genetic influences).

Plasminogen A substance that is important in the pathway to remove blood clots.

Plasticity The capacity of biological organisms to change, especially in relation to cell function and metabolism, as per the fetal origins type of hypothesis.

Polymorphism See mutagen.

Polyunsaturated fatty acids See also free fatty acids. These are fats with two or more double carbon bands which means they have capacity to carry more hydrogen (hence unsaturated, i.e. with hydrogen).

Population sciences A loose phrase for a number of research disciplines that examine groupings of individuals, e.g. epidemiology, demography, sociology, etc.

Postprandial After a meal. The word is common and important because blood glucose rises after a meal and the pattern and extent of the change is vitally important especially in diagnosing and managing diabetes mellitus type 2.

Prevalence The number of cases of a disease or other condition in a given population at a designated time. When this number is divided by the number of people in the relevant population we have the prevalence proportion, also commonly called the prevalence rate.

Procoagulant Substance that promote clotting.

Programming See fetal origins hypotheses.

Pulse wave velocity See arterial stiffness.

RNA (ribonucleic acid) See gene.

Saturated fatty acids These are fatty acids where nearly all the carbon atoms are joined by single bonds and the molecule is saturated with hydrogen.

Skinfold thickness A fold of skin is pinched by specially designed callipers and the thickness measured as an indication of the amount of subcutaneous fat.

SNP (single nucleotide polymorphism) See mutagen.

South Asian A person whose ancestry is in the countries of the Indian sub-continent (in terms of racial classifications, most people in this group probably fit best into Caucasian or Caucasoid but this is confusing and is not recommended). This label is usually assigned, for individuals rarely identify with it. (See also Indian, Indian Asian, Pakistani, Bangladeshi.)

Stroke See cerebrovascular disease.

Sphygmomanometer A device for measuring arterial blood pressure using an inflatable cuff (usually applied to the upper arm). The cuff is inflated until blood flow stops, then deflated until blood flow occurs when the heart beats (systolic blood pressure) and then occurs freely (diastolic blood pressure).

Subcutaneous/cutaneous The tissue just below the dermis, the inner layer of the skin, where there is much connective tissue including a substantial component of the body's fat. Cutaneous refers to the skin.

Sympathetic nervous system See autonomic nervous system.

Syndrome X See metabolic syndrome.

Systolic BP The blood pressure when the left ventricle is contracting.

Theory A system of ideas offered to explain and connect observed factors or conjectures. A statement of general principles or laws underlying a subject.

Thrifty gene A hypothesis that evolutionary adaptation has led to some population having particularly efficient eating patterns or metabolism (or both) that permits them to store energy as fat during times of plenty for use when food is scarce.

Thrifty phenotype A hypothesis that adverse environmental circumstances, especially around conception, fetal development, and infancy, alter metabolism to make it especially efficient in storing and utilizing energy in later life. See also DOHAD.

Thrombosis See clot/clotting.

Thrombus The clot.

Trans fatty acids Trans refers to placement of the hydrogen and other chemical groups (across from each other as opposed to along the carbon chain of the fatty acid). Trans fatty acids occur naturally but are produced in high concentration as polyunsaturated oils are hydrogenated to produce solid fats for the food chain, e.g. Vanaspati 'ghee'. Trans fats are associated with atherosclerosis.

Triglyceride There are three fatty acids attached to a glycerol molecule (hence triglyceride). This is a main constituent of fat.

Trunk/truncal The common name for the torso, i.e. the chest and abdomen, which has significance for cardiovascular disease and diabetes mellitus type 2 because fat here tends to be more active than that on the limbs.

Type A/type B personality A concept of personality type controversially linked to cardiovascular disease, where type A people, who are driven and competitive are said to be more prone than the less driven, more relaxed type B people.

Vanaspati A Sanskrit word that has been used for hydrogenated oils that have been formulated to be like ghee (see above). They have a great deal of trans fats.

Vasa vasorum The network of small blood vessels that supply the arterial blood to the wall of the artery, and convey the blood to the venous circulation.

Ventricular fibrillation See arrhythmias.

Very low density lipoprotein (VLDL) A lipoprotein carrying a large amount of triglyceride and cholesterol. See also lipoprotein and apolipoprotein.

Visceral (fat) Referring to the internal organs of the chest and abdomen including the intestines and in our context most often referring to visceral fat.

White European The term usually used to describe people with European ancestral origins who identify, or are identified, as White (sometimes called European, or in terms of racial classifications, the group usually known as Caucasian or Caucasoid). The word may be capitalized to highlight its specific use. The label is widely acceptable to the populations so described. The term has served to distinguish these groups from those groups with skin of other colours (black, yellow, etc.), and hence derives from the concept of race but is used increasingly as an indicator of ethnicity.

Chapter 1

Introduction to the causes of cardiovascular disease and type 2 diabetes mellitus, South Asians, and the structure and approach of this book

1.1 Chapter 1 objectives are to:

1. Briefly describe the nature of type 2 diabetes, stroke, and coronary heart disease with emphasis on their pathology and causes.

2. Introduce the heterogeneous population of about 1.7 billion people that is to be studied under the term South Asian.

3. Introduce the immensity of the problem arising from the susceptibility of South Asians to the above three interlinked chronic diseases.

4. Show how the experience of South Asians overseas, e.g. in the UK, has heralded the experience in metropolitan areas of South Asia, and in turn the experience in semi-urban and even rural South Asia.

5. Illustrate that standard knowledge of the causes of these three diseases is not sufficient to explain puzzling observations, e.g. Bangladeshis have low blood pressure but very high rates of stroke and low body mass index but high type 2 diabetes risk.

6. Outline the scientific puzzles that need explaining.

7. Introduce the key scientific explanations (hypotheses) relevant to explaining the puzzles.

8. Set out the concepts and methods used to produce this book, including the principles of epidemiology, the use of traditional literature review and discussions with key scholars.

9. Set out the aims (and structure) of the book, particularly to develop a causal synthesis that can help direct current interventions and guide future research.

1.2 **Chapter summary**

The definition of South Asians used in this book is people with ancestry in one of eight countries of South Asia, including those with such ancestry living overseas (the diaspora). Most of the research on the three interlinked diseases considered here has been done on Indians, Pakistanis, Bangladeshis, and Mauritians but the findings are likely to be generalizable to others, e.g. Sri Lankans.

Until the 1980s, coronary heart disease (CHD), stroke (especially of the ischaemic kind), and type 2 diabetes (DM_2) were seen as problems of Western lifestyle and modernity. On the basis of causal knowledge of that time South Asians would have been expected to be comparatively protected, e.g. by their lower rate of smoking, especially in women, higher rate of vegetarianism, and lower levels of obesity. Research on South Asians across the world, especially in the UK, showed the contrary was true nearly everywhere with an unusually high susceptibility to all three diseases. This susceptibility was not a phenomenon solely of migrant South Asians but also demonstrable in metropolitan South Asia. As lifestyles change, even in rural areas, this susceptibility is quickly manifest. Generally, the established causes of these diseases are also the causes in South Asians. Currently, however, whether examined individually or collectively the established causes cannot account for the comparatively high levels of cardiovascular disease (CVD) and DM_2 in South Asians(1, 2).

CHD and stroke, collectively known as CVD, are both primarily caused by narrowing and ultimately blockage of the arteries supplying the heart and brain, respectively. DM_2 is the disease whereby the quality and/or quantity of insulin are insufficient to maintain a normal blood glucose level. A long-term rise of blood glucose together with other biochemical changes in DM_2 cause numerous health problems, including CHD and stroke.

In this book South Asians are compared principally with people of North European ancestral origin wherever they live internationally, but sometimes with other groups such as the Chinese. The puzzling patterns include that body mass index (BMI), the best established marker of obesity, tends to be lower in South Asians than in European-origin people, but DM_2, though principally caused by obesity, is about three times commoner. Blood pressure (BP) in Pakistanis and Bangladeshis is comparatively low but stroke is more common. There are several other such puzzles. About ten major explanations have been proposed that can be grouped as genetic, developmental, lifestyle, and socioeconomic. None have yet resolved the puzzles.

The primary aim of this book is to undertake a thorough, critical review of explanations, and the research underpinning them, to produce a synthesis that can help guide prevention, clinical care, and research. I have been particularly keen to unite the literature on risk factors with that on more broadly based causal hypotheses. This task is done through utilizing the principles of epidemiology, the concepts underpinning ethnicity, and the methods of traditional literature review, all augmented by discussions with leading researchers in the field. Summaries of the discussions with leading researchers are in an appendix, and an overview of their observations is integrated into Chapter 9.

1.3 Introduction to the puzzle of South Asians' high susceptibility to CVD and DM_2 using an example from Scotland, and the aims of this book

Scotland is infamous as a top ranking nation for heart disease, stroke, and DM_2(3). These disorders are associated with modern lifestyles such as smoking cigarettes, eating large amounts of processed food with high fat, sugar, and salt, and low levels of physical activity. It is a shock, therefore, that South Asian populations living in Scotland have overtaken the long-settled White Scottish populations in relation to CHD(4) and more than matched them for stroke(5) and DM_2(6). Table 1.1 provides a few illustrative statistics. Scottish women of Pakistani ethnicity, for example, have nearly twice the rate of hospitalization or death from CVD outcomes, including chest pain, angina(7), heart failure(8), and South Asian women combined have about four times the amount of DM_2 compared to the White Scottish ethnic group. This is extraordinary because compared to White Scottish women, Pakistani women in the UK are much less likely to smoke cigarettes, have lower blood pressures, and similar cholesterol and weight in relation to height (BMI), to take a few key risk factors for CVD and DM_2(9–13).

South Asians' susceptibility to CVD and DM_2 cannot be explained easily by the stresses of the migration experience as Chinese women in Scotland with a similar migration background have much lower rates of CHD than do Pakistani women(4). It is not explained by the quality of health care either because there is no evidence that their care is worse, for example, once Pakistani women have a heart attack (myocardial infarction; MI) their survival is actually better than that of White Scottish women(4). This kind of puzzling susceptibility has been described over the last 50 years in several countries(14). South Asians overseas have a high susceptibility to CVD and DM_2, exhibited in high incidence rates of these diseases compared to other populations in their midst(14).

Box 1.1 lists a few of the puzzles that have preoccupied scholars in this field. There is another puzzle of low rates of many common cancers, such as those of

Table 1.1 Some recent Scottish data on CVD (SHELS data, age 30+ yrs)(4, 5, 7) and DM_2 (DARTS data, all ages) (4)

Outcome		White Scottish	Indian	Pakistani	South Asian recombined[2]
DM_2: age standardized prevalence (%) in Tayside, Scotland(6)	M	3%	–	–	10.5%
	F	2.4%	–	–	9.8%
Chest pain hospitalization or death: age standardized incidence rate ratio[3](7)	M	100	141.2[1]	216.2[1]	–
	F	100	148.6[1]	243.0[1]	–
Angina hospitalization or death: age standardized incidence rate ratio(7)	M	100	110.3	189.3[1]	–
	F	100	106.4	159.7[1]	–
MI hospitalization or death: age standardized incidence rate ratio(4)	M	100	121.2	142.4[1]	–
	F	100	123.5	129.3[1]	–
Stroke hospitalization or death: age standardized incidence rate ratio(5)	M	100	104.8	120.5	–
	F	100	76.5	107.1	–

Source: data from Bansal, N. et al. Myocardial infarction incidence and survival by ethnic group: Scottish Health and Ethnicity Linkage retrospective cohort study. *BMJ Open.* 2013;3(9):e003415. Copyright © 2003 BMJ.

[1]The 95% confidence interval excludes 100, the reference value. (Please see original publications for exact confidence intervals.)

[2]South Asians were identified by name analysis, which is not good at disaggregating subgroups.

[3]The ratio has been multiplied by 100 to be interpretable as a percentage.

the lung, breast, and colon/rectum, demonstrated in several countries including Scotland(15). Yet, the risk factors for these cancers overlap with those for CVD and DM_2, e.g. smoking, obesity, physical inactivity, and high fat, highly processed food. This paradox was pointed out as early as 1984(16). Attempts to explain these puzzles have led to many intriguing ideas, some expressed as scientific propositions that are scientifically testable (hypotheses). As yet, only one major hypothesis has been carefully tested and that revolves around insulin resistance as the underlying susceptibility factor(1, 17, 18). The empirical tests, however, have not backed this up as we will consider. The excess risk of CVD (and DM_2) is not a problem of poor health care or higher mortality after disease onset but in the occurrence of new cases, i.e. of disease incidence. Indeed outcomes after an MI are better in South Asians. This has now been demonstrated in several countries(4, 19–21).

Several new hypotheses have emerged and risk factor data have been accumulated from South Asian populations across the world. It is timely, therefore, to re-examine the evidence. The aim of this book is to examine the reasons why

---

Box 1.1 Some puzzling questions relating to CVD and DM$_2$ in South Asians compared to White Europeans

Body composition

South Asians have a high proportion of adipose tissue, and a low proportion of muscle mass. Why is this so and what are the consequences?

DM$_2$

Given adiposity, overweight, and obesity are the dominant causes of DM$_2$ why do South Asians have so much DM$_2$ even although their total body fat is no higher and BMI often lower (e.g. especially so in Bangladeshis) than in White Europeans?

CHD

Given they rarely smoke or use tobacco products why do Pakistani and Indian women, especially those living outside South Asia, have so much CHD?

Stroke

Why do Bangladeshi men and women, especially, have so much stroke even though their blood pressure, arguably the dominant risk factor, is much lower than in comparative European White populations?

South Asians get CVD and DM$_2$ far more frequently than we would expect on the basis of known risk factor patterns and to develop a coherent causal framework that sets out what we already know and what we need to know more about. Figure 1.1 illustrates the goal of this book, i.e. to put together a seemingly complex jigsaw of multiple causal hypotheses and risk factors into a new coherent, causal synthesis. This framework is then used to underpin recommendations for future research, prevention, and health care. While much of the research on South Asians' tendency to CVD and DM$_2$ has been done in South Asians living outside that continent, the findings are of relevance to those living in South Asia. The focus of the book is, therefore, South Asians globally, particularly to help prevent or at least slow the epidemics of CVD and DM$_2$ that are spreading so fast, especially to the urban and semi-rural parts of South Asia. The battle in the primary prevention of these diseases may, largely, have already been lost in the metropolitan areas of South Asia(22, 23). Nonetheless, the war can still be won. In Section 1.4 I will introduce the situation relating to CHD

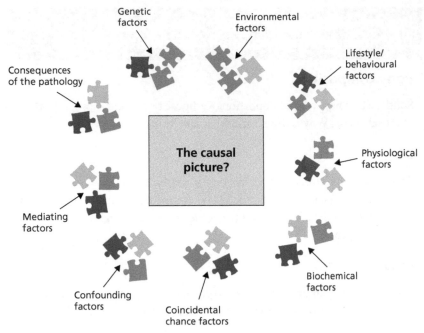

Genetic factors

Environmental factors

Lifestyle/ behavioural factors

Consequences of the pathology

The causal picture?

Physiological factors

Mediating factors

Biochemical factors

Confounding factors

Coincidental chance factors

Figure 1.1 The jigsaw puzzle analogy.

and DM_2 in India, as an example. I also discuss what I have meant by the terms South Asians and South Asia.

1.4 South Asians and South Asia: definitions and the issue of heterogeneity

South Asian is a term that is mainly used by scholars and is rarely heard in general conversation. It refers to people who can trace their ancestry to the countries of South Asia: the land that includes part of the Himalayas and southwards, i.e. the eight countries of Afghanistan, Pakistan, Nepal, Bhutan, Bangladesh, India, Sri Lanka, and the Maldives. In such discussions Mauritius is sometimes included, although it is an African country with a large proportion of people of Indian ancestry. These countries comprise more than 1.8 billion people, about one quarter of the global population. Most of this population is in India, Pakistan, and Bangladesh. In addition there are an estimated 30–40 million South Asians living outside South Asia, many in the UK, US, Canada, Mauritius, the Middle East, and South East Asia. This overseas population of emigrants and their descendants will be called the South Asian diaspora (a scattering) or just the diaspora for short.

South Asians comprise diverse populations in terms of religion, languages, diet, behaviours relating to health, economic development, and environmental circumstances, and indeed this applies to most of the individual countries, especially India. This population is living in a massive and highly varied terrain including the world's highest mountains, the Himalayas, deserts, vast coastlines, and subtropical forests. This is reflected in risk factor and disease patterns(24). It might seem a folly to consider such diverse groups in one book, especially when adding the South Asian diaspora. There are four reasons for taking this approach. First, the research evidence, admittedly mostly based on Indian, Pakistani, and Bangladeshi populations, indicates that despite their diversity, the susceptibility of South Asians to CVD and DM_2 is largely shared(14, 25). It would be good to find anomalies to this generalization, as we sometimes learn more from the exceptions that contradict our beliefs (following Karl Popper's philosophy of science(26)) than from confirmations. Second, population sciences including epidemiology work through the analysis of variation in both the exposure variables (risk factors) and outcome variables (CVD and DM_2)(27). By considering heterogeneous South Asians populations, we take advantage of diversity in exposure and outcome variables. Third, there is greater public health potential in taking this broad view as the findings are applicable to huge populations. Fourth, in practice, even though the heterogeneity of South Asian populations has been repeatedly emphasized, including by me(9, 28), and the implications shown empirically to be important, most research has reported using broad ethnic group labels. These groups might be captured under labels like Asian, South East Asian, South Asian, Indian, and Asian Indian. Even if were wholly desirable, it is not possible to undertake a full analysis that is specific, e.g. on Punjabi Sikhs, Muslims, or Hindus, given the literature available. Examining only the UK's South Asians, might have delivered many of the theoretical aims of this book and would have been easier, but the question would remain as to whether there is something particular to that population and whether the findings are relevant elsewhere. As the South Asians in the UK are already in the grip of the CVD and DM_2 epidemic(29), the potential for primary prevention is more limited and the strategies required are somewhat different to those required in South Asia, especially in the semi-rural and rural areas.

This book, however, places emphasis on the experience of the South Asian diaspora. The practical reason for this is that much of the causal research and theoretical analysis has been done or motivated by the need to understand the high rates of CVD and DM_2 in these populations(1, 14, 18, 30, 31). The UK has a large South Asian population and has led this work and is, therefore, considered carefully. The analysis here, however, is focused on its significance for South

Asians worldwide, and especially for those regions of South Asia where the CVD and DM_2 epidemic has not yet struck. Generally, findings in the UK have been replicated in metropolitan areas in other continents(30, 32, 33) and in South Asia(34), e.g. the high prevalence of diabetes in Southall(35) was echoed in a similar survey in Darya Ganj, New Delhi(36). In many places, whether whole countries such as Afghanistan, or areas such as the rural parts of Orissa, there is little or no published research. I have made an assumption that when the research is done the usual pattern of susceptibility in South Asians to CVD/DM_2 will be shown. Evidence from some (but far from all) rural areas of South Asia is already supporting this assumption, i.e. of an impending epidemic. I now consider the ancestral origins of South Asians and the main comparison population, White Northern Europeans.

1.5 Origins of South Asians and Europeans: implications for genetics

The origins of modern humans and their dispersal globally is a complex subject on which knowledge is growing fast because genetic mapping methods are adding to the evidence from paleontology, archaeology, and linguistics(37). The new genetic research supports traditional accounts with one major surprise, i.e. of reproductive success in matings between *Homo sapiens* and other species or sub-species of humans, including *Homo neanderthalensis*. This was a point of debate but is no longer so. *H. sapiens* and *H. neanderthalensis* mated and about 4% of modern humans' genome is estimated to be from this source. However, such admixture also took place elsewhere including in the Far East where the admixture seems to have been greater than in Europe. The data on such admixture are not available from India but it is speculated that it will be intermediate between Europeans and Far Eastern population. Admixture with other human species or sub-species is yet to be studied in depth although such mating with Denisovan hominins is established(38, 39).

All human species first evolved in Africa, including *H. sapiens*, from where they migrated. The migration route via the Red Sea to the Indian subcontinent was used by *H. sapiens* to leave Africa about 60–80 thousand years ago, perhaps even earlier(40, 41). From there humans went on further to the Far East, South East Asia, and Australasia. There were many subsequent migrations to India throughout history, including (reverse) migration from further east. Nonetheless, most modern Indians can trace their ancestry to ancient migrations from Africa. There is considerable heterogeneity in every way, including genetics, but there has been much admixture, even though caste and other customs have promoted endogamy, especially in the last two millennia(41, 42).

The migration route via Turkey and the Mediterranean was used by *H. sapiens* about 40,000 years ago. Over time people went both north and west into Northern Europe and east to India. Northern Europe was gripped by an ice age about 18,000 years ago forcing people to migrate south. When Northern Europe was re-colonized after the ice age about 10,000 years ago, farmers from the Southern Mediterranean also migrated northwards. As with South Asia, there was much admixture in Europe, including with non-*sapiens* species or sub-species of humans(43).

In more recent millennia there have been numerous movements of people relating to wars and trade with much genetic admixture. Other than a few small, isolated populations Europeans are—in genetic terms—very similar. On the Indian subcontinent there have been similar constraints on mating across major caste groups and between tribal and non-tribal groups creating some important genetic variation between populations(41).

Given the recency of the emergence as a new species of *H. sapiens* only about 150,000 years ago, the common historical origins and development of populations, and admixture, we would expect South Asian populations to be genetically similar to European ones. In Chapter 2 we will look at some of the genetic studies relating to CVD and DM_2, which mostly confirm this view. In Section 1.3 I referred to the Scottish scene where South Asians are very susceptible to CVD and DM_2 and I now look at India.

1.6 The immensity of the CVD and DM₂ epidemic in South Asia: the case of India

The volume of statistical data, review of such data, and analysis/commentary on the epidemic of CVD and DM_2 in South Asians is large and growing rapidly. It is not the purpose of this book to reiterate or summarize this literature as that would veer from the focus on explaining rather than describing the problem. In Section 1.3, I took the example of South Asians in Scotland as a forewarning of what might happen across South Asia. I now consider, albeit briefly, the case of India. This choice, rather than other South Asian countries, is justified by the size of India's population, and by its heterogeneity—the social conditions and environments in all the other South Asian countries have their equivalents in India(24). Furthermore, most of the recent research, review, and analysis on CVD and DM_2 in South Asia has been in India.

Srivastava et al.'s major review of the topic is summarized in Box 1.2 (p 33) (22). This illustrates how the Indian research community has intertwined the topics of CVD and DM_2. In doing so, it has followed both South Asian and UK researchers such as Haider et al. in Pakistan and McKeigue et al. in the UK(14, 44, 45). This path was, according to Reaven, proposed by Camus (published in French in 1966) and developed by Reaven (17) and is summarized in Box 1.3(p 36). Essentially, insulin, insulin-like molecules, and insulin resistance are seen as central to a wider range of metabolic abnormalities, including high blood pressure, that are important causes of CVD. Clearly, insulin resistance is important in causing DM_2 because it occurs despite high levels of insulin, which is not reducing blood glucose adequately, an insight attributed by Reaven(17) to Himsworth (1939). Insulin resistance is unlikely to be genetic but acquired as a result of rising adiposity and inadequacies in diet and exercise patterns. As early as 1989, McKeigue's systematic examination of the pattern of risk factors in White European and South Asian populations lead him to conclude that central obesity, insulin, diabetes, and postprandial triglycerides were the factors in common in South Asians(14).

Srivastava et al.'s comprehensive review combines an international and Indian perspective, while generating lessons for all South Asians(46). Though the paper is in a journal specializing in reviews of diabetes, the span is much wider. This reflects a view that has emerged since the late 1980s that CVD and DM_2, especially in South Asians, are best considered together, especially in relation to adiposity. The phrase cardio-metabolic diseases is often used for this constellation of problems. Srivastava et al. give many explanations for the high risk of CVD and DM_2 but these are mainly listed as risk factors. I reorganized them in categories as shown in Table 1.2. The causation of disease is not clear with such lists. Nonetheless, such lists reflect the complexity of the problem.

While there are few published data on CVD with slightly more on DM_2 from some South Asian countries (e.g. Afghanistan, Bhutan, Nepal) and it may well be that the epidemic is not so advanced there, that would be a complacent conclusion(47, 48). It is more likely that either these countries are yet to urbanize and enter fully into the demographic and epidemiological transition that precedes the CVD and DM_2 epidemics or that the studies have not been done. Pakistan(49) and Bangladesh(50) have already shown the signs of the Indian experience summarized in Box 1.2, at least in the metropolitan areas, but not yet in some rural areas(51, 52). While the epidemic is in urban areas, many of our insights, especially for prevention, will come from rural areas. Remarkably, in Yajnik et al.'s study in Pune, India, not one of 149 rural men who were 30–50 years old had DM_2 on an oral glucose tolerance t(53). DM_2 was common both in the nearby urban slum and in the urban middle class.

On the evidence already available from a range of South Asian countries it is reasonable to conclude that there is an epidemic of CVD and DM_2 there. When we say an outcome is high, or in epidemic form, we need some way of judging what is to be expected, and this is considered in Section 1.7.

Table 1.2 Factors implicated as potential or actual causes of cardiovascular diseases and/or DM$_2$ in India as given by Shrivasta et al. (organized by me into categories)(46)

Biochemical	High Apo B/Apo A-1 ratio
	Low HDL-cholesterol
	High total cholesterol/high LDL-C
	High triglycerides
	High level of small dense LDL-C particles
	Low adiponectin
	High fibrinogen
	High pro-coagulant activity
	Reduced tissue plasminogen activator level
	High plasminogen activator
	High inhibitor-1 s-CRP
Anthropometric	Ectopic fat in abdominal compartments
	High waist–hip ratio
Physiological	High blood pressure
	Low cardio-respiratory fitness
	Low capacity for fat oxidation
	Insulin resistance
Other health problems (co-morbidities)	Diabetes
	Non-alcoholic fatty liver disease
	Sub-clinical inflammation
	Infections
	Endothelial dysfunction
Foods (in excess)	Ghee
	Vegetable ghee (Vanaspati)
	Coconut oil
	Sugar/sugar sweetened beverages
	Refined cereals/polished white rice
	Milk and its products
Foods in deficit	Fruit and vegetables
Food constituents in excess	Saturated fatty acids
	Trans-fatty acids
Food constituents in deficit	n-6 polyunsaturated fatty acids
	n-3 poly-unsaturated fatty acids
	Mono-unsaturated fatty acids
Physical activity	Sedentary behaviour
	Low recreational physical activity
Tobacco	Smoking cigarettes and bidis, chewing tobacco, and sniffing tobacco

Source: data from Shrivastava U, Misra A, Mohan V, Unnikrishnan R, Bachani D. Obesity, Diabetes and Cardiovascular Diseases in India: Public Health Challenges. *Current Diabetes Reviews*. 2017;13(1):65–80. Copyright © 2017 Bentham Science.

1.7 Inferring high susceptibility and the emergence of epidemics—the role of reference populations for comparison

I have referred to South Asians' high susceptibility to CVD and DM_2 and the emergence of epidemics of these diseases but such inferences require a concept to underpin them. In population sciences, the inference of high susceptibility is based on comparison of risk factor patterns and their effects on outcomes with suitable reference groups(27).

In most research involving the South Asian diaspora the majority (or sometimes whole) population of the nation supplies the reference group. Since most research on diaspora South Asians has been in Northern Europe, Canada, and more recently in the US and Australasia, the reference groups usually have been of European ancestral origins(54). Such populations used to be called Caucasian, a term from the vocabulary and classifications of the biological concept of race(55). The more broadly founded concept of ethnicity is used in this book (except when referring directly to studies explicitly based on race) and such populations are usually referred to as European, European origin/ancestry, European White, or just White, the word white then being capitalized as an ethnic group label and not merely an adjective (after all no-one is actually the colour white)(54). Mostly, in this book I use European origin or White, e.g. White Scottish, to refer to these reference populations. This approach is following current conventions though it is obviously not ideal(54). Sometimes, the comparison of diaspora populations is with other groups, the choice depending on the country setting, e.g. in Malaysia the comparison is with Malays and Chinese(56), and in South Africa with Black Africans and White Africans(57). We can also compare South Asian subgroups, e.g. Indians, and Bangladeshis(58) (though such studies have been done on the Diaspora rather than on the Indian subcontinent), or Indians from Northern and Southern States(24). Comparisons involving different generations or amount of time spent abroad are also valuable.

In making such comparisons there is a difficult question, i.e. which group is 'normal'? There is a natural, but inappropriate tendency to treat the majority, reference population as normal and even worse, as ideal(55). This tendency makes the study population, here South Asians, abnormal. This is obviously wrong, especially in human biology and health where we do not know what the normal or ideal state is. For example, South Asians have, compared to White and several other reference populations, high insulin levels. Is that good for bad? We don't know. Such comparisons should be used for their reasoning potential for causal understanding and not to make judgements like good or bad (or healthy or unhealthy). Sometimes, however, it is obvious which is good or bad, e.g. in health outcomes such as a heart attack or even worse, death.

We should reflect on whether the study population (here, South Asians) is adversely effected or whether the reference population is protected. It is usual, for example, to conclude that South Asians have high rates of DM_2 compared with White Europeans. Perhaps, however, White Europeans have abnormally low DM_2 rates, while those for South Asians are normal. This is not merely of theoretical value but it also alters our search for explanations and interventions. If South Asians have abnormally high levels of DM_2 we are searching for damaging risk factors in them. If White Europeans have an abnormally low rate we are searching for protective risk factors in them. Comparisons with several ethnic groups, e.g. of South Asians, White Europeans, Africans, and Chinese help to choose between these two interpretations(4). If one population stands apart that one is probably abnormal.

The identification of comparison groups is more difficult in studies in South Asia. South Asian countries are ethnically diverse but it is not normal practice to study them through the lens of the ethnicity variable. Mauritius is an African country in the Indian Ocean and illustrates the potential. The South Asian population there has been compared to Creole and Chinese ethnic groups also living there(59). Sometimes researchers compare by region or religion. In theory, comparisons across the eight South Asian countries would be valuable but such work has not been done. Another valuable and practical approach is to compare rural, semi-rural, urban, and metropolitan populations(24, 53). In this approach we can assess whether South Asians are susceptible in their traditional agricultural contexts or only in new environments and lifestyles. Studies comparing South Asian diaspora populations with their counterparts in countries of ancestral origin are rare but powerful(60, 61).

I have stated that South Asians are in the midst of an epidemic of CVD and DM_2. An epidemic arises when the frequency of a disease is much higher than that expected based on the previous experience. It is clear that DM_2, CHD, and ischaemic stroke (but not haemorrhagic stroke) are becoming much commoner in South Asians than in the recent past. The explanation is not only that there is an ageing population, living longer than in the past, and hence more susceptible to diseases of older ages, such as CVD and DM_2. The epidemics of CVD and DM_2 are a result of demographic and other changes. These changes are the topic of this book and are largely around social and environmental circumstances and lifestyle. Fortunately, unlike in the wealthy, long-industrialized countries of Europe, North America, and Australasia, where these diseases are pandemic (affecting mostly everyone), in South Asia large numbers of people are not (yet) affected. For readers who are not already knowledgeable about

CVD and DM$_2$ in Section 1.8, I provide some background detail on their pathology and causes.

1.8 A brief introduction to CHD, stroke, and DM$_2$ and especially their known causes

Detailed accounts of these diseases from the general perspective of causation, pathophysiology, clinical presentation, and treatment are in other books. This brief account aims to give enough information to help readers, especially those who are not clinicians, to follow the later discussions, so it is focused on causes.

The causes and underlying pathology of CVD and DM$_2$ are quite well, though still imperfectly, understood(62). Our understanding permits us to devise effective interventions to bring these diseases under control in populations, at least in theory. The challenges arise from the resistance of societies and individuals to making the legal, environmental, and lifestyle changes required for prevention and control of CVD and DM$_2$, e.g. on blood pressure, smoking, and cholesterol reduction. There are, nonetheless, important unanswered questions from public health and epidemiological perspectives, such as the one under examination in this book.

CHD is also known as coronary artery disease (CAD) because the fundamental problem is that the arterial blood supply to the heart muscle is insufficient. I prefer CHD to CAD as the clinical disease, or dysfunction, is of the heart. Most people develop arterial atherosclerosis at some point. This insufficiency is, in most cases, due to narrowing of the arteries supplying the heart, most commonly caused by atherosclerosis.

In the development of atherosclerosis, lipid-rich materials are incorporated into the arterial wall. The process involves inflammation and results in fibrosis, which stiffens (hardens) the artery. The inner surface lining of the artery (endothelium) is also harmed in this process leading to endothelial dysfunction(63). In normal endothelium nitric oxide (NO) is produced and is important in dilating arteries and preventing atherosclerosis. NO is also produced in the skin on exposure to sunlight, potentially another benefit of sun exposure, other than vitamin D production. Chambers et al. found that the 26 Indians they studied in London had less endothelium-dependent vasodilation than Europeans (3.2% vs 5.9%)(64). Endothelial dysfunction and arterial stiffness co-exist and South Asians have evidence of both (see Chapter 8, Section 8.12). Boon et al. found South Asian newborns in the Netherlands had higher E-selectin levels than Dutch Caucasians (as well as higher C-reactive protein (CRP) and insulin) and inferred they had greater endothelial dysfunction at birth(65). Such endothelial dysfunction promotes inflammation, deposition of lipids (fats), fibrosis, and arterial spasm and narrowing, creating an unfortunate cycle of harm. Calcium is deposited, further hardening the artery wall and this is an indicator of adverse outcomes. Several studies have shown that South Asians are no more, and perhaps less, likely to deposit calcium than White European populations(66, 67). Also, they do not have more extensive atherosclerotic lesions.

Atherosclerosis is patchy for reasons that are not clear. The result is both narrowing due to atherosclerotic plaques and a tendency to form clots as the arterial wall is disposed to inflammation and damage, e.g. a crack forming on the endothelial surface of the artery which is repaired in a process starting with a blood clot. The most devastating outcome of atherosclerosis is a heart attack known clinically as myocardial infarction (MI). This results from the complete, or almost complete, blockage of one or more of the three major arteries that supply the heart. The blockage may arise from a blood clot inside the artery or the breaking up of an atherosclerotic plaque, or both. The result is serious damage to and even the death of part of the heart muscle supplied by that artery. There are small blood vessels and branches of major arteries that supply the heart muscle and these can become more extensive following atherosclerosis of the major arteries. These vessels are known as the collateral circulation. If a person survives an MI the collateral circulation may extend. MI is often the first sign of damage to the heart muscle caused by insufficient blood supply. It can cause severe chest and other pain and can trigger irregular heart rhythms (arrhythmias) which may be life threatening, e.g. asystole where the heart stops beating or ventricular fibrillation where the beating is uncoordinated and ineffective in circulating the blood. Death is a common consequence of these arrhythmias. When the patient survives, the heart muscle is partially repaired, usually with scarring and long-term impaired function, though some people return to full fitness.

The first symptom of arterial narrowing is sometimes chest (or other upper body) discomfort, chest pain, or breathlessness on exertion. This is known as angina pectoris or just angina. The underlying problem is the same as for an MI, i.e. insufficient blood supply to the heart muscle.

MI and angina arising from atherosclerosis are the main kinds of CHD that I consider in this book. There are rarer causes of CHD arising from non-atherosclerotic damage to arteries, whether from infections (e.g. syphilis) or autoimmune diseases (arteritis). These rarer causes are not the reason for the worldwide rise of CHD, and not of the epidemic in South Asians.

There are three major kinds of stroke that affect the arteries of the brain, called the cerebral arteries. The first kind is a bleed from the arterial wall, and this is called a haemorrhagic stroke. The second kind is from narrowing of the arteries of the brain from atherosclerosis, as described for the heart. Unlike the heart's simple blood circulation, the brain has a complex and interconnected system. The brain requires an extensive and constantly high blood supply and is exquisitely sensitive to any disruption. Fortunately, because of the interconnections of the arteries, minor disruptions in one artery can often be accommodated by blood flow from alternative routes. A third cause of stroke is an embolus (a travelling blood clot or other piece of tissue) that usually comes from the heart or its valves or the major arteries as they leave the heart, and that blocks the circulation to the brain. The consequence of stroke is often severe with paralysis, partial loss of vision or speech, or even death. In this book I am mainly considering atherosclerotic stroke, where the causes are similar to CVD.

The major causes of atherosclerosis are well established, even although the biological pathways are not always fully understood(62). In essence, many factors can disturb the surface walls of the artery. This pathway, via endothelial cell dysfunction (damage from inside the artery), is the main one that underpins the analysis in this book(63). However, another possibility that has recently been proposed is that the damage may start with the arterioles that supply blood to the large arteries, known as the vasa vasorum(68–75). According to this account, atherosclerosis starts as a disease of the microvasculature and occurs in arteries that have a vasa vasorum. The disruption to the blood supply to the outer wall of the artery is the trigger point for atherosclerosis. This alternative account has salience for South Asians who have more microvascular problems arising from their tendency to hyperglycaemia and diabetes. Of course, both pathways are possible. Figure 1.2 illustrates the two potential pathways to atherosclerosis.

The best understood of the reversible factors in the causation of atherosclerosis are listed in Table 1.3. The effects of these nine factors may be temporary or permanent as shown in the table. In addition to these agreed and well-established factors, there are literally hundreds of other associated factors that are not considered causal or are not currently agreed to be so, possibly because more research is needed(76). Quite likely, however, many of these factors are increased as a consequence of atherosclerosis, rather than being a cause or are coincidental. In addition there are important irreversible factors, e.g. age, sex, and family history. Although family history is a powerful predictor of CHD, it does not necessarily denote genetic factors. Although genetic factors are often involved in the causation of CHD, currently their role beyond their effects through the factors in Table 1.3 is considered to be small, and their capacity to explain ethnic variations is extremely small as we shall consider in Chapters 2–4.

The factors that cause the cerebral arteries to bleed are less well understood though high arterial blood pressure is one. Poverty, presumably through

1. Inside-out: endothelial dysfunction

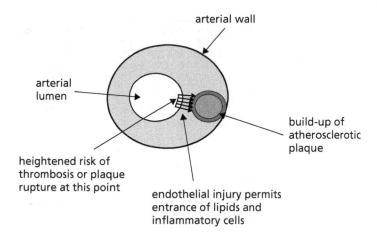

2. Outside in: damage to the blood supply of the artery

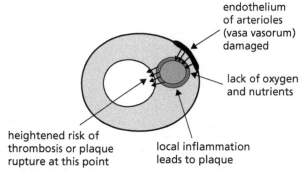

Figure 1.2 Two pathways to atherosclerosis.

nutrition, quite possibly in fetal and early life, is closely associated with haemorrhagic stroke. The role of poverty, and other socio-economic circumstances, is complex and clearly has different effects at different stages of the epidemics of CHD and atherosclerotic stroke, which first appears in relatively wealthy populations, and later in relatively poor ones, particularly as they develop socio-economically(23).

In DM$_2$ there are numerous biochemical disturbances but the defining feature is high blood glucose(77, 78). High glucose levels damage the small arteries (microcirculation). How might these effects occur? It is possible that the damage occurs directly as a result of glycation, the production of glycation

Table 1.3 Risk factors widely agreed as causes for CHD, and their presumed pathway and timing of effects

	Factors	Presumed pathway	Effect over time[1]
1	High BP	The higher pressure leads to greater intrusion of materials into the artery through endothelial dysfunction causing atherosclerosis. Very high pressure leads to arterial thickening and also increased risk of haemorrhage from small arteries including those in the brain.	While in most cases the effects are slow, in some causes of hypertension the BP can rise dramatically causing damage rapidly.
2	Tobacco, especially when inhaled as cigarettes or bidis	Components of tobacco are absorbed into the blood-stream causing inflammation of linings of arteries, promoting thrombosis, and accelerating deposition of lipid-rich deposits in the arteries.	Long-term and partly reversible by ceasing tobacco use, some of the CVD-related benefits occurring quickly.
3	Poor quality diet with few fruits and vegetables and many processed foods especially with high salt, sugar and fat	This is highly controversial but presumably some foods promote endothelial dysfunction and speed up atherosclerosis while others (fruit/vegetables) counter these tendencies.	These are long-term effects on atherosclerosis but it may be that acute events are superimposed by acute endothelial dysfunction caused by, e.g. high fat, high processed food.
4	Obesity, as defined by BMI thresholds	Obesity increases BP and blood lipids, and through fat deposition in the liver, insulin resistance. The effects may be through these paths and not direct.	The effects are long term. Reduction of weight reduces risk of DM_2 but not clearly of CVD.
5	Physical inactivity	The ways that physical inactivity affects CVD and DM_2 are not well understood but is likely to be through the pathways above, i.e. endothelial function, obesity, and hyperglycaemia.	The effects arise and disappear rapidly, e.g. exercise reduces insulin resistance quickly, and physical inactivity reinstates it fast.
6	Hyperglycaemia, especially at the levels defined for diabetes and impaired glucose tolerance	Hyperglycaemia may have direct effects in the glycation of proteins but it may be that the cluster of biochemical changes accompanying DM_2 is the key factor.	Very long-term and reducing hyperglycaemia does not translate into early demonstrable reductions in CVD.

Table 1.3 Continued

Factors	Presumed pathway	Effect over time[1]
7 High levels of lipids, especially LDL-C and triglycerides in the blood	Circulation of lipids reflected in LDL-C, presumably in the presence of factors that cause arterial wall damage, promote atherosclerosis.	Very long-term damage that is slowed, reversed, or halted by very low fat diets or treatments such as statins.
8 High levels of trans-fatty acids	Endothelial dysfunction leading to atherosclerotic and other changes	Population risks change rapidly when trans-fatty acids are removed from diets suggesting non-structural mechanisms are important
9 Psychosocial factors especially depression	The pathways are poorly understood and the effects may be through other risk factors. Direct pathways may be though the autonomic nervous system	The effects are long term.

[1]Rapidly means days or even less.

Quickly means months or a few years.

Long term means several decades.

end-products, or through damage to proteins and nucleic acids. Other harms may occur from the disturbances of lipid metabolism. The processes leading to obesity that in turn leads to DM$_2$ are well understood but the mechanisms of their action are not. DM$_2$ has a tendency to run in families and, clearly, there is a strong genetic influence on the biochemistry and physiology of glucose metabolism and the function of the beta cells of the pancreas.

The tendency to develop DM$_2$ is profoundly accelerated by gain of fat, especially if there is also a physically inactive lifestyle. Glucose levels do not rise until beta cell function declines by about 70%. Beta cell dysfunction starts long before—perhaps 10 years or more—a diagnosis of DM$_2$(79). The usual reason given for this is insulin resistance, which we will return to in Chapters 7 and 9. The accumulation of lipids in muscle, liver, pancreas, and other tissue may underlie this. Taylor, in addition, proposes that low oxidative capacity in the mitochondria is the problem that reduces oxidation of fatty acids, allowing lipid accumulation(79). (In Chapter 2, Section 2.7, I consider a related hypothesis— mitochondrial efficiency—to explain South Asians propensity to adiposity.) Glycation of mitochondrial proteins may alter function. Lipid in the muscle is clearly associated with insulin resistance in Europeans but this was not found in South Asians(80–82). Lipid accumulation is common in the liver in South Asians(83). Nonetheless, it is not clear that this is the key underlying pathology.

Another possibility that has been considered over prolonged periods, and usually set aside, is of direct pathology of the pancreas, e.g. pancreatitis. Indeed, this concept lead to a now discredited view that there was a distinct form of DM_2 called tropical diabetes, affecting South Asians(84). Currently, most opinion is that the pathology of DM_2 in South Asians is the same as in other populations and the explanation around tropical diabetes is not deemed valid.

The known factors influencing the occurrence of DM_2 are in Table 1.4. In Section 1.9, I consider briefly the role of such factors in South Asians' susceptibility to CVD and DM_2.

Table 1.4 Risk factors widely agreed to be causes of type DM_2

	Factors	Presumed pathway	Effect over time
1	Genetic predisposition	Genetic products influence the capacity for glucose metabolism (including its distribution) such that there is variation in production and function of key substances such as insulin.	Traditionally, it was thought to be long term with the genetic predisposition to DM_2 showing itself in middle age but increasingly it is seen in children and younger adults.
2	Weight gained as adipose tissue	The effect of adipose tissue seems to be depot-dependent with ectopic fat, especially in the liver, most noticeably impairing glucose metabolism.	The effect is long-term even though it is sometimes seen in the development of DM_2 in children. Loss of weight can rapidly reverse and even cure DM_2.
3	Physical inactivity	Much of the glucose load is utilized by muscle so inactivity may lead to storage of excess glucose as fat— see above.	The effect on glucose metabolism is fast.
4	Tobacco use, especially as inhaled cigarettes	The mechanism of action is not clear but it may be that tobacco products act as toxins in the glucose metabolism paths, e.g. on the pancreatic beta cells.	Long term.
5	Adverse development as reflected in low birthweight[1]	It is postulated that the adverse developmental circumstances reflected in low birthweight may mean lesser capacity in organs such as the pancreas.	Long term.

[1] As discussed in Chapter 5 this mechanism is also thought by many people to be important for CVD but it does not tend to be emphasized.

1.9 Explanations for the susceptibility of South Asians to CVD and DM$_2$: outline

Undoubtedly, the causes of CVD and DM$_2$ affect all populations, including South Asians(85) though some refinements to our understanding are needed. For example, obesity measured by BMI is not a good indicator of CVD risk in South Asians so we should use other measures that place emphasis on central fat, e.g. waist or waist/hip ratio(86). There are also important questions about the thresholds at which the adverse effects of risk factors arise and the shape of risk factor–outcome relationships. Much, perhaps even most, of the occurrence of CVD and DM$_2$ in South Asians can be explained well. What is left is the question of why, given the risk factor patterns are no worse, sometimes even more favourable, South Asians get more CVD and DM$_2$ than expected as reflected in comparisons with reference populations (as already discussed, usually, but not always, White European origin groups). This question will preoccupy us in the next eight chapters. Table 1.5 sets out some of the explanations offered in the research literature and states which chapter they will be considered in. Explanations are usually framed as general hypotheses or focused on specific risk factors.

Conceptually, South Asians are either more susceptible (sensitive) to the causes, the primary focus of this book, or have more exposure to the causes(29, 87). The former implies there are other unknown factors, perhaps

Table 1.5 Explanations to be explored by chapter

1. Greater sensitivity to the known causal factors	
Explanations	**Chapter**
Thrifty genotype	2
Drifty genotype	2
Mitochondrial efficiency	2
Adipose tissue distribution	3
Variable disease selection hypothesis	3
Neurobehavioural hypotheses (soldier-to-diplomat)	4
Developmental origins	5
Intergenerational effects	5
Adaptation/dysadaptation	5
High heat cooking hypothesis	7

(continued)

Table 1.5 Continued

2. Postulated factors	
a) General explanations	**Chapter**
Socio-economic development	6
Demographic and epidemiological transitions	6
Psychosocial environments	6
Psychological health—stress (including racism) and depression	6
Exposure to infections/causes of inflammation	6
b) Specific explanations	
Tobacco and other drugs	7
Blood pressure	7
Diabetes, hyperglycaemia (for CHD and stroke)	7
Diet (glycaemic load, calories, fats, fruit/veg, dairy products red meat, processed foods, high-heat cooking)	7
Physical inactivity	7
Cholesterol/Lp(a) and other lipids	7
3. Other explanations	
Micronutrients (vitamin D, vitamin B_{12}, folate)	8
Thyroid function	8
Coagulation etc.	8
4. Integrating explanations into a coherent whole	9

acting as co-factors, enhancing the adverse effects of the known factors. An alternative is that the modification of the effect of known risk factors in the presence of other known risk factors is greater in South Asians than in reference populations, i.e. there is effect modification or in statistical terms interaction[27].

There are three other general explanations that I consider briefly below but that are not a major focus of this book, i.e. data artefact, competing causes, and health care access.

1.10 **Data artefact: an improbable explanation**

The view that South Asians have unexpectedly high risks of CVD and DM_2 is largely based on epidemiology (see Section 1.14 for more on this topic).

Epidemiology is the population science that studies the patterns of diseases and other health outcomes in populations, comparing and contrasting whenever possible, and seeking explanations for the differences observed(27). The patterns are first studied by counting the outcomes of interest and relating them to the size and age/sex structure of the population. Errors in such counts and calculations arise. When an outcome is slightly different from the expected, or reference, value it is not wise to place too much emphasis on it, at least not until it is rigorously replicated. When the difference is large, and demonstrated in different places, times, and subgroups, and by using a variety of comparison populations, an artefact is an unlikely explanation. The latter is the case for CVD and DM_2 in South Asians. That said, studies to show the statistics are correct are rare because such validation studies are difficult. One common source of error is death certificate (mortality) statistics. Errors can be made in both population counts, required for calculating rates and numbers and causes of death. Sufficient studies of different kinds show that miscounts in population sizes are not the cause of the excess CVD mortality in, for example, UK South Asians. A rare study reviewed the death certificates of 315 Indian Asians and Europeans dying in London between 2002 and 2011, showing that there were some errors but these were similar in Indian Asians and Europeans so could not explain the differences in CVD mortality(88).

The high risk of DM_2 in South Asian populations is not unique, and it is even higher in some small populations such as Pima Indians(89). The risk in South Asians is, however, much higher than in our primary comparison group—European origin people. Traditionally, the diagnosis of DM_2 was made using the oral glucose tolerance test, whereby 75g of glucose is given to a fasting person and the rise and fall of blood glucose is observed, and the interpretation of this confirms or refutes the clinical diagnosis. The question is whether a 75g dose might be too much for some populations, e.g. in Bangladeshis who are much shorter and lighter than White Europeans(90). This kind of artefact is subtle compared to errors such as undercounts or overcounts of cases, and should be borne in mind. The excess of DM_2 in Bangladeshis is not, however, simply an artefact arising from this diagnostic test as it can be shown by other tests (fasting glucose, glycosylated haemoglobin) and by clinical observations of the complications arising from high blood glucose. I shall consider the possibility of artefact throughout but I don't see it as a major explanation of the phenomenon under study here. Data artefacts can exaggerate differences but, we should remember, they can hide or underplay differences too. I consider in Section 1.11 the competing causes explanation.

1.11 Competing causes: potentially important in examining patterns of death but not usually of morbidity

If the appearance of one disease (say X) influences the development of another disease (Y) then there is effect modification or an interaction between them. One disease may stimulate the occurrence of another, especially if the mechanism of occurrence is similar. For example, a heart attack can increase the risk of a stroke through the development of blood clots, emboli, and poor circulation of blood. DM_2 increases the risk of both CHD and stroke. Sometimes the occurrence of disease X may block the occurrence of Y. This, obviously, is important for studies of the cause of death. If a person dies of a stroke then he/she has not died of DM_2 or CHD even though these diseases may be at an advanced stage. This is an example of the competing causes phenomenon. The interpretation of death statistics, especially, requires attention to competing causes. This is less of a problem in studies of non-fatal disease (morbidity). Given competing causes the outcomes that occur later in life are most likely to be underestimated. For example, in places where infections are major killers, diseases such as CHD, which tend to kill in middle or old age, may not be common in death statistics. Where CHD is very common the potential risk of deaths due to cancers of older age may be underestimated. As the excess of CHD/DM_2 in South Asians can be demonstrated even more clearly with morbidity than mortality data, and especially so in younger age groups, the competing causes explanation is unlikely and therefore not a focus of this book. Nevertheless, awareness of this concept is required.

Might the explanation for the differences in CHD and DM_2 lie in health care? This unlikely scenario is considered in Section 1.12.

1.12 Health care access: critically important to progression of CVD and DM₂ but not to their occurrence

Differences in access to, and the amount and quality of, health care are critically important to the progression of CVD and DM_2 but not to the likelihood of their occurrence in the first place. For these diseases, mostly, health services become involved after the disease is diagnosed. There are, however, some ways that health services do influence occurrence too. First, health services run health education and health promotion activities. Second, they have screening activities. Third, they have risk factor control (behaviour management) services, e.g.

smoking cessation drives. Differential uptake and impact of such services could potentially explain some of the observed ethnic group variations. Such population level activities, however, do not have a strong impact on disease incidence.

There are effective interventions important to those who already have CVD such as smoking cessation services, drugs such as statins to reduce cholesterol, and drugs to reduce blood pressure. Control of DM_2 helps in preventing CVD.

A few studies have been done on the quality and quantity of health care for South Asian populations in the UK context. Although the results are sometimes in conflict, especially between older and newer studies, health care does not seem to be critically important in explaining South Asians' susceptibility to CVD and DM_2(91–93). Currently, health care providers seem to be sensitized to the high risk of DM_2 and CVD in South Asians and therefore are making appropriate diagnoses and providing comprehensive health care. Health care is a potential solution to, rather than a cause of, the problem.

1.13 The book's approach to the acquisition and synthesis of evidence: literature review and discussions

I am focusing on explanations in the scientific research literature for South Asians' susceptibility to CVD and DM_2. The primary material is, therefore, papers and books on causal hypotheses and risk factors generally agreed as casual. Some papers are summarized by me in boxes based on the authors' exposition and occasionally others' critiques or updates.

I have also examined many reviews. These generally discuss a wide range of causal and non-causal risk factors, rather than hypotheses, in relation to the frequency and pattern of disease. Hypotheses and review papers usually emphasize the close relations between CHD, stroke, and DM_2. Indeed, the most common explanation offered by reviews of CVD in South Asians is the high frequency of DM_2 and insulin resistance. In reviews of diabetes in South Asians, the high risk of subsequent CVD is usually a major feature. General hypotheses are not usually considered in detail. When mentioned, the reference is most usually to the thrifty genotype considered in Chapter 2 (94) or thrifty phenotype considered in Chapter 5(95).

Some of this literature offers causal diagrams, mostly trying to link up the many risk factors. These causal diagrams tend to be for CHD, stroke, or DM_2, not the three combined. The causal diagrams are mostly of the logic diagram type, whereby relationships between factors are set out. They are not usually constrained by the formal rules (e.g. one-way causal direction) of techniques such as directed acyclic graphs. I have examined several published causal diagrams, with the goal of moving towards a single comprehensive, yet comprehensible, framework and causal model. I have created many simple, conceptual causal diagrams using the textual explanations of the primary authors. I have also used the metaphor of the jigsaw, with the pieces shown in this chapter, and then put together in Chapter 9.

There is a large literature examining the frequency of CVD and DM_2 in South Asian populations worldwide, including comparisons with other populations. Summarizing or synthesizing this literature in a descriptive way is not my purpose. Sometimes, this literature is used to set the background and as a means of assessing the fit between the explanations and the empirical data as exemplified in my paper on a four-stage model explaining the high risk of DM_2 in South Asians(96).

This book is based on a traditional literature review. The breadth of the subject inhibits, and my goals do not require, new systematic review or meta-analysis. However, I do emphasize systematic reviews and meta-analysis that are already published. In addition to accessing my own collection of papers and books acquired over 33 years of study of the topic I have searched for the most relevant literature carefully, including examining the citation lists relating to major hypotheses and review papers. As a way of adding value to the work, and ensuring inclusion of unpublished ideas, and checking whether the direction of the argument aligns with other's views, I discussed the topic with 22 leading researchers and scholars across the world. Their thoughts are reflected in the text, integrated in Chapter 9, while the summaries of discussions are given in the appendix.

The book aims to summarize knowledge to create a causal synthesis and framework to guide both future research and practical action. It also aims to strengthen the theoretical foundations of this area of scholarship to help progress towards a general theory. My perspective is that of a medical public health epidemiologist and the core ideas of this approach are summarized in Section 1.14.

1.14 The scientific perspective of the book and its author: introducing epidemiology as a clinical, social, environmental, and public health science

The quest for explanation and understanding cannot be limited by artificial, methodological, or disciplinary boundaries. Some of the greatest causal discoveries in medical and public health sciences have arisen in the imagination, which we can call armchair science! Others have been sparked by a fortuitous observation. Mostly, however, advancement in causal understanding comes from scientific reasoning and empirical investigation of hypotheses and theories. This book will reflect all these kinds of domains of knowledge.

I aim to consider all causal ideas that might answer the central question: why do South Asians have an unexpectedly high susceptibility to CVD and DM_2 especially in urbanized settings? This question arises from a population health perspective. The primary scientific discipline for the investigation of population health is epidemiology(27). The question of interest sits squarely in the fields of ethnicity (including the concept of race), migration, and health(54). For details on these two domains of study, readers might wish to consult other writings, possibly including my books *Concepts of Epidemiology* and *Migration, Ethnicity, Race and Health in Multicultural Societies*. In this section my goal is to introduce some of the core concepts needed to follow the reasoning in this book.

Epidemiology studies the patterns of diseases and other health outcomes in population settings. The primary measurement for this is the incidence rate of disease, i.e. the number of new outcomes in a given time in a population. This fraction is multiplied and typically expressed as, for example, 100 cases per 100,000 population per year. Such measures, of which there are many, can allow comparisons over time, between places, and by characteristics of persons (population groups). For example, time might include seasonal variations or disease trends over some decades or centuries. Place of disease studies might be comparing urban and rural areas, regions, nations, continents, and possibly migrating and non-migrating populations. Studies of persons, or strictly population groups, may compare populations of different ages, sexes, ethnicity, or social class. These kinds of studies often show interesting and unexpected variations. It is these kind of studies that have shown that CVD and DM_2 have risen in incidence in urbanizing and migrating South Asians and that in the early stages of the epidemic (but not later) the wealthy classes are affected more than the poor.

Having made such observations, and given the human desire for understanding, the next step is to propose an explanation stated in a way that can be tested using quantitative data. This proposed explanation is a hypothesis. Quite often hypotheses are not made explicit but are implicit in the data actually collected. The most popular and compelling hypothesis for high CVD rates in South Asians over the last 30 years, as we have noted, is the one involving insulin resistance. (Box 1.3)

Empirical data are collected by epidemiologists within the framework of tested study designs. The most commonly used study designs are case series (including those on whole populations, e.g. disease registers) and cross-sectional studies. In a case series, as the name implies, a list of people with the disease is created and relevant data collected on them, usually from the clinical case notes. Such case series have traditionally been assembled by clinicians, who notice features in common among their patients that might offer causal clues. When all the cases in a population are put together then we can call it a population case series or population register, e.g. all cases of MI in a city or nation. Much, if not most, of the research on CVD in South Asia is based on case series usually from hospitals. It is obvious that clinical case series are of highly selected populations.

A cross-sectional study is usually of a sample of the population at a particular time and place. The general characteristics, risk factors, and diseases of the sample are measured. Associations between these characteristics may be studied though the primary output is the prevalence of risk factors and disease in the population. Cross-sectional studies are common in the field of CVD and DM_2 in South Asians, because they are, relative to other studies excepting case series, easier and cheaper to do. There are excellent designs for measuring the amount of disease and risk factors in a population but causal knowledge from them is usually considered preliminary and for hypothesis generation for later hypothesis testing using other study designs.

Two study designs are commonly used for hypothesis testing, the case–control study and the cohort study. In the case–control study a group of people with the disease are compared with an appropriate control group, most if not all of whom are disease-free. In the differences observed between case and control groups lie clues that might explain the causes of the disease. The case group could be a population of people with existing CVD, e.g. of South Asians, and the control group of CVD cases from another ethnic group, e.g. White Europeans. This kind of comparison was done by Chambers et al., who also made the traditional comparison of people with and without the disease(97).

The most important epidemiological study design for causal reasoning is the prospective cohort study where populations are characterized at baseline including measures of potential risk factors, then followed up, sometimes for decades. The association between risk factors and disease outcomes is studied. There are numerous such studies but few include South Asian populations(98). Some cross-sectional studies have added a follow-up component, one example being the cross-sectional Southall and Brent Studies subsequently followed up as the cohort known by the acronym SABRE that is summarized in Box 7.1 in Chapter 7(99).

The most rigorous causal design is the trial, which is an experiment. This examines the causal effect of an intervention. The most rigorous trials are randomized, blinded, and controlled. This means that two or more groups are randomly allocated to receive the intervention or not. Those who do not receive it may be given an alternative, placebo, or best alternative, as a substitute for the intervention under test. Blinded means that the participants, professionals, and researchers do not know who has received the test intervention or the alternative. Controlled just means there is a control group. Trials to try to explain ethnic differences in CVD and DM_2 do not exist so our interest in them is more general, i.e. in understanding the validity of causal claims made for risk factors.

The Mendelian randomization study takes advantage of an experiment of nature, i.e. the inheritance of genes and gene variants is, effectively, random. Where a gene variant alters a risk factor we can compare people with and without the gene variant to see the association with disease outcome. This is an emerging field of study but one that has already found application in examinations of South Asians' tendency to cardio-metabolic disorders(100).

The interpretation of epidemiological data is difficult. Errors are easily made in measurements, which are often made on thousands and even hundreds of thousands of people. People invited to participate often decline to do so leading to selection biases. The groups compared are often very different leading to invalid inferences on the role of a risk factor, the phenomenon called confounding. A simple example of confounding would be a study showing rising CHD incidence in a South Asian city, say Karachi, in 1961, 1971, 1981, 1991, 2001, and 2011. It may be that CHD incidence is rising but it may also be that the people living in Karachi in 2011 are much older, on average, than in 1961 and the rise is explained by ageing rather than some underlying change in the disease. This would be called confounding by age. Summary statistics are adjusted to take into account for variables (such as age) that we are not specifically and currently interested in as causal factors.

Epidemiology uses quantitative data on associations between variables to support or refute hypotheses. The data are interpreted using causal frameworks, models, and guidelines. Causal guidelines, for example, include interpreting the data using questions, e.g.

- Does the supposed cause precede the disease? (Temporality or timing of the association)
- Does exposure to the supposed cause raise the incidence of the disease? (Strength of the association)
- Is the association between supposed cause and diseases limited in range? (Specificity of the association)
- Is the association seen across studies and population groups? (Consistency of the association)
- Does altering the exposure to the supposed cause change disease frequency? (Experimental confirmation of the association)

◆ Is the way the supposed cause acts understood biologically? (Biological plausibility of the association)

Causal reasoning goes beyond statistics. It is not easy to apply this kind of causal reasoning to ethnic group differences. Most studies of ethnic group differences focus on the strength of the association. This is usually measured using the summary statistic called relative risk, which is the incidence rate in the group of interest (here, South Asians), divided by that in the comparison population. This ratio is above 1 if the disease is more common in South Asians and less than 1 if the disease is less common. If so we would say there is association between South Asian ethnicity and the disease outcome. Typically the risk factors that are potentially explanatory of why there is an association are entered into the statistical model, usually using regression methods, as we see in the SABRE study (Chapter 7; Box 7.1). The model adjusts the relative risk to take these into account and we can see how it changes.

There are efforts to go beyond this level of causal reasoning. Firstly, there is increasing attention to integrating data on various levels from genome to environment. Secondly, there is integration of data from different disciplines including population and laboratory sciences, and experiments on tissues, animals, and humans. Thirdly, there is a move to utilize causal graphs, both to make the writers' thinking explicit but also to guide and subsequently interpret data analysis. The aim of Chapter 9 is to produce a theory based causal graph that integrates our knowledge on the question at hand.

Science goes beyond data and empiricism. Data do not give the answer. We have to interpret them, especially on whether they help evaluate and modify our prior hypotheses. Even more importantly, science moves from hypothesis to theory. A theory is a system of ideas to connect observations and is usually stated in terms of general principles, themselves based on hypotheses and relevant data. There are many hypotheses and studies but these could not be described as theories on South Asians' susceptibility to CVD and DM_2. In Chapter 9 I will summarize the 'state of the art' and assess the potential for a causal theory.

This brief introduction to epidemiology portrays it as a broad, inclusive population health science that is goal orientated. This book's goal to understand the epidemic of CVD and DM_2 in South Asians will be based on epidemiology but will be inclusive of findings from many other relevant disciplines.

1.15 **Structure of the book**

The book's structure is evident from Table 1.5. I move from general and fundamental biological explanations to more specific socio-economic, psychosocial, cultural, and lifestyle ones. There is an allure to genetic explanations and they deeply influence both scientific and public discourse. The genetic explanation is usually the first to come to mind in thinking of human differences especially between groups. Genetic factors are also potentially of great importance, and thus enjoy prominence in scientific research. The thrifty genotype hypothesis relating to energy acquisition, storage, and utilization is the archetype of the evolutionary, genetic idea in this context(94), and it and some other related genetic hypotheses are discussed in Chapter 2. To help people who are not familiar with genetics understand such hypotheses a small amount of background is provided.

Chapter 3 cover genetic hypotheses that relate to body shape and composition focusing on body size especially at birth, adipose tissue, and muscle mass. An example is the adipose tissue compartment overflow hypotheses(101).

Chapter 4 is on complex, genetically driven neurobehavioural hypotheses, an example being the behavioural switch (soldier-to-diplomat) hypothesis(102).

In leaving genetic hypotheses for other ideas, we must carry over the concepts because all health outcomes arise from an interplay between genes and other non-genetic factors, for simplicity usually called the environment. The genome influences how the environment exerts its effects, and also the genome adapts its functions in relation to the prevailing environment through the process called epigenetics. This idea of gene–environment interplay is particularly important in fetal and early life development, which may have lasting influences throughout life including on CVD and DM_2. The suite of hypotheses in Chapter 5, widely known as the thrifty phenotype (95), can be aptly described by the phrase adaptation–dysadaptation. The fetus/infant is prepared (or programmed) by environmental factors, perhaps influenced by genes, for a particular kind of metabolism that seems to be required. When some other kind of metabolism is required in later life, because the environment is different, the individual is mal-adapted, giving rising to CVD and DM_2. This is an appealing hypothesis, which fits within the developmental origins of health and disease (DOHAD).

Chapter 6 is largely on environmental explanations. We start with general explanations relating to socio-economic and psycho-social factors, including their possible role as environmental triggers of inflammation. One general issue arising is that South Asians' susceptibility is part of a phenomenon described as the demographic and epidemiological transition(103, 104). Populations in poverty in childhood tend to have high rates of CVD and DM_2 in later life, an observation that underpinned early work on the developmental origins of adult health and disease research in Chapter 5(105). In Chapter 6 we also consider more specific explanations including air pollution.

Chapter 7 turns to the established risk factors (as summarized in Tables 1.3 and 1.4). I especially consider how they might exert more than their usual effects in South Asians given the susceptibility factors discussed in Chapter 2–6. Amongst the ideas to be considered are that adaptation–dysadaptation may lead to an unexpected change in a risk factor (say blood pressure or total cholesterol) and it is the level of change rather than the absolute level of the risk factor that matters. This concept of change is a general idea within a chapter on specific explanations(106). Another general idea is the recently articulated high-heat cooking hypothesis, which is a dietary hypothesis unrelated to specific dietary components(107). The role of diabetes and less severe forms of hyperglycaemia as the susceptibility factor for CVD in South Asians has been dominant and deserves special scrutiny. Insulin and glucose are closely governed by genetic and fetal development and the links between them and this insulin resistance hypothesis is examined. As this hypothesis has dominated our topic for the last 30 years, as a prelude it is summarized in Box 1.3 (p 36) and Figure 1.3.

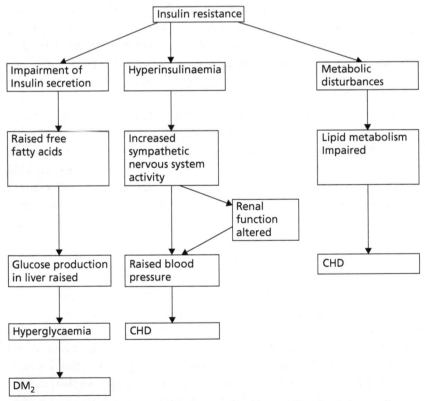

Figure 1.3 My diagram to summarize the insulin resistance hypothesis (Reaven).

Many other ideas have been mooted, sometimes without evidence or detailed backing, and these will be considered, mostly briefly, in Chapter 8, not least to avoid missing an important ingredient that in future may be shown to be critical. Amongst the ideas here that deserve closer scrutiny are micronutrients, especially vitamins D and B_{12}, given South Asians are known to have comparatively low levels of these(108–110).

Chapter 9 provides an explanatory framework, discarding weak causal candidates, emphasizing strong ones including promising new ones, and highlighting gaps in knowledge. This chapter also integrates the discussions with scholars across the world. These ideas are then developed as both causal diagrams and as a causal story.

In Chapter 10 I draw the practical lessons from this causal synthesis. The questions that are asked and answered are whether our current policies and strategies for preventing CVD and DM_2 in South Asians are soundly based and whether they need adjustment, especially given international strategies(111). Then I consider the role of services, particularly preventive and other public health services, in countering the epidemics of CVD and DM_2 in South Asians. I also consider what kind of community action would align with the findings here. Finally, especially relating to the gaps in the causal framework in Chapter 9, I set out a research and scholarship agenda to advance our understanding beyond the current state-of-the-art.

Box 1.2 The immensity of the case of India

Shrivastava U, et al. Obesity, diabetes and cardiovascular diseases in India: Public health challenges. Current Diabetes Review. 2017;13(1)65–80(46).

My introductory remarks

In much of the developing world, including India, the emphasis of social and public health policy has been on the problems of poverty, infectious disease, nutritional deficiencies, and maternal and child health. The rapid emergence of CVD and DM_2 has provided additional, unwelcome, and conflicting demands. Whether public policy should change is a controversial matter, not least because the newer epidemics are affecting the relatively well-off first. This review draws attention to the immensity of the challenge at hand.

Summary of paper(22)

Of 284 articles and reports found by searching three databases and relating to CVD, diabetes, obesity, and their risk factors in India, 123 were selected

---

Box 1.2 The immensity of the case of India (*continued*)

by the authors. The results, set out in seven substantial tables illustrated with 12 figures, back the key message of an impending crisis. The Indian scene is set in the global context where non-communicable diseases are a dominant and increasing cause of disease, disability, and death. The decline in death rates, with increased lifespan, is seen as the key driver of this change. Non-communicable diseases are estimated by WHO to contribute to 52% of deaths in South Asia's 1.7 billion plus population, projected to increase to 72% by 2030. Some of the facts presented were extracted by me into Table 1.6, with observations on the urban and rural contexts.

Obesity

The problem of overweight and obesity is large and increasing though the 12 studies tabulated in the paper cannot be compared because of different methods and cut-offs for the measures used to define obesity. In Table 1.6 I have taken an illustrative statistic from North India. The cut-off of a BMI of more than 25 Kg/m^2 as denoting obesity (not 30 as globally using WHO

Table 1.6 Key statistics from Shrivasta et al. review of obesity, diabetes and cardiovascular diseases in India(22)

Burden of disease		Rural[1]	Urban[2]	Total
Obesity	Men			24.3%
(ICMR-INDIAB-3 Study) BMI > 25	Women			38.7%
Diabetes		8.3	14.2	
(ICMR-INDIAB-3 Study)				
CVD mortality per 100,000		75–100	360–430	
Acute MI	Males			141
mortality per 100,000	Females			136
Low HDL-c				72.3%
High triglycerides				29.5%
High LDL-c				11.8%
(ICMR-INDIAB Study)				
Hypertension-age-standardized				26.3%
(ICMR-INDIAB Study)				

Source: data from Shrivastava U, Misra A, Mohan V, Unnikrishnan R, Bachani D. Obesity, Diabetes and Cardiovascular Diseases in India: Public Health Challenges. *Current Diabetes Reviews*. 2017;13(1):65–80. Copyright © 2017 Bentham Science.

[1]Nagaland, Meghalaya, Himachal Pradesh, and Sikkim.

[2]Andhra Pradesh, Tamil Nadu, Punjab, Goa.

Box 1.2 The immensity of the case of India (*continued***)**

guidelines) is in line with Indian guidelines. Obesity is very common. The problem is compounded by a relatively high fat content (adiposity) of the Indian physique at any BMI (see Chapters 3 and 7) and tendency to deposit central abdominal and hepatic ectopic fat, which is especially harmful from the CVD and DM_2 perspective.

Diabetes mellitus

The prevalence of diabetes has soared from 1–2% of the population in the 1960s to 10–20% in urban areas and 5–10% in rural areas, as demonstrated in a tabulation of 10 studies. The figures for Chandigarh in Table 1.6 from a 2011 publication illustrate both the huge scale of the problem and that there is still great scope to prevent it in rural areas (3% in rural Jharkhand, East India). The more recent CARRS studies gave a prevalence of DM_2 of 25.2% in N. India and 16.3% in Karachi. India is estimated to have 69 million people with DM_2 already. The problem of DM_2 is compounded by early onset and severe cardiovascular complications.

CVD

Mainly the focus of the paper was on CHD rather than stroke. The acute MI mortality rate in Table 1.6 is estimated as nearly double that in the US and China.

Causes

A multiplicity of causes were highlighted and were re-categorized by me and listed in Table 1.2. In some of the analysis, the authors referred to studies on South Asians in the UK or the US for lack of Indian data.

My concluding comments

In one relatively short article (given its scope) the authors have implicated at least 39 factors, which are quite often components of a broader category of cause (e.g. lipids or diet quality). It is hard, but important, to make sense of such an assembly of factors and that requires a theoretical framework.

It is also notable to see what the authors have not emphasized and that includes genetics (mentioned in passing) and the developmental origins of disease. The paper, in the style of most such reviews, does not emphasize the hypotheses or theories that might underpin explanations. There are many reviews of this kind, and also many hypotheses papers. These spheres of activity have not yet been synthesized. That is, therefore, a task for this book.

Box 1.3 The insulin resistance hypothesis

Reaven GM. Role of insulin resistance in human disease. Diabetes. 1988;37(12):1595–607(17).

My introductory remarks

The insulin resistance hypothesis has dominated discussions of South Asians' tendency to CVD and DM_2 for more than 30 years. This is the defining paper on the subject. It pinpoints the key consequence—a syndrome that Reaven called Syndrome X but which came to be known as the metabolic syndrome. I have summarized the hypothesis in Figure 1.3.

Summary of the paper

The paper opens by claiming that insulin resistance is central in the pathogenesis of several diseases. The paper first focuses on non-insulin dependent diabetes (NIDDM), that we now call type 2 diabetes mellitus and abbreviate in this book to DM_2, and impaired glucose tolerance (IGT). Insulin resistance is proposed as necessary though not sufficient, alone, to produce DM_2. Insulin resistance is said to set off other changes, even without hyperglycaemia, that increase hypertension and coronary artery disease (called CHD here).

Insulin resistance leads to reduced uptake of glucose by tissues such as muscle but it does not determine plasma glucose. Further, in normoglycaemic people, insulin resistance varies greatly. The similar glycaemic response is maintained by differential insulin secretion. This points to the role of the pancreatic beta cell. A concept is introduced of the beta cell being stressed by the need to produce insulin. The assumption is then made that in DM_2 hyperinsulinemia cannot be maintained long term so blood glucose levels tend to rise.

The paper considers free fatty acids (FFAs) observing that small differences in insulin can lead to large differences in circulating FFAs (and more so than glucose). The inference is that insulin resistance reduces the expected suppression of plasma FFAs. The train of events proposed is that the loss of ability to control FFAs then leads to hyperglycaemia. The favoured mechanism for this is that hepatic production of glucose is increased when plasma FFAs are high, and presumably reaching the liver. (The biochemical mechanisms for this are outlined in detail in the paper but are not necessary

Box 1.3 The insulin resistance hypothesis (*continued*)

here.) Experimental evidence for this in rats is given. The rise and reduction of blood glucose associated with FFAs is not, itself, via insulin.

Even when plasma glucose and FFAs are normal, because of hyperinsulinemia, there is harm through hypertension. Hypertensive people are relatively insulin resistant, with higher glucose and insulin following a glucose stimulus. Evidence that insulin, per se, may raise blood pressure is provided and mechanisms via catecholamines (via the sympathetic nervous system) or the kidney are discussed. The causal connection for human health is portrayed cautiously as most of the evidence is from rats.

Finally, Reaven turns to CHD and identifies both hypertension as above and lipid abnormalities (especially hypertriglyceridaemia but also VLDL and/or HDL) as the mechanisms, both promoted by insulin resistance and high insulin levels. So these variables are seen as clustering and this is named as Syndrome X, and proposed as of enormous significance for CHD. Insulin resistance is the hypothesized underlying factor in common. Genetic and lifestyle factors (obesity, physical activity) are seen as underlying Syndrome X.

My concluding remarks

The potential significance of this paper for the epidemic of CVD and DM_2 is immediately obvious, i.e. insulin resistance as the underlying linking factor. In the text, especially in Chapter 7, we consider the extent to which the hypothesis is now considered explanatory. Of course, it still raises the unanswered question of why some individuals and populations are insulin resistant and others are not. This fundamental question preoccupies several of the hypotheses we will consider.

Chapter 2

Genetic explanations 1: the thrifty genotype and its variants

2.1 Chapter 2 objectives are to:

1. Describe and discuss the long-established thrifty genotype hypothesis and more specific but related ideas, e.g. the mitochondrial efficiency hypothesis.
2. Evaluate the validity of the hypothesis as an explanation for South Asians' susceptibility to CVD and DM_2.

2.2 Chapter summary

There is a family of interrelated hypotheses, the best known of which is the thrifty genotype. The concept is that populations susceptible to CVD and DM_2, such as South Asians, have been subjected to intermittent serious food shortages, including large-scale famines, such that they have evolved genetically to cope with these conditions. One proposed genetic adaptation for coping, for example, makes them comparatively insulin resistant. This means their glucose is not readily entering the muscle to be used there but is preferentially used by the brain and liver. In the liver glucose is converted to fat then transported and stored in adipose tissue for times of food scarcity. This thrifty state is not beneficial in modern times where food is plentiful.

This hypothesis has caught the imagination of researchers and health professionals and remains a central and much-discussed explanation. It raises questions such as whether the kind of famines seen in South Asia in recent times actually occurred in evolutionary time scales or whether they are a modern phenomenon. Why is a thrifty genotype not also seen in Northern Europeans, e.g. the Irish, who endured one of the worst famines ever? Further, there is the question of which genes were affected and whether thrifty gene variants can be demonstrated. Overall, the evidence in support of the hypothesis is not in line with its' appeal. It has, however, sparked off related ideas, e.g. the mitochondrial efficiency hypothesis, that make a similar evolutionary argument but on the basis of living in warm climates rather than chronic food shortages.

Recently, the thrifty genotype hypothesis has lost support, mostly because of lack of confirmatory empirical data, especially from genetic studies. The development of more attractive, alternative hypotheses has also diminished support for the thrifty gene hypothesis. Future research should aim to pinpoint specific mechanisms, e.g. mitochondrial function. The practical implications of these hypotheses, even if correct, are related to lifestyle, rather than genetics.

2.3 Introduction to genetic hypotheses and to their appeal

When differences are shown between populations, especially in their physical characteristics, including health status, there is a tendency to turn first to genetic explanations(54, 112). This is particularly so when we show differences between the sexes and between ethnic (or racial) groups. This approach was probably at its height in the 19th century, when many differences between populations, including in intelligence, were attributed to innate, inherited factors, i.e. genetics, even though at the time the mode of inheritance was only understood vaguely(113, 114). (Section 2.4 provides information that readers without much knowledge of genetics may find helpful.) In the 19th century the link between genetics and population level differences, say between nations or continents (loosely interpreted as race related), was deeply ingrained.

Genetic factors are important in explaining many human characteristics at the individual level including intelligence and health status. A person may have an extremely high risk of CHD because of, for example, a genetic condition called familial hypercholesterolaemia, whereby cholesterol levels may become dangerously high(115). The genetic mutations causing this were discovered in 1973, but the problem was described by Carl Muller in 1938. This person's and the family's high risk can be attributed to genetic mutations pinpointed to three genes on the 19th chromosome. The inheritance is dominant in the sense that of the two copies of each gene each person has, only one has to be affected to cause the problem. So, if we discover a family, or a small community, with a great deal of CHD, especially under the age of 65 years, this genetic condition would be a potential cause.

It is a small step to extend this logic to large populations, including South Asians. If a higher percentage of South Asians have genetic conditions such as familial hypercholesterolaemia than other populations such as Northern Europeans and the Chinese, then the mystery we are investigating in this book might be solved. This is not, however, the case as familial hypercholesterolaemia is relatively uncommon in South Asia(116, 117).

On first principles, and on our knowledge of genetic structure in human populations and historical migration patterns, we would expect the genome of South Asians to be very similar to other human populations, especially in Europe and China, though less so than in populations in Africa. As considered in Chapter 1, Section 1.5, our species originated in East Africa about 150–250,000 years ago, some members migrating from there about 60–80,000 years ago, heading East to India and beyond. In a second wave of migration about 40–50,000 years ago people colonized the Mediterranean area some heading North in due course but others going East including to India. Admixture has been commonplace over the last 4000 years(37).

The key point is that 150,000 years is a short time for major genetic differences to appear and become common unless there was a marked benefit in terms of survival and reproduction. In that time human subpopulations have differentiated in many ways, including skin colour, hair type, facial features, and the ability to produce intestinal lactase throughout life to digest milk. To some extent, though not wholly, we have understood the benefits of some such changes, e.g. the lighter skin in Northern climates increases the capacity to produce vitamin D in the skin, which is necessary as solar ultraviolet B radiation is reduced as we move away from the Equator(118). The ability to digest milk into adulthood confers an advantage to populations that herd animals that produce milk that humans can drink(119). If there are genetic differences that explain the high risk of CVD and DM_2 in South Asians, the question is of the advantage they conferred and/or still confer that allowed them to accumulate through natural selection. Most common mutations (polymorphisms) are ancient and are often present in non-human primates and other mammals. We would not expect these to vary much, if at all, by ethnic group in *H. sapiens*. We will shortly consider some hypotheses that propose there were such mutations and infer the potential advantages.

The similarity of the genetic make-up of human populations is demonstrable by genetic modelling and genetic mapping studies that show that more than 99.9% of the human genome is shared across populations, leaving little room for differences–most genetic variation is within, not between, populations(120). Nonetheless, because there are 3 billion nucleotides in the human DNA, a 0.1% difference across populations means 3 million differences and even if it is only a tenth of that, 300,000 differences. The exploration of these differences is incomplete but the results to date are not promising for explaining ethnic differences in either CVD or DM_2 including in South Asians. For example, INTERHEART examined 1536 single nucleotide polymorphisms (SNPs) but only 13 were associated (statistically significantly) with CVD and 11 were related to Apo B/A1 levels, an association which we already knew about(121). The Apo E gene is one of the most important in CVD. If South Asians had a high prevalence of the high risk variant (E4/4) that would be explanatory but Chhabra et al. found the opposite(122). Kooner et al. did a genome-wide association study in three large South Asian study samples but only six new SNPs were found, associated with insulin secretion and signalling(123). Hopewell et al. (2016) concluded from their study of gene variants in 15,000 South Asian and European CHD cases and 15,000 controls that there were no clinically meaningful differences in genetic susceptibility between these populations(124). The empirical data supports the long-standing view that specific genetic differences cannot be the cause of ethnic variations in modern diseases.

Genetic studies are also finding that gene variants associated with high disease risk in European origin populations do not necessarily raise risk in South Asians(125). This kind of observation raise doubts about the causal validity of such variants. Genetic variants that do cause high risk of diseases are generally too rare to explain the extent of disease, and especially variation between groups in modern populations, as shown for the calpain 10 gene variants(126).

Occasionally, a gene variant conferring risk is found to be commoner in South Asians than Europeans, but even then the differences tend to be modest. For example, Chambers et al. reported that an SNP (rs12970134) associated with a 0.82 kg greater weight and 2 cm greater waist size was present in 30% of South Asians compared with 27% of Europeans. The odds ratio associated with this variant was only 7% higher per allele(127). Another study found no differences of importance between South Asians and Europeans in relation to gene variants for obesity(128).

Recent research has shown more variation between populations in the DNA that does not code for proteins than in DNA that does. The non-coding part was previously described as 'junk' DNA but that label is proving incorrect as its functions become understood. Another twist is the increasing evidence that *H. sapiens* interbred with other extinct humans including *H. neanderthalensis*. The important point is that such admixture may have affected different human populations differently. The evidence on this topic is scant but growing. At present, however, there is no evidence that such interbreeding was different in South Asia compared to, say, Europe or China(38).

A genetic explanation for the susceptibility to CVD and DM_2 of South Asians requires reasons why differences might have evolved and empirical evidence that differences exist. We start with the archetype of genetic hypotheses— the thrifty genotype, which arose as an explanation of why DM_2 might be so common but has been generalized beyond this to other metabolic disorders including cardiovascular diseases(94). As a prelude, Section 2.4 gives introductory information on genetics, and the origins of South Asian population.

2.4 A brief introduction to some elements of genetics relating to evolutionary hypotheses for chronic disease in individuals and populations

I have outlined the key issues relating to genetics and epidemiology in greater detail in *Concepts of Epidemiology*(27). The genome comprises of DNA and all associated elements, e.g. genes containing the codes for assembling proteins, non-gene/non-coding DNA, and RNA. DNA comprises a double strand of chemicals called nucleic acids that provide a code for assembling a sequence of amino acids to make proteins. So, DNA provides a code for making proteins. The genome can be thought of as the recipe book for biological development. There are about 20,000 genes in 23 pairs of chromosomes in the nucleus of each human cell (with the exception of reproductive cells or cells that do not have a nucleus). There are a small number of genes in the cellular structures called mitochondria which can be thought of as the batteries of the cell, storing energy and generating heat. Mitochondria are in the main body of the cell and not in the nucleus.

Changes in the number and structure of the chromosome usually lead to severe problems that need not concern us as they do not explain CVD and DM_2 epidemics. The chromosomes comprise an equal mixture of DNA from each parent. The mitochondrial genes are, essentially, from the mother as the sperm does not pass on any mitochondria when it fertilizes the ovum..

In the process of forming the male's sperm cell and female's egg cell, the ovum, there is a mixing of the original pair of chromosomes, one originally inherited from each parent, in a process called meiosis. One pair of these mixed up chromosomes is discarded in the formation of sperm from precursor cells so when the ovum is fertilized by the sperm it contains 23 pairs of chromosomes, one set from the sperm and the other from the ovum. (It is this process that underlies the concept of Mendelian randomization studies.)

The nucleic acids that make up genes are nearly identical in all humans but there are some differences that are a result of mutations which are caused, for example, by radiation. Such mutations during an individual's lifetime are important in causing cancers, but are not important causes for CVD and DM_2. If, however, mutations occur in the germ cells (sperm/ovum and their precursors) they can be transmitted across generations. Mostly such mutations are harmless. If harmless, then the mutation will not become common in large populations because there will be no (natural) selection for them across generations. If they are harmful they will be selected out by evolution as they are likely to reduce reproductive success. If a mutation improves function, it could improve survival and reproduction and hence become common in the population across many generations. The commonest kind of genetic variant is a change in one nucleic acid and is called the single nucleotide polymorphism (SNP). There are some other kinds of genetic variation including epigenetics (see Chapter 5 for a brief introduction to this process).

If 1% or more of the population has a gene variant (say a SNP), that is considered common. If the advantage conferred by a mutation is large, the variant can even become the commonest version, e.g. the variant of the lactase gene that permits production of the digestive enzyme lactase, usually only found in the early years, has become the norm in Northern European adults giving them the capacity to digest substantial quantities of milk sugars throughout life. The survival and reproductive advantage of this mutation, especially when food is scarce in winter and it is hard to hunt or gather food, is evident.

The mutant variant version of the gene may be present on none, one, or both of a pair of chromosomes. The variant can be dominant or recessive meaning that it is preferentially expressed, or not so, respectively. If the variant is recessive the individual will need to have it on both chromosomes for the effect to occur, whereas if it is dominant its presence on one chromosome will produce the effect. For example, the SNPs causing sickle cell disease are recessive (so the effect occurs only if the variant is on both of the pair of chromosomes) while those causing familial hypercholesterolaemia are dominant (so the effect occurs even if the variant is only in one of the two chromosomes). It is usually difficult to pinpoint the advantages of such variants that allow them to become common but sometimes we understand them. The sickle cell mutation offers protection from malaria(129). We do not know the evolutionary advantage, if any, of the familial hypercholesterolaemia variant. This latter mutation is, fortunately, quite rare at about 0.4%.

Common gene variants are usually a result of very old mutations as it takes many generations for them to accrue in the population. The lactase gene variant has accrued exceptionally fast in only 7000 years. The advantages of such mutations that were present in ancient times may not apply in modern times, e.g. the sickle cell variant is of no value to South Asians or Africans living in countries where there is no malaria.

While familial hypercholesterolemia is a classic example of SNPs causing CVD, this kind of genetic variation is too rare to explain population level differences in CVD. As no SNPs have been discovered that potentially do this, current interest is in the role of multiple genes acting together with environmental factors in a complex, multifactorial way.

CVD and DM_2 usually 'run in families' but no common, simple genetic mechanisms have been discovered to explain this. The inheritability may arise from the effects of many genes together (gene–gene interactions), genes and environmental factors together, or largely the effects of the environment alone. Gene variants have not been selected through evolution to either increase or lower CVD and DM_2 as these are diseases of modern times. However, gene variants alter anatomy, biochemistry, immune function, and physiology to change the person's or populations' susceptibility to diseases. The changes may alter, for example, metabolism, the endothelial lining of the arteries, or the structure and vasculature of the beta cell of the pancreas.

There must, obviously, be genetic control on the level of biological risk factors. This control, as a minimum, must be on the lowest level compatible with life, e.g. the lowest BP or cholesterol. There must be genetic controls on the optimum level and mechanisms for maintaining homeostasis, e.g. keeping the diastolic BP at rest between 60 and 80mmHg. The capacity for homeostasis is genetic. Allostasis is the capacity to alter, semi-permanently if not permanently, the set-point of a biological characteristic, e.g. in some people the BP changes, say from 80mmHg at rest to 90mmHg at rest. The reasons are not usually discovered. Clearly, however, we have the genetic capacity for such change. Some populations may have looser allostasis or homeostasis than others, so permitting a more rapid or greater change in response to environmental change. If so, these differences must have evolved and been selected for. It is this kind of thinking that has sparked several evolutionary, genetically based hypotheses to explain, firstly, human susceptibility to CVD and DM_2 and, secondly, differences in susceptibility between populations.

Evolutionary hypotheses have considerable potential value in: 1) understanding the fundamental reasons why gene variants that increase the risk of diseases may become common; 2) understanding within and between population variations in disease patterns; 3) interpreting empirical research evidence, e.g. on why obesity is becoming common and why it is related to DM_2; 4) contributing to a causal framework; 5) setting directions for empirical research; 6) providing additional, arguably deeper, insights into the prevention and control of diseases, especially across generations. We first consider the highly influential thrifty gene hypothesis.

2.5 The thrifty genotype hypothesis

This hypothesis was articulated in detail by James Neel in 1962 and has maintained its hold to this day, and it has led to modifications, developments, and new directions(94, 130). Whether genetic or otherwise, the concept of thriftiness has become central in the fields of CVD and DM_2, perhaps especially as related to South Asians. For example, in their review of risk factors in childhood Prasad et al. (2011) pick out the thrifty genotype and genetic susceptibility as of particular relevance(131). This is commonplace in the literature on DM$_2$ and CVD in South Asians, even although Neel has first modified and then pointed to weaknesses in the data supporting this hypothesis(130, 132).

Box 2.1 (p 52) summarizes Neel's paper with my introductory and concluding remarks. Figure 2.1 is my summary of the hypothesis as a simple causal diagram. Neel's paper sets out to explain the high prevalence of DM$_2$. His remarkable concept is that the mechanisms that lead to DM$_2$ in modern life were an adaptation that permitted survival and reproduction in the hunter-gatherer state that our species spent most of its history in. Twenty years later Neel updated the hypothesis, acknowledging that his 1962 version was wrong in detail, especially on the role of anti-insulins, but may still be right in principle. The core concepts remained much the same though he introduced a new detail— that high levels of insulin during fasting prevent loss of glucose in the urine and hence conserve calories. The main difference is his differentiating between insulin (now type 1) and non-insulin (type 2) dependent diabetes and offering at least three alternatives to why high levels of insulin cause insulin resistance and extra pressure on beta-cells in the pancreas. Two of the explanations relate to insulin receptors (function and number) and the third to lipid accumulation in fat depots, particularly the liver, that increase insulin resistance. Overall, the revision of the hypothesis is about the mechanisms and not the core concept.

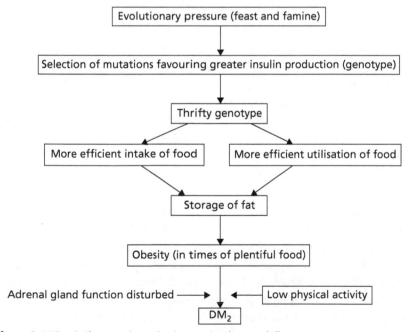

Figure 2.1 The thrifty gene hypothesis: my simple causal diagram.

If the hypothesis is correct then we should find evidence for its central predictions including that individuals and populations predisposed to DM$_2$ should:

♦ Have had stronger evolutionary pressures to adapt in this way i.e. more exposure to feast or famine than other populations at lower risk

♦ Have greater intake of food or be able to utilize it more efficiently (thrift), both for genetic reasons

♦ Should survive and reproduce better

♦ Have high insulin production that is genetically determined (not secondary to other factors e.g. obesity).

Table 2.1 summarizes some evidence for and against this and related hypotheses. The assumptions underpinning the hypothesis have been questioned and criticized. The criticisms have included the broad one that the hypothesis follows a tradition of biological determinism that seeks causes in genetic factors when they actually lie in social, environmental, and lifestyle ones(133, 134). More specific criticisms include that the state of feast or famine was, probably, a universal one in most of human history and would be expected to be most extreme in places where the winter was harshest and not in warm climate countries(135, 136). The pattern of DM$_2$ and insulin resistance syndromes shows these problems are, however, commonest in warm climate populations including South Asians and least in Northern Europeans evolving in cold winter climes(137). Ireland, among many countries, has suffered from severe famines but its population does not have a severe predisposition to DM$_2$. The argument that South Asians were subjected to famines is strong but possibly not so on evolutionary time scales, with many of the most severe ones, e.g. the Bengal famine of 1943, occurring in recent centuries and being especially hard hitting in colonial times, i.e. the last few hundred years(138). The evidence that people at high risk of DM$_2$ have greater 'thrift' in acquisition or metabolism of food is not strong and we will return to this in the mitochondrial efficiency hypothesis below.

The hypothesis explains that storage of energy as fat is the key to survival and reproductive success. Adipose tissue has a multiplicity of important, even vital, functions and this concept cannot be set aside. Obesity, however, with large amounts of additional adipose tissue, reduces reproductive success, and obese people do not survive starvation conditions better than others(135, 136).

Ultimately, however, a genetic hypothesis needs support from genetic studies. Obesity-related genes have not been shown to have functions that might provide other survival and reproductive advantages(135). The genes that relate to higher risks of DM$_2$, tend to be about appetite, glucose, pancreatic function, insulin, and other aspects of metabolism rather than obesity itself(139). Gene

Table 2.1 Evidence for and against the thrifty genotype, drifty genotype

Hypothesis	Evidence and arguments in favour	Evidence and arguments against
1. Thrifty genotype	Thrifty variant gene affecting BMI found in Samoans(143).	Biological determinism is emphasized when the important causes are social and environmental(134).
		Famine/feast would have occurred in all populations but especially where winters are severe(136).
		Famine in Indian Subcontinent is a recent phenomenon, exacerbated by colonialism(138).
		Survival in obese people not necessarily better in starvation(135, 136).
		Obesity reduces fecundity(135).
		Gene variants not found where expected, e.g. Pima Indians and Oji Cree(133).
		Obesity-related genes show no properties to indicate an adaptive advantage.
		Thrifty gene in Samoans protects against DM_2(144).
2. Predation release/drifty gene	A model is provided that fits reasonably well with the observed distribution of BMI(145).	Biological determinism. Explanatory power is in explaining why humans are susceptible to obesity but not why this susceptibility might differ across ethnic groups, e.g. South Asians.
3. Mitochondrial efficiency	Generalizes explanation to warm climates. One study provides an independent test the hypothesis (Nair) (151).	Biological determinism. Explanatory power limited to explaining how energy is conserved so it can be stored as fat. Genetic evidence limited.

variants with thrifty properties have been difficult to find in populations at high risk of DM_2, including in South Asians. Tabassum et al. reported a study of 12,535 Indians. The loci linked to DM_2 were associated with 7.65% of the risk. Nearly all the loci were already identified in non-South Asian populations(140). Kooner and colleagues have found a few extra susceptibility loci for South Asians(123).

An important transferable message for South Asians can be derived from the observation that the gene variants associated with CVD, explored in 68 papers, made no contribution to explain the pattern of CVD in African and White Americans(141). It is likely this conclusion will apply to the analogous work on South Asians and White Europeans, with some evidence to this effect already(121), even although some variants have been found(142). A gene variant in Samoans does have the properties associated with thrift but it is, for reasons that are yet to be explained, protective against DM_2(143, 144).

Currently, the thrifty gene hypothesis in itself is a weak candidate in explaining the high risk of DM_2 (and indirectly CVD) in high risk populations such as South Asians. Other closely related ideas are also unlikely to be strong candidates but we will take a brief look at three ideas developed in response to the thrifty genotype, i.e. the predation release, drifty phenotype, and mitochondrial efficiency.

2.6 The predation release and drifty genotype hypotheses

The predation release/drifty genotype hypotheses are an alternative interpretation of the human tendency to obesity and subsequently diabetes where the evolutionary forces are unrelated to feast and famine(135, 145, 146). Box 2.2 (p 54) and Figure 2.2 summarize the predation release and closely related drifty gene hypotheses. The reasoning is that there are separate genetic controls on the lower and upper levels of BMI. The selection pressures to maintain a minimum BMI are influenced by factors such as the need for females' reproduction success and male and females' immune function and these have continued over time. The evolutionary pressure to avoid a high BMI has diminished since the risk of being chased and possibly maimed or killed by predators has declined. These controls from predation are ancient and long predate the arrival

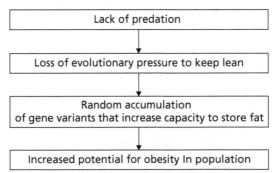

Figure 2.2 Predation release and drifty genotype hypothesis of Speakman: my simple causal diagram.

of *H. sapiens*. Although it is a fascinating hypothesis, at present, I cannot see how it might explain ethnic group variations, specifically South Asians' susceptibility to CVD and DM_2, but we will reconsider it in the explanatory models in Chapter 9. It is interesting, however, that South Asian women tend to have reproductive success at very low BMIs, possibly because of fat preservation—a matter we will return to.

We now turn to another related idea that considers the evolutionary pressure to control body temperature in warm climates.

2.7 **The mitochondrial efficiency hypothesis**

The potential importance of mitochondria in the causation of metabolic disorders including DM_2 has already been highlighted in Chapter 1, Section 1.8. Taylor, for example, postulates that a mitochondrial function impairment allows lipid accumulation in cells leading to insulin resistance, subsequently leading to beta cell damage(79). Other perspectives on the role of mitochondria include the mitochondrial efficiency hypothesis which tries to explain why South Asians have a tendency to accumulate fat(147). I have placed the hypothesis in this genetic hypotheses chapter, because it offers an evolutionary perspective. Mitochondrial function, however, can also be affected in non-genetic ways, perhaps in line with the DOHAD hypothesis. In Chapter 5 (DOHAD) and in Chapter 7 (diet) I also return to mitochondrial in relation to maternal diet.

Box 2.3 (p 55) summarizes this hypothesis and Figure 2.3 gives my explanatory, simple causal diagram. The thrifty gene proposes there might be more efficient

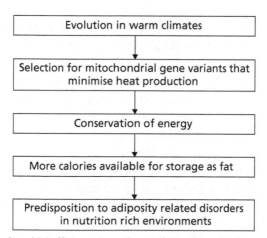

Figure 2.3 Mitochondrial efficiency hypothesis of Bhopal and Rafnsson: my simple causal diagram.

utilization of food. But how so? That is not clear. In this hypothesis the core idea is that there is less use of energy in maintaining body temperature. The idea here provides a potential mechanism for conserving energy that might then be stored as fat. The idea is that over evolutionary periods, driven by the needs of living in a warm climate, the cellular 'batteries', the mitochondria, have become more thrifty in conserving energy in the form of the molecule ATP (adenosine triphosphate) rather than using energy via the alternative mechanism of releasing it as heat.

The hypothesis would predict that the basal metabolic rate of people with such efficiency would be comparatively low. There is not strong evidence for a comparatively low metabolic rate in South Asians though it is true for Africans, and there is a clear relationship between increasing obesity and diminishing basal metabolic rate(148–150). Measuring basal metabolism is very difficult and there have been few studies including South Asians.

In their 1991 review of equations to predict basal metabolic rate in the tropics Henry and Rees conclude that this has been overestimated by about 13% in Indians and 22% in Ceylonese (now called Sri Lankans)(149). This is greater than previous studies that also indicated an overestimation. If this is correct, whether as a result of muscular or thyroid function (as the authors speculate), or more adipose tissue/less muscle or mitochondrial function (as here) the point is that nutritional guidelines may be overestimating South Asians' caloric needs.

Direct studies of mitochondrial function in South Asians are also few(151, 152). Cassel et al. examined the association between the basal metabolic rate and mitochondrial uncoupling protein predominant in skeletal muscle (UCP3) in 85 South Indian and 150 European parent–offspring pairs (one of them at least with DM_2) and 455 community-based South Indians(152). The dysfunctional variant of MCP3 associated with reduced thermogenesis was associated with a raised waist/hip ratio in females but not with other outcomes. Nair et al. studied 13 young South Asian people with and 13 without diabetes and compared them with Northern European origin Americans (see Box 2.3, p 55). Their study, done after this hypothesis was proposed, but completely independently, showed evidence for the hypothesis(151). Martinez-Hervas et al., in a 2011 paper, found genetic variants associated with tight coupling, i.e. efficiency as above, were associated with a higher waist circumference and increased abdominal obesity in the Spanish population(153).

The explanatory power of this hypothesis in relation to the CVD and DM_2 epidemic is limited but it could be an underlying component for several hypotheses and risk factors: mitochondrial efficiency, low physical activity, and rising calorie intake(147).

2.8 **Conclusions**

The thrifty gene and related hypotheses are ingenious and have captured and retained attention. They propose evolutionary forces of one kind or another that make it possible to store additional fat, a tissue with many purposes in addition to being an energy reservoir (see Chapter 3, Section 3.4 for the roles of fat). If these hypotheses are partially correct they help to explain why humans are susceptible to becoming overweight and even greatly obese. This would, potentially, partly explain the rise in insulin resistance (secondary to fat deposition) and connect us to CVD and DM_2 via the metabolic dysfunction that accompanies insulin resistance as in Reaven's ideas that were considered in Chapter 1 (Box 1.3, p 36).

There are three important obstacles to these kinds of hypotheses as explanations for the susceptibility of South Asians to CVD and DM_2. First, the empirical evidence backing the hypotheses is limited despite more than 50 years of research. Paradoxically and surprisingly, in 2016 a thrifty gene was found in Samoans but while it was associated with extra weight it was also associated with less risk of DM_2(143, 144). Second, theoretical criticism of the basic assumptions of the thrifty genotype hypothesis have accumulated(134–136). Third, the evidence that being overweight or obese, the key outcome considered in these hypotheses, is a risk factor for mortality and possibly even CVD in South Asians populations is weak(154–156). Weight gain in South Asians undoubtedly contributes strongly to DM_2 and its precursor conditions(78, 157). In many studies in populations worldwide the relationship between all-cause mortality and CVD outcomes and overweight and even mild/moderate obesity has been hard to demonstrate. This has been called the obesity paradox, and it is also seen in South Asians. This is a controversial area of ongoing debate but in my view it is most likely that there are methodological reasons why it occurs, and that in reality being overweight/obese is not beneficial with few exceptions such as infections. I will consider adiposity, overweight, and obesity in much more detail in Chapters 3 and 7.

Despite the above criticisms, it would not be wise to discard from our causal synthesis in Chapter 9 a potential role, albeit a modest one, for the thrifty genotype family of hypotheses. The hypotheses here could explain generalized overweight and obesity, yet we know fat accumulation in particular places, especially intra-abdominally and in the liver, is more the problem. In Chapter 3 we consider two genetic explanations related to body shape and size, where the pattern of fat distribution is emphasized.

Box 2.1 The thrifty gene

Neel J.V. Diabetes mellitus: A 'Thrifty' genotype rendered detrimental by 'Progress'? American Journal of Human Genetics 1962;14:353–62(94).

My introductory remarks

This paper set out a captivating hypothesis that has held centre stage in many discussions of population variations in obesity, diabetes mellitus, and their sequelae, including CVD. The hypothesis has been subjected to criticisms on first principles and is currently buffeted by unsupportive genetic empirical research as we will discuss in the text. It remains popular even though Neel was lukewarm about his hypothesis in later publications(132). Imitation is flattery, and is reflected in the naming of later hypotheses to echo this one, e.g. the thrifty phenotype and the drifty gene. I have created a simple causal diagram, Figure 2.1, using the textual descriptions in the paper, which is summarized below.

Summary of the paper

The paper opens with the question of why non-insulin dependent diabetes mellitus (DM, now called type 2 diabetes mellitus and DM_2 in this book) is common even though it has a strong genetic basis, and, therefore, we would expect it to be selected out by evolution, e.g. because the disease would be expected to reduce reproductive success. Neel's hypothesis offers an explanation starting with the observation that some people are predisposed to DM from birth. Further, he notes that mothers with DM are more likely to have large babies. Neel postulates this is not just the effect of the mother but also the predisposition of the baby. This predisposition is to a thrifty genotype, making the person efficient in intake and/or utilization of food. He offers mechanisms on how thriftiness might operate, i.e. more prolonged or more rapid secretion of insulin leads to (relative) hypoglycaemia, leading to sensation of hunger and greater food intake.

Neel then makes a key assumption that humans evolved mostly in states of feast or famine when they were hunter-gatherers. If so, the ability to secrete extra insulin would be valuable in permitting the storage of excess energy as fat to be accessed during famines. Babies born to mothers with DM handle a glucose load better than other children and this may not just relate to maternal factors but the baby's genotype.

Box 2.1 The thrifty gene (*continued*)

Neel questions how a state of insulin excess, which he observes is also seen in pre-diabetics and those with mild diabetes, turns in later stages to a disease characterized by an insulin deficit. He dismisses exhaustion of the pancreas, where insulin is produced, as an explanation. He postulates the discrepancy is a result of an overproduction of anti-insulins.

He explains the modern rise in DM, firstly, as a result of increasing obesity, preceded and accompanied by high levels of insulin and then of anti-insulin. Secondly, he invokes a disturbance in the response of the adrenal cortex in releasing adrenaline. Thirdly, as in modern societies adrenaline release is not followed by physical activity as much as in past societies, the glucose mobilized by adrenaline leads to an insulin and insulin antagonist response. He includes DM as one of the stress diseases.

In short, Neel proposes that genetically driven insulin overproduction is the first phase in most diabetes, followed by overproduction of anti-insulins. This overproduction of insulin was, purportedly, an asset in hunter-gatherer times. Neel then suggests that people with less severe variants (in his words heterozygotes) may also have a thrifty genotype without the disadvantages of developing DM. This then is the advantage that allows the selection of mutations that underpin the thrifty genotype. Neel optimistically forecasts this hypothesis will be easy to test.

My concluding remarks

This is a wide-ranging paper with many matters considered including the eugenic implications of the hypothesis. Neel's ideas are based on a relatively simple genetic basis to DM, akin to Mendelian inheritance, whereas we now know that it is a multifactorial disorder with complex genetic influences. The central idea is of intrinsic, enhanced, early life capacity to secrete extra insulin to help store intermittently available, excess energy as fat for use in times of food shortage. It is especially interesting to note his seldom cited observation on adrenal function as a contributor, his inclusion of DM among the stress diseases, and also his view that DM is not a result of pancreatic exhaustion. The thrifty gene concept has been widely generalized including to South Asian populations, and to related disorders including cardiovascular diseases.

Box 2.2 Predation release hypothesis and the drifty gene

Speakman JR. A nonadaptive scenario explaining the genetic predisposition to obesity: The 'predation release' hypothesis. Cell Metabolism. 2007;6(1):5–12(146).

Speakman JR. Thrifty genes for obesity, an attractive but flawed idea, and an alternative perspective: the 'drifty gene' hypothesis. International Journal of Obesity. 2008;32(11):1611–17(145).

My introduction

Predation release is one of several alternative explanations for the increased tendency to obesity in humans and it, in essence, follows the argument of the thrifty genotype hypothesis but offers an alternative to feast and famine, i.e. release from the fear of predation by wild animals (my comment—possibly humans as well). The arguments here were later developed to articulate the drifty gene hypothesis. My simple causal diagram for this hypothesis is Figure 2.2.

The papers and the hypothesis

The author accepts that obesity has strong genetic underpinnings and also the importance of evolutionary forces and then explains why famine was not the key factor. The underpinning evolutionary force is hypothesized to be release from predation. The genetic variations accumulate through genetic drift, not positive selection, hence the subsequent description the drifty genotype. The difference is that genetic drift, rather than positive selection, would explain why the variants favouring fat storage are not already nearly universal—even in the US only a little more than 60% of people are either overweight or obese.

In wild animals, body weight is tightly controlled and highly resistant to changes in the availability of food. In humans living as hunter gatherers or in subsistence agriculture communities, the BMI is about 18–22 kg/m². The level of fat at such BMIs is important to female reproduction, and to countering the dangers of temporary food insecurity. Using the example of the small mammal, the vole, he shows that the presence of predators influences body size, keeping it small. The point is that small, lean animals can escape predators easier than large fat ones.

Box 2.2 Predation release hypothesis and the drifty gene (*continued*)

In the period of human development 2–6 million years ago, predators were more common. Banding together socially, using fire and making tools among *Homo* species occurred about 2 million years ago and would have been strong defences against predators. Mutations leading to increased body size would accumulate randomly in the absence of predation (which would select for smaller body size). There will be an asymmetry because the pressures to maintain a minimum BMI will remain for reproduction and immune function but the pressure for the BMI not to rise have diminished as predation risk declines.

My concluding remarks

The predation release hypothesis proposes both different timescales and evolutionary pressures for the genetic susceptibility to obesity compared with the thrifty gene hypothesis. Unlike the thrifty genotype, however, this one is universal to all modern day human populations, so it cannot explain differences between them, and specifically, South Asians' predisposition to adiposity-related problems. It is directly relevant, however, as it takes attention away from famine and ideas such as the thrifty genotype that have been closely associated with South Asian populations.

Box 2.3 The mitochondrial efficiency hypothesis

Bhopal RS, Rafnsson SB. Could mitochondrial efficiency explain the susceptibility to adiposity, metabolic syndrome, diabetes and cardiovascular diseases in South Asian populations? International Journal of Epidemiology 2009;38(4):1072–81(147).

My introductory remarks

As the instigator of this hypothesis, developed with my colleague Snorri Rafnsson, I was trying to integrate ideas around thriftiness of energy metabolism (thrifty gene, thrifty phenotype) and those around climate adaptation, a feature that I had thought important in the adipose tissue compartment overflow hypothesis (see Chapter 3). If energy is being conserved, I reasoned it would be through mitochondria, the cellular battery.

Box 2.3 The mitochondrial efficiency hypothesis (*continued*)

The paper

The paper sets the scene of South Asians' high rates of CVD, DM_2, and related metabolic disorders, the inability to explain the excess using traditional risk factors including insulin resistance and dysglycaemia, and four major hypotheses: 1) thrifty genotype, 2) thrifty phenotype (Chapter 5), 3) adipose tissue overflow (Chapters 3 and 4) and variable disease selection (Chapter 3). These hypotheses all propose conservation of energy as fat including creating a deep visceral fat store. The question posed is of how South Asians might have conserved energy to make this possible. The hypothesis here is that this is done by reducing the heat production function of mitochondria. The underlying evolutionary forces were assumed to be adaptation to a warm climate, limited food supply and as a response to infectious disease (so conserving energy for the use of the immune system).

This paper then explains the nature of mitochondria, which number about 10 million billion in the average person, with 300–400 per cell. Their role is either to use dietary energy to produce potential energy stored in the molecule ATP (adenosine triphosphate) or to produce heat. The efficiency with which dietary energy is converted to ATP is related to the efficiency of a biochemical process called oxidative phosphorylation (OXPHOS). When efficiency is high there is high ATP production and low heat production. Such mitochondria are said to be tightly coupled and to have high coupling efficiency.

Of the 80 or so proteins involved in OXPHOS, 13 are encoded by mitochondrial DNA, the rest by nuclear DNA. The mitochondrial DNA variants correlate with latitude indicating climate, among other forces, has been important in their evolution. Mitochondria are almost entirely transmitted from mother to child through the ovum as the sperm cell does not pass on any mitochondria during the process of fertilization.

There are several uncoupling proteins (UCP). UCP_1 is in brown fat and favours dissipation of energy as heat. UCP_2 and UCP_3 are widely distributed in tissues. UCP polymorphisms are associated with basal metabolic rate and fat mass in African American women. This paper reported no evidence of this kind for South Asians, and only one directly relevant study was found, that of Nair et al.(151). They compared 13 non-diabetic Asian Indians in the US and 13 Northern European Americans, matching for age, sex, and BMI. Similar comparisons were made for South Asian and North European people with diabetes. Asians Indians with and without diabetes had similar

Box 2.3 The mitochondrial efficiency hypothesis (*continued*)

mitochondrial function but higher OXPHOS activity than their Northern European American counterparts. Our hypothesis was first written in 2006, 2 years before Nair's paper, and completely independently so we took this to be in support of our prior hypothesis.

High OXPHOS implies tight(er) coupling and use of energy for purposes other than heat generation. One important result of energy saved is more energy available for fat storage. This potentially valuable trait may become maladaptive in modern times.

The mitochondrial efficiency hypothesis offers a mechanism for the effects of thrifty genotypes and phenotypes, and a way of conserving energy to be stored in fat depots. The paper, therefore, emphasized the value of the hypothesis for connecting ideas, including on modern lifestyles. The paper notes the potential relevance to all warm climate populations.

Concluding remarks

The paper pointed to a fundamental biological mechanism through which a general tendency to metabolic disturbances might be explained. Remarkably, there was only one study on South Asians to test it and it was published long after we started work so it was an independent test of a prior hypothesis.

Chapter 3

Genetic explanations 2: adaptations in body size, shape, and composition

3.1 Chapter 3 objectives are to:

1. Discuss the core ingredients of hypotheses that relate to body size, shape, and composition especially those focussing on adipose tissue mass and distribution, and muscle mass. These hypotheses include the adipose tissue overflow hypothesis and the variable disease selection hypothesis.
2. Summarize the evidence relating to these hypotheses.
3. Critically evaluate the validity of these hypotheses as explanations for South Asians' high susceptibility to CVD and DM_2.
4. Explore potential links between these and the hypotheses in Chapter 2.

3.2 Chapter summary

Observations on the differing body shapes of populations worldwide such as length of the limbs in relation to the trunk, usually attributed to the influence of climate, have been further developed in relation to South Asians' health. The distribution of body fat has been studied as central body fat has been shown to be metabolically harmful unlike peripheral fat. Two recent hypotheses—the adipose tissue (compartment) overflow hypothesis, and the variable disease selection hypotheses—aim to explain why South Asians tend to have a high proportion of their fat tissue on the trunk and intra-abdominally. The former proposes it results from a small primary, superficial subcutaneous fat compartment especially in the lower limbs, so excess energy is deposited as fat in other compartments. The evolutionary forces leading to this are presumed to be climatic. The latter proposes central fat deposits in South Asians as an evolutionary adaptation to gastrointestinal infections. There has also been an interest in the amount and function of brown fat in South Asians.

South Asians' also have small muscle mass, and small hips, for which there are no well-defined hypotheses. The small size at birth of South Asians may be relevant to all these observations. These differences in abdominal fat distribution and differences in skeletal structure with a small pelvis could explain a tendency to central (apple-shaped) obesity which has more adverse cardio-metabolic effects than generalized or peripheral obesity (pear-shaped). These differences are, most likely, driven by genetic and developmental factors. Overall, the evidence for these explanations is small but expanding. The possible overlaps with the genetic explanations in Chapter 2 and the developmental explanations in Chapter 5 are considered.

3.3 **Introduction**

Of the major cardiovascular and DM_2 risk factors (Tables 1.4 and 1.5) that are widely agreed as causal the only one that relates to body size and shape is obesity and particularly central obesity(158). Yet, there are empirically demonstrated associations between several other measures of body size and shape and both CVD and DM_2. Among these are height, leg length, and waist-to-hip ratio as a measure of both hip and waist size, and muscle bulk and strength(159). Populations vary considerably in these measures in ways that seem relevant to CVD and DM_2. These variations are often not genetic, even although they may wrongly be assumed to be. For example, socio-economic development has led to a large gain in height in just one or two generations, a change that is demonstrable globally but especially in populations generally thought to be innately small, e.g. Bangladeshis, Chinese, and Japanese. In this chapter we will concentrate on genetically orientated explanations, and defer developmental (Chapter 5), socio-economic (Chapter 6), and risk-factor-related (Chapters 7, 8) explanations until later. Bodily dimensions are related to climate and these relationships are changing over time, given trends in height and adiposity(160).

Genetic factors are important though understanding their role in relation to non-genetic factors is difficult. The most obvious example is the difference between males and females in height, weight, muscle-mass, fat mass, and fat distribution. Obviously, these characteristics are modifiable by the environment but genetic factors underlie the male–female differences. Some of the difference in height, muscle mass, and fat between ethnic groups might also be partly genetic, but environment is a big player. In this chapter, I will concentrate on adipose tissue and muscle mass as both are clearly important for CVD and DM_2. The story is complex as multiple genes are involved in the pathway to obesity. Some genetic variants associated with promoting obesity are, surprisingly, associated with less disease, including DM_2 and CVD(161). The explanation may be that these variants make it easier to store excess energy in subcutaneous, rather than intra-abdominal, fat stores, which links well to the discussion in Section 3.4 on fat distribution.

The gene variants that are most clearly linked to obesity are related to appetite control(139). The most clear cut of these is genetic leptin deficiency, and we do find ethnic differences in this hormone(162). Leptin is a hormone produced by adipose tissue that was discovered in 1994. Leptin signals satiety to the brain and its absence signals hunger. Leptin deficiency causes severe obesity because appetite cannot be regulated normally. Fortunately, these kind of genetic abnormalities are very rare but they inform us about biological pathways to obesity. There is an interplay between genetic and developmental fetal and child factors in determining fat and muscle mass and distribution (Chapter 5). The issues in this chapter also relate to the insulin resistance hypothesis (Chapter 1) and to the thrifty gene family of ideas in Chapter 2. These links will be integrated in Chapter 9.

3.4 The distribution of body fat and why it matters

The traditional, lay view of body fat is that it is healthy to be plump, especially as a baby and child, and it is unhealthy to be skinny and even to be lean, although views are changing over time and vary by ethnic group and generation(163, 164). This is almost universal, especially in South Asian societies as reflected, for example, in the near equivalence of the Hindi and Punjabi word for good health (*atchi seth*) with not being skinny but plump. I was a plump baby and child and this characteristic was widely admired in my family, until I lost most of my childhood fat in adolescence. This lay view is important both for its potential truth and for designing culturally acceptable health promotion. There may be some wisdom in lay views, not least in relation to general indicators of health including mortality, and they need to be respected.

A low BMI, say less than 18.5 kg/m^2, is associated with higher mortality, and a raised risk of infections, especially of the respiratory tract including tuberculosis (154, 165). This kind of adverse association has usually been interpreted as a result of a lack of fat and hence impaired immune function but BMI is also reflecting lean tissue, especially muscle. In one study a low percentage of body fat was not associated with high mortality while a low BMI was, suggesting lean tissue is important in explaining the association. Being excessively and obviously obese has not been associated with good health, at least in the modern era, and this has been confirmed in multiple studies(166–168). Speakman's hypothesis that we discussed in Chapter 2 presumes that the threat of predation, and the need to flee from predators fast and nimbly, was a deterrent to obesity over evolutionary time scales(146). It is reasonable to assume that excessive fat was never, or rarely perceived as good although there are ancient, prehistoric statuettes of extremely obese people, usually women, thought to be celebrating fertility.

The traditional medical view, one that I was taught as a medical student in the 1970s, was that fat was a relatively inert, energy storage tissue with a low metabolic rate. Despite this, the medical view that being overweight, and especially being obese, was harmful is longstanding and backed up by extensive epidemiological research(166, 168). One of the recent surprises in this research, however, has been that being modestly overweight has little or no measureable adverse effect on all-cause death rates and very small effects on CVD death rates, especially in South Asians (the adverse effects on DM_2 are, however, clear-cut even with small gains in weight)(154, 155, 168, 169). This topic has become very controversial with several huge, contradictory, meta-analyses. Obesity is discussed in detail as a classic cardiovascular and DM_2 risk factor in Section 7.8 in Chapter 7 and some readers might find it helpful to read that section as background to the hypotheses to be discussed here. I have also summarized some of the functions of adipose tissue in Tables 3.1 and 3.2.

In 1956 Jean Vague published a now classic paper on male and female patterns of obesity. He proposed that the female pattern—called gynoid obesity—only caused mechanical problems(170). The male pattern—called android obesity—lead to metabolic disturbances, and he identified these as contributing to premature atherosclerosis and diabetes. He estimated that this pattern

Table 3.1 Functions of adipose tissue and examples of products produced by fat cells

1	Endocrine organ producing hormones including leptin, resistin, adiponectin, and cytokines
2	Immunity including triggering molecules and macrophages (e.g. we observe high TB rates in thin people)
3	Energy storage mostly as triglyceride
4	Heat production (especially but not exclusively from beige and brown fat)
5	Protection (physical barrier between skin and internal structures)
6	Insulation from cold and heat
7	Sexual attraction especially in female secondary sexual characteristics
8	Regulation of appetite through the release of hormones, especially leptin
9	Energy expenditure regulation
10	Triggering menarche and in maintaining fertility in females
11	Maintenance of social status as larger size is associated with more status

Table 3.2 Adipose tissue types and compartments and their properties

Compartments	Characteristics and products
All fat	Leptin (appetite regulation), low metabolism tissue (except brown fat), and adiponectin (insulin sensitizing and anti-inflammatory protein)
	Interleukins lead to increase in inflammation, e.g. as shown by CRP
	Regulates metabolic rate via thyroid hormones and catecholamines
White fat	Few mitochondria
	As BMI rises brown fat declines
Brown fat (beige fat is intermediate between white fat and brown fat)	Small amount in humans but more can be induced
	Found mostly in neck and upper thorax
	Mitochondria are many and express uncoupling protein (heat production)
	Originate from muscle cells
Superficial subcutaneous	Not associated with increased CVD risk (possibly protective, especially if in lower limbs)
	Essential depot for energy storage
	Especially important source of leptin
Deep subcutaneous	The effects depend on location. The fat on the trunk (especially the back) is deleterious in South Asians.
Intra-abdominal/omental	Clearly associated with CVD and DM_2 risk
	Promotes atherosclerotic pattern of lipids (LDL-c concentration and particle size)
	Produces much more resistin than other depots. Products go to liver directly via portal circulation.
	Most sensitive to catecholamines
	Promotes inflammation
Muscle	Energy source for muscle
	Intramuscular fat correlates with insulin resistance but not in South Asians
In and around specific organs	
Liver	Strongly related to insulin resistance but may have benefits, e.g. fat around the heart has been reported to produce chemicals that dilate the arteries. The role of pancreatic fat is unknown.
Heart/pericardium	
Pancreas	

of obesity is the cause of diabetes in the adult in 80–90% of cases. He proposed that over-activity of the pituitary–adrenal axis was the cause of android obesity. In hindsight, this account seems remarkable. In the 60 years since, adipose tissue has been shown to be not one but several tissues with different anatomy, physiology, biochemistry, functions (see Table 3.1), and adverse effects. In a recent experiment Shadid et al. gave radiolabelled free fatty acids to men and women. In men abdominal subcutaneous fat took up more of these fatty acids than femoral leg fat depots. In women femoral depots took up more than subcutaneous ones(171). This experiment underlines the veracity of Vague's concept, and his emphasis on abdominal subcutaneous male/female differences in adipose tissue. This is a rapidly developing area of knowledge. Table 3.2 lists several fat types and compartments with some of their products and properties.

In 2014 Chau et al. showed that the embryological origins of fat compartments are different(172). The visceral fat compartments have different embryological origins than the subcutaneous or brown fat ones. Usually visceral fat is considered as one compartment but Chau et al. list six: omental, mesenteric, retroperitoneal, renal, gonadal, and epicardial. There may be different kinds of brown fat, including some brown fat cells that have an embryological origin in common with myocytes (muscle cells). Brown fat utilizes glucose and free fatty acids to produce heat through the mechanism discussed in Section 2.7 (mitochondrial efficiency hypothesis), and there is a small amount of contradictory research studying this in South Asians(173, 174). People with high levels of fat tend to have low levels of brown fat. The role of brown fat in South Asians in relation to CVD and DM_2 is unclear at present. This kind of advance heralds new ways of thinking with, as yet, unclear consequences. These may be very subtle effects, e.g. Veilleux et al. reported that omental adipocyte enlargement was associated with high triglycerides in the blood, but this was not true for subcutaneous adipocytes(175). We cannot think of body fat as simple or as one organ. We now discuss distribution related hypotheses that focus attention on South Asians and other populations at high risk of CVD and DM_2.

3.5 Explaining South Asians' tendency to high levels of adiposity in general and abdominal obesity in particular

Compared to White Europeans South Asians have relatively more fat as a percentage of body mass and a higher proportion of this fat is on the torso and in intra-abdominal compartments(83, 86, 176–179). This has been shown in South Asia and South Asian babies and adults across the world including in Bangladesh and in Surinam where Indians settled more than 100 years ago(180, 181). The strong association between intra-abdominal fat and lipid-related risk factors is also demonstrable. It is important to emphasize, however, that the total amount of fat is often similar, or even lower, in South Asians. The main reason for the higher body fat percentage is that South Asians have lower lean tissue, especially muscle mass than White Europeans. (82, 182).

This pattern is established at an early age, perhaps even in the fetus and hence it is demonstrable at birth(182). In London, Stanfield and colleagues measured body composition in 30 each of South Asian and White European infants at 6–12 weeks. Fat-free mass was lower by 0.34 kg but fat mass was 0.02 kg higher in South Asians(178). The cardiometabolic consequences of fat deposition depends on where it is, with a rough rank order for associated metabolic dysfunction being: liver and other organs; visceral/intra-abdominal; central deep subcutaneous; intramuscular; superficial subcutaneous on the torso; and limbs, with some evidence of cardiometabolic benefits from lower limb fat(101, 183–185). Visceral fat is intraperitoneal and its veins drain into the portal circulation which goes to the liver first. This might give such fat special importance in metabolic disorders(186).

The high level of relative adiposity of South Asians is clear in comparison with White Europeans but not with many other populations, especially in the Middle East, South East Asia, and Polynesia(187–189). The explanation for this is under study. It may be related to nutritional and developmental factors and we will explore these this later (Chapter 5 especially but also Chapters 7 and 8). It may be genetic, e.g. if fetal insulin and fetal growth are regulated mostly genetically this could be the mechanism as insulin promotes proliferation of fat cells and deposition of fat(190). South Asians have comparatively high levels of insulin at birth and, by inference, during fetal development(191). They are also born small for gestational age compared with most other populations (see Chapter 5) which is associated with higher body fat, relative to other tissues, though again not in absolute terms. This has led to the concept of fat sparing (really, preference) during the process of fetal development leading to the thin-fat Indian baby a phrase coined by Chittaranjan Yajnik to make the point that such a baby may look thin and scrawny but has a high fat composition(192). This thin-fat pattern is typical of South Asians through life. Explanations for this will be considered in Chapter 5. In this chapter we focus on potential genetic explanations of why South Asians might deposit, preferentially, their fat centrally, rather than peripherally. We start with the adipose tissue (compartment) overflow hypothesis.

3.6 **The adipose tissue (compartment) overflow hypothesis**

Box 3.1 (p 71) and Figure 3.1 summarize this hypothesis(101), which has gained increasing interest, because empirical data have been generally supportive, not just in studies of South Asians but also in studies of other kinds, e.g. in premature babies(193–196). The central idea is that South Asians have comparatively low storage capacity in a relatively inactive (and even potentially beneficial) fat compartment, i.e. the superficial subcutaneous layers of fat, especially in the lower limbs(183–185). Most fat in normal weight people is in the superficial subcutaneous compartment. This low capacity in South Asians is postulated to lead to excess calories being deposited in other, more active fat compartments.

There was little evidence that this anatomical proposition was correct available before the hypothesis was published but it has accrued. The evidence in White European populations on the inverse association (potentially protective) between lower limb fat and metabolic disorders is quite

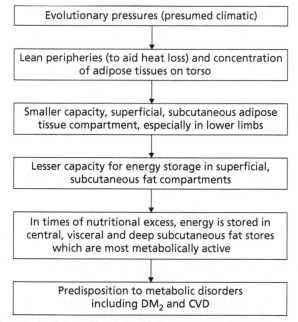

Figure 3.1 Adipose tissue overflow hypothesis.
Source: data from Sniderman, AD. Why might South Asians be so susceptible to central obesity and its atherogenic consequences? The adipose tissue overflow hypothesis. *International Journal of Epidemiology*. 36(1), 220–5. Copyright © 2007 OUP.

extensive(183–185). Sniderman et al. were unaware at the time of publication of the hypothesis but McKeigue et al. had reported the hypothesized pattern in South Asians in Southall, UK(197). Every skinfold was greater in South Asians compared with White Europeans except for the two on the lower limbs, i.e. suprapatellar and thigh, which were similar. Rush et al. observed in 19 Indians in New Zealand that while thigh fat was greater than in Europeans, as a proportion of the total it was less (8.9% vs 9.5%)(198). Kohli et al. found that at similar BMI and waist circumference South Asians in Canada had more fat in the upper body than White Canadians but lower body fat was similar(199). There was evidence that South Asians deposit more deep than superficial subcutaneous fat. The stronger association between lipid-related cardio-metabolic risk factors and intra-abdominal than subcutaneous fat has been shown in South Asia(200). This was also seen in Chinese populations in the US(201). Okosun et al. showed lower birthweight was associated with higher subscapular skinfold in White, Black, and Hispanic populations(202).

Whether this pattern is a result of genetic, developmental, or other environmental factors remains unclear, although it is unlikely to be merely genetic. Ali et al. have hypothesized that insulin resistance occurs fat compartment-by-compartment(190). They propose that as the subcutaneous compartment increases so does insulin resistance there, thus inhibiting further deposition of triglycerides. Triglycerides are then deposited in another depot (e.g. intra-abdominal) until that also becomes insulin resistant and then they go to other ectopic fat depots. They link this evolutionary mechanism to the need to avoid fatty limbs to stay mobile, an idea that reminds us of the predation release hypothesis(135). Sniderman et al. favoured climate-related reasons, even although they did not discuss this in detail(101). Sellayah et al. and Horvath et al. have also emphasized adaptation to climate in their recent hypotheses to explain the human propensity to obesity(137, 203).

The critical question is whether this hypothesis, in itself, is a strong contender to explain South Asians' susceptibility to CVD and DM_2? A tendency to central adiposity and ectopic fat deposition is undoubtedly important although, in itself, unlikely to be the whole explanation. Body fat distribution clearly needs to be considered alongside other factors of which one is lean mass, especially skeletal muscle. Lear et al. showed that when both fat mass and lean mass were considered simultaneously, differences in insulin resistance measured by HOMA-IR between Indigenous (Canadians), Chinese, Europeans, and South Asians were removed(204). We will return to this idea in Chapters 7 and 9, but below we examine an alternative explanation for the same observed phenomenon, i.e. a tendency to central adiposity.

3.7 **The variable disease selection hypothesis**

Jonathan Wells has published many theoretical discussions directly or indirectly relevant to the epidemic of CVD and DM_2 and some of these are considered in this book(138, 188, 205–207). His variable disease selection hypothesis is a way of explaining why South Asians have a tendency to central obesity(207). It is summarized in Box 3.2 (p 73) and Figure 3.2. In essence, Wells proposes that a tendency to central adiposity is an evolutionary adaptation arising from exposure to high levels of gastrointestinal infections and the need for local depots of adipose tissue to provide both immunity and energy to combat these.

This hypothesis both provides an explanation for central deposition of fat and for the pro-inflammatory effects of central fat deposits. South Asians, without doubt, have a relatively pro-inflammatory state and this has been related to central obesity—a matter we will discuss in Chapter 8(208). Wells has emphasized gastrointestinal infections in South Asians(207) but they are also unusually exposed and prone to tuberculosis, not only of the respiratory tract but also of the lymphoid tissue whether in the chest or elsewhere including the gastrointestinal tract. Adipose tissue is a major component of the immune system. The point of the hypothesis is that South Asians' central adiposity may be an adaptive and favourable state, at least in the past, when gastrointestinal infections were very common.

Earlier I noted that the higher relative but not absolute fat in South Asians results from a lower fat-free and especially lower muscle mass, which I consider next.

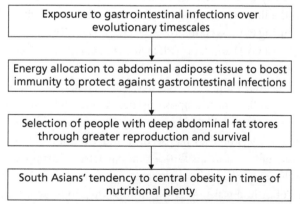

Figure 3.2 Variable disease selection hypothesis: my simple causal diagram.
Source: data from Wells, JCK. Ethnic variability in adiposity and cardiovascular risk: the variable disease selection hypothesis. *International Journal of Epidemiology*. 38(1), 63–71. Copyright © 2009 OUP.

3.8 **Fat-free mass and the role of muscle**

Adipose tissue and its distribution, and the consequences for glucose and lipid metabolism, have been dominant in the quest for understanding CVD and DM_2. This interest has been accelerated by the developmental origins of health and adult diseases hypothesis, discussed in Chapter 5, which emphasizes the relative adiposity of the small Indian baby(192). Large hips and thighs are associated, in White Europeans, with lower risk for CVD and metabolic dysfunction (185, 209, 210). Large hips and thighs reflect a combination of more muscle and more fat.

South Asians, from birth and across the life-course, have a deficit of fat-free mass, also known as lean tissue, compared to White European populations with differences in muscle function and fitness(204, 211, 212). McKeigue's study in Southall, UK showed that in males but not females both hip circumference (2.6 cm less) and thigh girth (1.3 cm less) were smaller in South Asians than Europeans(197). The reason this did not apply to women was they had a higher BMI than European women (1.8 BMI units) while the two groups of men had similar BMIs. In the UK, Elitisham et al. found that South Asian adolescents had a higher BMI and were bigger than Europeans except in the thigh circumference(213). Chahal et al. provided data showing that Asian Indians in London aged 35–75 years of age had lower lean body mass (6 kg less in men) than Europeans even though their BMIs were similar(214). Most of this lean tissue is bone and muscle. Maintenance of strong bones requires exercise and good nutrition and muscles in all populations including South Asians.

Physical activity and muscle are topics that have, until fairly recently, been neglected in the literature on South Asians in comparison with other factors potentially causing the susceptibility to CVD and DM_2. The discussion of physical inactivity as a CVD and DM_2 risk factor is in Chapter 7, so here I consider why low muscle mass might be important.

Muscle is potentially important in three ways. First, it is a tissue with a high metabolic rate, unlike most adipose tissue. A body with low muscle mass and high adipose tissue will use less energy at rest so more energy is potentially available to be stored as fat. Second, muscle utilizes glucose as a fuel (as well as fat) but it is an insulin-dependent tissue. Insulin resistance will inhibit muscle from using blood glucose. A low muscle mass, especially in the presence of insulin resistance, will promote hyperglycaemia and resultant hyperinsulinaemia, which, in turn, will promote the use of glucose as a fuel for-insulin-independent tissues and for storage as fat. Third, in the regulation of appetite, weight gain and weight regain muscle plays an important part. Fat-free mass, of which muscle is a dominant component, is a powerful determinant of energy intake normally and after physical activity and after weight loss(215). There are signalling mechanisms that are still to be clarified that maintain homeostasis of fat-free mass even when weight has been regained as fat. Indeed, there is a concept that excess fat acquisition may be 'collateral fattening' arising from an increased appetite as the body strives to regain its normal free-fat mass(215). Physical activity, especially anaerobic exercise, increases muscle mass and sedentary lifestyles reduce it, and that latter state might, paradoxically, increase appetite.

The South Asian phenotype is characterized by a comparatively low weight and fat-free mass at birth with rapid catch up growth. This catch up leads to generalized weight gain including adipose tissue but fat-free mass remains comparatively low. Muscle contains fat which is used as a fuel. In White Europeans, muscle fat is associated with insulin resistance but this is not so in South Asians(80, 81, 212, 216).

Misra and colleagues have been in the vanguard in stressing the importance of anaerobic exercise, e.g. using weight training, in South Asians(217, 218). Given the sparse evidence on this issue it is not possible to be sure but it may be more important than so far recognized in relation to CVD and DM$_2$ in South Asians. Future research and scholarship should consider adipose and muscle tissue together, and not separately as has mostly been the case hitherto.

3.9 Other anatomical measures in relation to CVD and DM$_2$

There are many measures that have been related to chronic disease outcomes. Some of them have been considered at length in the general literature, e.g. height and leg length in relation to the length of the torso(219). Height is strongly dependent on both genetic and environmental factors. While boys and girls are of similar height, on average, men are taller than women as girls stop growing at a younger age. Height is related to chronic diseases but weakly. For example, taller people, on average, have more cancers but less stroke and CHD. The differences in height in men and women are not reflected in these disease patterns. The association between height and CVD is clearer when we look at leg length or sitting height/leg length ratio, which reflect childhood circumstances and the effects on growth(160, 220).

Longer legs are a sign of good nutrition and socio-economic well-being in the growth period before adolescence. Height and leg length are not, in themselves, causes of CVD or DM_2 but possibly markers of other causes. People born in South Asia are generally shorter than White Europeans, and Bangladeshis are especially so, as reflected clearly in UK studies(9). However, South Asians born and raised in the UK have similar height, weight, and BMI to White Europeans even in childhood, even though they are born smaller, reflecting the role of the environment(179). Is this relevant to the epidemic of CVD and DM2 in South Asians? If low height in those born in South Asia reflects adverse development, possibly because of poor nutrition and stunting, then it would certainly be expected to increase haemorrhagic stroke. The potential effects on atherosclerotic CVD and DM_2 could be through a mismatch between early life, prepubertal, and adult life circumstances. This mismatch would align with the thrifty phenotype hypothesis considered in Chapter 5.

Waist circumference in relation to hip, height, and other measures has been examined particularly carefully(85). I will consider waist in relation to other measures, especially hip, when I discuss obesity in Chapter 7. I will discuss cardiovascular anatomy and physiology in Chapter 8.

3.10 Conclusions

Soon after South Asians' propensity to CVD and DM_2 was confirmed by a consistent body of evidence in the 1980s, the spotlight turned on insulin and insulin resistance and that was closely linked to adiposity as a mechanism(17, 221). As the perception of the importance of insulin and insulin resistance has diminished, the focus has shifted to other functions of adipose tissue including inflammatory processes (1, 208) The knowledge that the functions of fat are complex and vary by bodily location has given new impetus to describing the distribution of fat in South Asians, and further, explaining why it is distributed relatively centrally where the cardiometabolic effects are most adverse. This chapter has focused on two relevant hypotheses. In the course of such studies, the role of fat-free mass, especially relatively low muscle mass, has emerged. Together, these observations, albeit inconclusive as yet, seem important in explaining South Asians' susceptibility to CVD and DM_2. We will examine their role, especially as potentiators of the effects of classic risk factors, in Chapter 9.

Box 3.1 The adipose tissue overflow hypothesis

Sniderman A et al. Why might South Asians be so susceptible to central obesity and its atherogenic consequences? The adipose tissue overflow hypothesis. International Journal of Epidemiology 2007;36:220–5(101).

My introduction to the paper

In 2004 I listened to Allan Sniderman speaking about lipid transport from varying adipose tissue compartments and in a post-lecture discussion I shared with him my anecdotal observation that many Indian and Pakistani people I knew had both pot bellies (abdominal obesity) but also scrawny lower limbs. I shared with him my speculation that this could be a climatic adaptation, possibly over evolutionary time-scales. We resolved to write this paper.

The paper

The paper opens by observing that in vascular diseases the developing countries may not only be following the path of developed countries but overtaking them, with the example being CHD in South Asians. The problem was identified as dyslipidaemia and dysglycaemia being manifest at relatively low body fat levels. The paper first observes that South Asians are highly prone to the atherogenic effects of adiposity and to developing abdominal adiposity and then attempts to explain these.

The paper emphasizes that adipose tissue is not uniform but has three major compartments: superficial subcutaneous, deep subcutaneous, and the visceral intra-abdominal. The superficial and deep subcutaneous compartments are separated by fascia (Scapa's membrane) and are functionally different. The paper designates the superficial compartment as the primary adipose tissue depot. Abdominal computed tomography scans are shown of these compartments and a table presents their characteristics. The superficial compartment is the least active and least associated with atherogenic dyslipidaemia and dysglycaemia. The visceral compartment is the most active in this way, with deep subcutaneous fat being intermediate. The largest depot for superficial adipose tissue is in the lower limbs, while deep subcutaneous fat is mostly in the torso.

The adipose tissue cells (adipocytes) work differently too, with superficial subcutaneous cells having less transfer (called flux in the paper) of fatty acids into and from the circulation in response to biochemical stimuli from food

Box 3.1 The adipose tissue overflow hypothesis (*continued*)

intake or lack of food. Circulation of fatty acids from adipocytes leads to the liver producing triglycerides, cholesterol, and Apo-B particles, which are released into the circulation, causing dyslipidaemia, including with small, dense LDL cholesterol particles. The point relevant to the hypothesis is that this pattern is the result of highly active adipocytes, which are not characteristic of superficial compartment adipocytes.

The paper then hypothesizes that the susceptibility of South Asians to the effects of obesity is a consequence of a low storage capacity, compared to White Europeans, in the superficial subcutaneous fat compartment. The proposition is that excess nutritional energy is converted to fat and deposited first in the superficial compartment and then when storage capacity there is depleted, into the other more metabolically active stores. This depletion of capacity in the superficial compartment is hypothesized to occur earlier in South Asians than in other populations such as Europeans.

The paper then reviews the evidence that, at a comparable BMI, South Asians (most data are on Indians) have more visceral fat than White populations and thicker truncal skinfolds. Truncal fat is, relative to other tissues, high in Indian babies, as measured by subscapular skinfold thickness. Observations of similar kinds are also seen in children, adolescents and adults in various countries. (This paper did not cite data on thinner lower limb skinfolds but subsequently I found data supporting the hypothesis in work by McKeigue et al(197)).

The paper alludes to climate as a fundamental factor in shaping this adipose tissue distribution but as direct evidence was lacking such discussion was curtailed (at the request of referees).

Ideas for testing the hypothesis are provided, and the hypothesis is summarized as follows: "... South Asians have a lower fat storage capacity in their primary adipose tissue compartment than Whites. As this compartment's capacity for storage is approached fat is stored in the more metabolically active compartment."

My concluding comments

There is a growing literature on this topic and the hypothesis has found a niche. While the paper was written on the assumption that the described adipose tissue pattern was genetic, driven by evolutionary forces, subsequent work has led to broader interpretations incorporating the role of development and dietary factors, matters which will be discussed in Chapter 5 and Chapter 7.

Box 3.2 The variable disease selection hypothesis

Wells J.C.K. Ethnic variability in adiposity and cardiovascular risk: the variable disease selection hypothesis. International Journal of Epidemiology 2008; 38: 63–71(207).

My introductory remarks

If a genetic trait is to become common in large populations, it must confer evolutionary advantages that exceed the disadvantages. So, there is a challenge to find the reason for such a trait to be selected, i.e. favoured. This paper starts on the evolutionary path of preceding hypotheses but takes an entirely new turn-off.

The paper

The paper focuses on South Asians' propensity to CVD and in doing so it mainly examines the central deposition of adipose tissue. Perhaps unusually in the CVD and DM_2 literature, Wells emphasizes that fat is not just an energy store but an endocrine organ, and particularly one with immune functions. Wells highlights eight functions for adipose tissue. The hypothesis is that the pattern of adipose tissue distribution has been shaped, evolutionarily, by exposure to particular infectious disease.

The concept is that there are trade-offs in the allocation of energy and these depend on the needs in relation to the environment. The goals of energy trade-offs are to maximize survival and reproduction. Males and females, for example, have different trade-offs, which vary over the lifespan, e.g. young females allocate energy preferentially to peripheral, subcutaneous depots. Severe malnutrition leads to loss of peripheral stores more than deep lying stores, e.g. visceral fat. Wells formulates the view that immune function is one of the two core roles of fat during a period of energy shortage. The adipose tissue hormone leptin is important in immune function and many other pathways relevant to CVD. Famines don't just kill through starvation but through infection. So allocating energy to maintain and augment visceral fat might protect against infections. When energy is not required by physical activity, pregnancy, and lactation it is, preferentially, allocated to central abdominal fat. Excess of this fat leads to a pro-inflammatory state, as seen in South Asians. The hypothesis proposes that the deep fat depots, rather than superficial ones, meet the needs of the immune system best and the

Box 3.2 The variable disease selection hypothesis (*continued*)

distribution of fat evolves according to the type of infection. Fat deposition is postulated to be close to the part of the body affected.

The metabolic cost of an infection includes the energy needs of the infecting microorganisms, the immune system, and the repair of tissues. The hypothesis proceeds to identify gastrointestinal infections as the primary selective force in the distribution of adipose tissue in South Asian populations, and fevers (e.g. due to malaria) as the selective force for Africans. Malaria leads to glucose metabolism and lipogenesis. In populations subjected to malaria, the adipose tissue might be deposited in muscle to help 'fund' fever (each 1°C rise in temperature increases metabolic rate by 15%). In malnourishment arising from diarrhoea the intestinal epithelium is affected. Visceral adipose tissue may help to protect it, and be preferentially stored near the intestinal tract to counter such infections. Over generations, this hypothesis proposes, evolution selects for people with this capacity. This kind of storage pattern may not be an asset when the pattern of infection changes.

My concluding comments

This interesting hypothesis is not overturning other hypotheses but is an adjunct, and an example of how genetic variants favouring a particular adipose tissue distribution might arise. So the thrifty genotype emphasizes famine, the adipose tissue overflow hypothesis emphasizes climate, and this one emphasizes the historical pattern of infections and particularly gastrointestinal infections as the basis of a centralized fat deposition pattern.

Chapter 4

Genetic explanations 3: neurobehavioural explanations

4.1 Chapter 4 objectives are to:

1. Discuss other genetic hypotheses, especially those that are behavioural and relate to cognition, e.g. the behavioural switch hypothesis.
2. Evaluate the validity of these hypotheses as explanations for South Asians' high susceptibility to CVD and DM_2.
3. Explore potential links between these and other genetic hypotheses.

4.2 Chapter summary

These hypotheses propose brain and behavioural evolution as the driver of the adaptations that are now leading to CVD and DM_2. Of these, the behavioural switch hypothesis, also known as the soldier-to-diplomat hypothesis, is the best developed. The idea is that as humans moved from hunter-gatherer to settled agricultural lives, complex changes occurred to support this lifestyle, e.g. reduced aggression, more resources to nurture fewer children, and preferential use of glucose by the brain rather than by muscle. Insulin resistance is seen as a secondary, once beneficial (adaptive), manifestation underlying this complex change. This hypothesis implies insulin resistance is valuable and it also provides an explanation for South Asians' reduced muscle mass. Similar ideas have been proposed on longer evolutionary timescales, e.g. the aggression control hypothesis. These complex ideas are conceptually different to other genetically based hypotheses, but there are overlaps. For example, the thrifty gene hypothesis also sees insulin resistance as valuable in different environmental circumstances, and the predation release hypothesis sees a change in previously required physiques, such as leanness for agility, as triggering higher prevalence of obesity. As with other genetic hypotheses, however, there is a fundamental question of what precise genetic changes underlie these explanations. At present, the evidence from these hypotheses does not explain South Asians' particular susceptibility to CVD and DM_2. The hypotheses do, valuably, point to the brain's central role in glucose metabolism.

4.3 **Introduction to neurobehavioural explanations**

The appeal of genetic hypotheses remains strong, but at least amongst scholars and researchers, perhaps less so the public, the case for the now classical, evolutionary-based explanations, such as the thrifty genotype discussed in Chapter 2, has weakened. The newer set of evolutionary explanations based on differences in adipose, and less so muscle, tissue composition and distribution considered in Chapter 3 are still too novel to evaluate but look promising as a partial explanation. The increasing uncertainties combined with an undiminished interest in genetic evolutionary mechanisms (206) has led to a fresh set of ideas that we can describe as neurobehavioural explanations(102, 136, 222).

These ideas have been most clearly articulated by Watve and colleagues working from Pune, India(136). Watve is a biologist and not an epidemiologist or a physician, and this is reflected in the breadth of his perspective and especially in his combining observations in animals and humans. The ideas are complex enough to merit a 380-page book called *Doves, Diplomats, and Diabetes*(136). The book's title reflects Watve's view that the hawk–dove dichotomy in animal behaviour is analogous with the soldier–diplomat opposition in humans.

Box 4.1 (p 82) and Figure 4.1 introduce the behavioural switch hypothesis as first published (102), and Box 4.2 (p 85) and Figure 4.2 move to developments of the ideas in the aggression control hypothesis(222).

While the neurobehavioral hypotheses are more complex than the others in this book, they can be simplified to a core idea. Changing patterns of behaviours in societies are accompanied, influenced, or caused by changes in brain and nervous system function that themselves are caused by hormonal and nervous system changes. These hormonal and nervous system changes lead to alterations in cardiometabolic function, e.g. in the metabolism of glucose, insulin, lipids, testosterone, and steroids, and these changes can cause disease.

In the soldier-to-diplomat hypothesis changes were hypothesized to occur in the timescale of the evolution of *Homo sapiens*, and indeed mostly around the transition from hunter-gathering to farming. In alternative recent accounts around aggression, the same concepts are set in the evolutionary history of primates, with the nervous system and hormonal changes being related to status and role within society. In this latter form, the hypothesis links to the role of psychosocial factors discussed in Chapter 6. Behavioural patterns are of two kinds: those emphasizing physical matters and hence muscle function and those emphasizing cognition and brain function.

There are two levels at which we can assess these ideas. First, are they potentially important in any population in explaining the occurrence of CVD

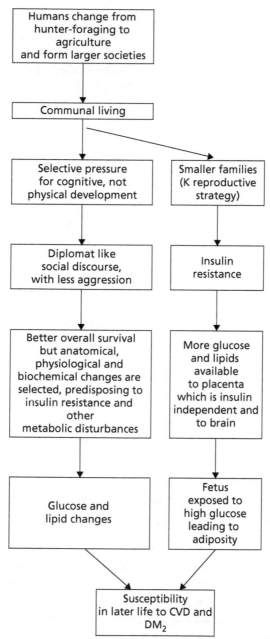

Figure 4.1 The behavioural switch (soldier-to-diplomat) hypothesis: my simple causal diagram.

Source: data from Watve, MG. et al. Evolutionary origins of insulin resistance: a behavioral switch hypothesis. *BMC Evolutionary Biology*. (7)61. Copyright © 2007 Watve and Yajnik; licensee BioMed Central Ltd.

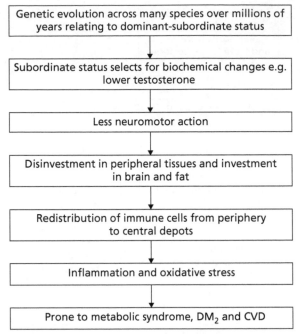

Figure 4.2 Aggression control hypothesis: my simple causal diagram.
Source: data from Belsare, PV. Metabolic syndrome: aggression control mechanisms gone out of control. *Medical Hypotheses*. 74(3):578–89. Copyright © 2010 Elsevier.

and DM_2? Second, do these hypotheses explain why South Asians have particular susceptibility to CVD and DM_2? It is the latter that I am particularly interested in.

4.4 Some reflections on the behavioural switch hypothesis (Box 4.1, p 82)

While the authors reject other hypotheses I see common ground. The thrifty gene hypothesis, e.g., also sees value in high levels of insulin and insulin resistance, i.e. in fat storage, whereas the behavioural switch sees benefits in improved brain function. This hypothesis offers a third explanation for central adiposity to add to those in Chapter 2, i.e. the soldierly life needs adipose tissue in the peripheries for physical protection and immune function but for the diplomatic life, this is less important.

The value of a hypothesis does not merely rest on whether it is right, which is rare, but on its capacity to spur development of new concepts or re-examination of old ones. This work is unusual in two respects, i.e. repositioning insulin and insulin resistance as assets even in modern times, not pathologies, and promoting the brain and brain function as the primary driver of blood glucose levels. Leaving aside the detail, these conceptual contributions alone are valuable. That said, there are many questions to answer before we can accept that this hypothesis helps explain South Asians' susceptibility to CVD and DM_2, which is a core question for Watve as for us.

The idea that South Asians have, somehow, evolved from the soldierly state to the diplomat/scholar state faster than other populations, especially White European populations, is questionable, and although it should be possible to provide historical evidence for this, the authors make no attempt to do so.

The hypothesis also implies that with their higher insulin and circulating glucose (possibly because of insulin resistance) South Asians should have better brain function than other populations without these assets. Again, this is improbable and the authors provide no data on it. If, on the other hand, the argument is that in the midst of nutritional disadvantage the adaptations have permitted adequate brain growth function—which is plausible—this is in accord with the thrifty phenotype hypothesis, which the authors try to refute.

There are other implications of this hypothesis that do not fit our general observations, e.g. that the South Asians' diplomat phenotype leads to lower fertility and more resources per child. This does not square with South Asia's historically large population size despite very high death rates in infancy and childhood.

One of the criticisms of the thrifty gene hypothesis, levelled by many, including Watve, is the lack of gene-level evidence underpinning it. The same is true of this hypothesis, though admittedly it is much newer. We should be able to demonstrate that gene variants associated with the diplomat phenotype, especially relating to the brain, are more common in South Asians than in comparison populations. Evidence for this is not presented.

This hypothesis was soon accompanied by another also involving Watve, which focused on aggression and social status, thus placing the core concepts on a much longer evolutionary time scale(222). There have also been other ideas that I will not go into but can be accessed in Watve's book(136).

4.5 Reflections on the aggression control hypothesis

The observations of Belsare et al. (Box 4.2, p 85, and Figure 4.2) are also fascinating(222). The role of social status in setting the levels of hormones, especially corticosteroids, and in influencing the autonomic nervous system are also central to socio-economic and psychosocial explanations. Mostly, other hypotheses do not emphasize physical aggression, and focus on social stress, but the concepts are similar.

Humans are, undoubtedly, the most domesticated of all animals and most of us have lost our aggression, probably because of social rather than biological factors. Yet, Belsare et al. are surely right that the physiological and hormonal changes in different behavioural states (here aggressive/passive) are ultimately under genetic and hormonal and, hence, evolutionary control(222).

The question, for our purposes, is whether this reasoning helps explain South Asians' susceptibility to CVD and DM$_2$, and not just whether the reasoning is relevant to all populations. Is it plausible that South Asians are less aggressive as a population than other populations, say Northern Europeans? Even if innately their aggression is similar, might it be that South Asians' behaviour is, in practice, less aggressive? The authors do not present evidence on these core questions, even though their work is motivated by the quest to understand South Asians' tendency to cardiometabolic diseases.

There are two widely confirmed observations that accord with this hypothesis. First, South Asians, compared to Northern Europeans, have low participation in physical activity, something that starts in childhood(223, 224). In South Asia, people tend to be active because of limited public transport and car ownership, and participation in organized leisure-time physical activity, muscle strengthening exercises, and sports is limited, as we will discuss in Chapter 7(217). These kind of activities, especially team sports, are recognized by Belsare et al. to be closely aligned to aggressive behaviours(222). The difficulty is to separate out the effects of physical activity and the independent, ostensibly aggressive component associated with it. Mental aggression is another matter, but as we will see in Chapter 6, aggression of that kind is, if anything, detrimental and not beneficial to CVD.

The role of overcrowding as a trigger to reducing aggression is noteworthy and considered by the authors. Might it be that over long timescales South Asians have been more overcrowded than other comparable populations? This seems possible but the authors do not provide the evidence. There is no evidence, however, that people living in rural areas, where the standard of living is comparable to urbanized areas as it tends to be in Europe, enjoy an advantage from a CVD and DM$_2$ perspective.

Overall, while the ideas in this hypothesis stretch our thinking, and the link between a wide range of signalling molecules and insulin—glucose metabolism, as considered in detail in the paper by Belsare et al. (222), is fascinating, it seems unlikely that South Asians' susceptibility to CVD and DM$_2$ is explicable by their non-aggressive lives (if, indeed, they do lead less aggressive lives than Europeans).

4.6 **Further concepts and implications of the neurobehavioural hypotheses of Watve and colleagues**

The papers in Boxes 4.1 and 4.2 are different from most hypotheses papers in their embrace of complexity, although Watve has pointed out to me that complexity is in the mind of the beholder. I cannot do full justice here to the richness of the arguments in these papers and in the related book. There are, however, some other points that may be important in understanding cardiometabolic diseases generally and perhaps in South Asians specifically.

The role of the brain, rather than the pancreas, in regulating glucose metabolism was, according to Watve, demonstrated by Claude Bernard, but largely forgotten(136). He redresses the balance by giving the brain a central role. As already stated, in this conception, insulin resistance is a mechanism for maintaining high levels of glucose and insulin for optimal brain function (and in the fetus and early life, for brain development). Watve sees DM_2 as the consequence of the brain trying to keep glucose high, possibly because of vascular dysfunction that impairs the supply of glucose to the brain.

Obesity is seen as one of the consequences of the switch to a diplomat lifestyle, but there are also other changes that are seen as critically important, including in the hormonal control of leptin, cholesterol, corticosteroids, and testosterone. He emphasizes macrophage distribution and its role in angiogenesis and he de-emphasizes glucotoxity as a cause of beta-cell dysfunction(136).

He links the diplomat strategy to the DOHAD hypothesis (Chapter 5), in that when faced with intrauterine growth problems the fetus is better adapted to thrive with the diplomat (brain-orientated) than soldier (muscle-orientated) phenotype.

Watve highlights many questions to which answers are required including how the brain influences peripheral glucose, and discusses some contrary observations, e.g. while testosterone seems to be beneficial (at least for metabolic syndrome) in men, it is not so in women.

The potential implications of the hypothesis are many including that the nature of the recommended physical activity should be specified to make it mimic aggression. Among the many molecules he singles out for attention is adiponectin, which is considered briefly in Chapter 8.

4.7 **Conclusions**

The set of hypotheses and detailed discussion and data in the two papers discussed here and in Watve's book are moving us into new territory. It is not possible, at present, to judge the practical value, as opposed to the research stimulus (considerable). The principles arising, e.g. the role of the brain in glucose metabolism and insulin resistance, are likely to be generalizable. It seems implausible that these principles apply especially to South Asians. Similarly, neurobehaviourally induced changes in aggression molecules are unlikely to be specific to South Asians. My judgement is that these ideas will help us understand cardiometabolic disorders better, including in South Asians, but they will not explain why South Asians are especially susceptible to CVD and DM_2.

These hypotheses have been placed squarely as evolutionary hypotheses. It is imperative, therefore, that before these ideas are promoted widely, the genes and genetic variants that underlie the behaviour changes are identified in humans and not just in animal models. We must avoid a repetition of the past where evolutionary hypotheses were accepted too readily.

It is possible, though not emphasized by the authors, that a change in behaviour achieved purely by social means, e.g. overcrowding, also alters brain function in much the same way as postulated in these hypotheses. If so, an evolutionary change would not be central to the argument. This area of enquiry would then merge with the set of psychosocial explanations in Chapter 6.

Box 4.1 The behavioural switch hypothesis

Watve M.G., Yajnik C.S. Evolutionary origins of insulin resistance: a behavioural switch hypothesis. BMC Evolutionary Biology 2007;7:61(102).

My introductory remarks

According to the philosophy of science of Thomas Kuhn, the frameworks of thought, often called paradigms, that scientists work with are those that are successful in solving current problems, and these paradigms are illustrated by exemplars(225). When it is clear that a paradigm is not solving problems, new ideas are generated, and a competition ensues whereby the new ideas might become the prevailing paradigm. The family of so-called thrifty hypotheses together with the underlying phenomenon of insulin resistance and ensuing cardiometabolic diseases, which they tried to explain, had prevailed for a long time but without increasing their empirical or theoretical strengths—rather the opposite(1, 18). This paper is one of the new, revolutionary ideas generated as a result.

Box 4.1 The behavioural switch hypothesis (*continued*)

The paper

The authors remind us that the insulin resistance syndrome hypothesis propounded by Reaven (originally as Syndrome X or, as it was later renamed by others, metabolic syndrome) refers to a cluster of cardiometabolic impairments(17). They examine Neel's thrifty gene hypothesis as the core hypothesis on why it occurs so commonly, and also evaluate the alternative thrifty phenotype hypothesis(94, 95). They find little evidence that there is, actually, thriftiness, i.e. conservation of energy with preferential deposition of conserved energy as fat in people prone to insulin resistance and diabetes.

Rather than insulin resistance leading to obesity, the authors propose that obesity leads to insulin resistance. They discuss climate, observing that insulin resistance is less common in cold-climate adapted populations where they predict feast and famine is more likely and more than in warm climate countries—a contestable though sensible point.

Watve and Yajnik then turn to their neurobehavioural explanations, introducing the key observation that insulin has many roles including in immunity and brain function. The brain cells (like red blood cells and the placenta) are not dependent on insulin. So they see insulin and insulin resistance as a way of allocating energy preferentially to critically important tissues, especially the brain. In this regard, the concept that there is a good reason for insulin resistance is aligned with Wells' variable disease selection hypothesis where the preferential allocation of energy is to the immune system and Neels's thrifty gene hypothesis where energy is stored as fat.

The behavioural switch hypothesis proposes that insulin resistance is an evolutionary adaptation that promotes: 1) small families where children are cared for carefully rather than large ones, so more investment is given per child (r to K strategy in evolutionary terms) and 2) where brain function is promoted above muscle function (smarter not stronger, and hence diplomat not soldier). Insulin is seen as the key molecule that allows this. Gestational (pregnancy-related) insulin resistance permits glucose to be diverted preferentially through the placenta, which does not require insulin for glucose uptake, to the fetus. This increases maternal nutritional investment in the fetus. Insulin resistance also reduces ovulation and hence fertility. These changes are said to support the diplomat life.

Insulin resistance means more glucose is available for the brain. Moreover, the brain responds to insulin directly and also itself synthesizes some

Box 4.1 The behavioural switch hypothesis (*continued*)

insulin. Neural development and aspects of cognition are stimulated by insulin. Leptin and cholesterol also affect cognitive function. The hypothesis develops the idea that in evolving a brain-centred lifestyle, increased insulin is required, but to prevent hypoglycaemia, detrimental to the brain, peripheral insulin resistance is needed. So, insulin resistance is seen as a necessary and positive adaptation that permits high insulin and yet adequate, even high, glucose levels.

The fetus that is facing nutritional challenges avoids impairment of the brain by preferentially diverting nutrition to it at the cost of other tissues including muscle, and again this is an adaptation that favours a brain-orientated life. Chronic malnutrition also leads to insulin resistance, presumed to be a way for the brain to ensure adequate nutrition even in these circumstances. A brain-centred life allows social manipulation to gain nutritional resources and ensure survival of offspring, thus permitting smaller families

So, in this hypothesis insulin resistance is not a disorder but an adaptation to permit a new way of communal life (a behavioural switch). The link between adiposity and insulin resistance is, on this hypothesis, explained as: 1) as the brain is mostly fat, adiposity is a vital resource to promote the switch; 2) fat signals high social rank, necessary to the K reproductive strategy; and 3) abdominal fat sends a signal that the individual is not of an aggressive predisposition.

The explanation for the pathology associated with this adaptation in modern times is focused on the release of inflammatory molecules from abdominal adipose tissue. The authors also point to a redistribution of adipose tissue from peripheral (needed there as fuel and protection for the soldierly life) to central depots. Other issues raised by the authors include the role of testosterone, social hierarchy, relative rather than absolute nutritional status, overcrowding, and the effects of insulin resistance on different tissues. The authors conclude with some thoughts on testing the hypothesis.

My concluding remarks

This is a complex hypothesis and paper with many concepts and facets. At its core, however, is the idea that insulin and insulin resistance are important in reducing fertility/family size and directing nutrition (glucose) to brain and placenta. Insulin itself is seen as important to the brain. The hypothesis proposes that the harm of insulin resistance is secondary to inflammation from central fat stores. We will examine the arguments further in the text. It is worth noting, in passing, that if there are high levels of insulin high levels of adiposity are inevitable as the hormone promotes deposition of fat(190).

Box 4.2 The aggression control hypothesis

Belsare P et al. Metabolic syndrome: aggression control mechanisms gone out of control. Medical Hypotheses 2010;74:578–589(222).

My introductory remarks

This paper develops the neurobehavioural hypotheses proposed in the behavioural switch hypothesis (soldier-to-diplomat) but now set in a much longer timescale.

The paper

Soldier-to-diplomat type changes are relatively recent, i.e. in the period of transition to settled agriculture and the postulated evolution is so fast that it may not be plausible. The authors present evidence for similar ideas but in longer-established behaviours. The hypothesis is developed in animals, especially primates, where subordinate individuals have different neurophysiologic and metabolic states to dominant ones. Subordinate individuals have comparatively low testosterone, high cholesterol and glucocorticoids, and high serotonin signalling. This metabolic state is said to be related to a strategy to reduce aggression. The raised serotonin leads to insulin resistance and other effects including the formation of new blood vessels (angiogenesis).

The dominant–subordinate dichotomy in the animal kingdom arises from competition for females and food. Winning such a competition requires aggression. Nonetheless, submissive individuals can also enjoy success by applying alternative strategies, e.g. sneaking mating or eating opportunities while the dominant males fight each other. The submissive individuals avoid confrontation. They do not enjoy access to the best sites for food so they need a thrifty metabolism and the capacity for storage of energy as fat.

This kind of dichotomy is ancient, unlike the soldier-to-diplomat dichotomy. The hypothesis is that loss of physical aggression, through the biochemical changes needed for that, induces: insulin resistance, a shift in energy from muscle to brain, and disinvestment in peripheral immunity in adipose tissue where it is needed less because wounds are less likely. The effects of this change on glucose control and cardiovascular function are compounded by the modern lifestyle. High population density also reduces aggression further, compounding the effects described.

Box 4.2 The aggression control hypothesis (*continued*)

Loss of aggression leads to disinvestment in bone and muscle strength. Changes in phagocyte distribution also occur, and this may matter as phagocytes are a major source of free radicals and oxidative stress that potentially damage tissues including the pancreatic beta cells.

The paper includes a review of chemicals (twenty-six in detail, and many others) involved in aggression and their roles in insulin resistance, insulin secretion, pancreatic regeneration, oxidative stress, obesity, sexual and reproductive function, inflammation, and angiogenesis. Many pro-aggression factors were insulin sensitizing and associated with less obesity.

The authors reported a trial in people with DM_2 of motor movements that mimic Stone Age hunting or combat. The exercises were taught in a 4-day camp and participants were asked to continue them for 3 months. They reported benefits, although whether these were a result of aggression or simply a change of scene and physical activity is unclear.

My concluding remarks

This hypothesis is complex. In essence, however, it proposes that an adaptation that helps animals, including humans, succeed in the subordinate, low-aggression state has become maladaptive in the modern world. The ties to the behavioural switch hypothesis are clear, but this one relates to ancient biological processes that are found across many animals, and not just recent changes in humans.

Chapter 5

The thrifty phenotype
and related developmental
hypotheses

5.1 Chapter 5 objectives are to:

1. Describe the core ingredients of several closely related hypotheses that contribute to the developmental origins of disease hypothesis, principally, the thrifty phenotype and adaptation–dysadaptation.

2. Evaluate these hypotheses as explanations for South Asians' high susceptibility to CVD and DM_2.

3. Consider how these developmental origins hypotheses might be related to other genetic hypothesis (e.g. through birthweight) and lifestyle/socio-economic hypotheses.

5.2 Chapter summary

The developmental origins of health and disease (DOHAD) hypothesis places emphasis on fetal and early life. Birthweight and similar indicators have been linked to CVD and DM_2 in numerous studies, including in South Asia. The DOHAD hypothesis is a highly favoured explanation for the CVD and DM_2 epidemic in South Asians.

The hypothesis proposes that impairment of fetal and infant development leads to lasting, perhaps permanent, changes in organ structure, body composition, and metabolism, i.e. there is programming of future anatomy, physiology, and biochemistry. The critical factor, however, is thought to be dysadaptation, whereby the environmental circumstances in later life do not match those the person is programmed for. This kind of mismatch is particularly likely in migrant populations leaving rural parts of South Asia (where nutrition is sometimes limited) and settling in affluent, nutrition-rich countries. The rapidity of change may be important.

South Asian babies are born small but with relatively well-preserved fat depots, especially on the torso and intra-abdominally. Nonetheless, the fat depots are still slightly smaller than in the usual Northern European reference populations but not as small as expected on birthweight. This relative central preservation of fat is a characteristic that remains through life. Rather than attributing this pattern to evolutionary and hence genetic factors, as the hypotheses in Chapters 2–4 do, the thrifty phenotype and related hypotheses attribute it to fetal and early life growth and development. The reasons may relate to parental, especially maternal, characteristics or lifestyle/behaviours, especially in nutrition. These differences, at least partially, may also relate to genes, e.g. those governing birthweight.

The evidence on birthweight and early life growth in South Asians is supportive of the general tenets of the hypothesis. Genetics, epigenetics, lifestyle, and socio-economic circumstances are intertwined in the causal pathways to chronic diseases in this hypothesis. While both fascinating and relevant, on the current evidence, I have judged lower birth weight and related factors to be no more than a small contributor to the epidemic of CVD and DM_2 in South Asians.

5.3 The scope and focus of this chapter

The topic is large and expanding fast and there is much to learn but it has found an important place in the life-course perspective on diseases. In this chapter, I will focus on the potential importance of this perspective for South Asians and also on the research on South Asians. There are two major studies, both in India, that have been particularly important that I will highlight: the Pune prospective birth cohort and the Mysore retrospective birth cohort. First, we will examine the thrifty phenotype hypothesis and developments thereof. Given the importance of the ideas, and the lack of quantitative reviews of the topic, I have made an exception in my approach and tabulated much of the evidence.

5.4 Introduction to the fetal and developmental origins of disease hypotheses

The idea that the circumstances in which organisms, including humans, are conceived, give birth, develop, and mature have important consequences for health and well-being in adulthood is a long-standing pillar of biology(226). The concept that there are critical periods during early life when normal development is triggered by a combination of genetic and external stimuli is also well established. In many animals these stimuli are very important. A classic study in pigeons is illustrative of the concept in relation to CVD(227). Pigeons exposed to dietary cholesterol early in life had a decreased atherogenic response to dietary cholesterol later in life. We don't know if this is the case in humans.

The potential of this kind of concept in explaining the CVD epidemic in human populations that are undergoing a nutritional transition is self-evident. Until recently our understanding of the importance of early life was based, in humans, on outcomes such as hearing, language, cognition, and vision. In the last 50 years or so, however, research has shown that these kinds of concepts are also important for a wide range of human diseases including CVD and DM_2. These ideas have now been widely disseminated and the sense of wonder, even disbelief, which originally accompanied them, is historical.

In the 1990s, the main ideas relating these hypotheses to chronic diseases were badged as the Barker hypothesis after David Barker who until his death in 2013 was the most powerful advocate, scholar, and researcher in this field in the 20th and 21st centuries(226, 228). It was originally called the fetal origins of adult disease (FOADS) hypothesis and with increasing recognition of the importance of events after birth it became the developmental origins of health and disease (DOHAD) hypothesis. It seems hard to believe that fetal and infant development could be relevant to the occurrence of a stroke, heart attack, or DM_2 at 70 years of age, especially as the major adulthood risk factors for these diseases had mostly been discovered by the 1980s when the work in this field accelerated.

Early work in population health was based on analysis of vital statistics, for example, the observation by Barker and colleagues that infant death rates were clearly associated with ischaemic heart disease (IHD) mortality rates in England and Wales, i.e. in places where infant death was high in the 1920s, IHD was high in 1968–1978. Barker and Osmond suggested the interpretation, i.e. poor nutrition in early life reflected in infant mortality, increases susceptibility in later life to the effects of the kind of diets associated with affluence(229). As is often the case in research, others had made similar observations. Barker and Osmond's (1986) paper refers to a 1977 paper by Forsdahl (who had published similar ideas and data in 1973 in Norwegian)(105, 230).

Forsdahl's studies in Norway had shown that adverse socio-economic circumstances in childhood were associated with high rates of CHD in adulthood. Forsdahl's conclusion was that poverty in childhood/adolescence followed by prosperity is a risk factor for arteriosclerotic heart disease. He speculated that the specific factors could include nutrition, e.g. a reduced tolerance to fat, or even a tendency to smoke cigarettes. Between Forsdahl and Barker's contributions, Bradley was making similar observations but put the emphasis on parental, particularly maternal, physique, e.g. adiposity and muscle mass(231–233) (Bradley's ideas did not gain prominence).

These kinds of observations were preceded by many similar ones but the study of the concept was re-established. These area-based studies were used to generate testable hypotheses. Barker and colleagues placed emphasis on maternal nutritional status as the critical issue and low birthweight as the main indicator of this. A series of studies across the world demonstrated a clear association between low birthweight and high risk of CVD and DM_2 (the latter was also associated with high birthweight), including much work in India(234, 235).

The DOHAD hypothesis was subsequently articulated and refined as, in essence: fetal and infant development leads to lasting, perhaps permanent, changes in organ structure, body composition, and metabolism. This was described as programming of anatomy, physiology, and biochemistry. According to Barker and his teams, the most important influence on such programming was the mother's nutrition with poor status leading to small, disproportionate babies at future risk of chronic diseases(228). The concept of programming fits well with biological observations on the plasticity of cells and organs and imprinting(236, 237). Another phrase that might be better than programming for human biology is environmental induction, i.e. biological changes are induced according to the environmental stimuli. One useful and commonly used analogy is of a weather forecast given by the mother to the fetus. The fetus is then prepared accordingly. If the weather turn out differently the newborn is ill-prepared. Poor maternal nutritional status would signal to the fetus to prepare (via programming) accordingly, i.e. for a nutrition-sparse future. Saben et al. have examined diet induced changes in mitochondrial function in mice. Exposure to a high-fat/high-sugar diet from conception until weaning in the female mouse had effects including on insulin signalling and mitochondrial function detectable in the third generation in the offspring, even though they were fed a normal diet(238). Whether this kind of observation can be replicated or has analogous effects in humans is yet to be demonstrated but it illustrates the concept and a potential mechanism. Even more remarkable results in rats over 50 generations need replicating before they can be evaluated(239).

As we will see, there have been critiques of this and related concepts.

5.5 Birth weight, size, and shape: implications for the thrifty phenotype hypothesis

The optimal birth weight, size, and shape is not known and, except at the extremes, may not be important, given the amount of human adaptability (plasticity) there is(237). As with most normal or reference values, much of the data on birthweight come from well-off nations, especially Northern European and North American populations, even though this is now changing(240, 241). The result is that average birthweights of about 3.4 kg have been widely accepted as normal. In South Asian countries average birthweights are typically under

3 kg and commonly around 2.7 kg in rural areas where traditional agricultural practices continue, as seen in the Pune studies(242). The WHO definition of a low birthweight baby is 2.5 kg. Applying this WHO definition in South Asia, in many places 30–50% of babies may be officially categorized as low birthweight. Given national and international health targets to reduce low birthweight this topic has led to much attention.

Clearly, birthweight is governed by both genetic and environmental factors. The most important outcome in the evolutionary success of a species is the birth of a healthy baby and the survival of the mother. The baby's size and shape must be commensurate with the mother's pelvic capacity and the pelvic outlet must permit the passage of the baby's head(243). In much of South Asia, there are cultural customs to restrict food intake in later pregnancy to avoid a large baby with a subsequent difficult birth. This strategy might not be helpful as the baby's head is the most difficult to deliver and it's circumference is similar in babies of 3.5 kg and 2.7 kg, because of the phenomenon known as brain sparing, whereby the fetal brain's development is prioritized above other organs, even in the most adverse circumstances(192). The implications for obstetrics and child health are not our focus, which are the consequences for CVD and DM_2. Birthweight and related attributes are hard to alter as there are innate determining factors. For example, the birthweight can only be raised by a small degree by nutritional supplementation, and the consequences for later life tend to be subtle and variable(244–247). Studies of trends in birthweights in many countries, both those with relatively high and low birthweights, show little change even as populations within societies became affluent and develop antenatal and other services(248, 249).

The low birthweight of the typical South Asian baby has gained a central place in explaining CVD and DM_2 because of the DOHAD hypothesis. Understanding birthweight is, therefore, important in the evaluation of the implications of the hypothesis. The central question is whether the typical birthweight in South Asians of 2.7–3.1 kg is abnormally low and if so whether steps should be taken to raise it to the European value of about 3.4 kg. The main strategy for this is socio-economic improvement. Supplementation of diet before and during pregnancy has modest, and sometimes no, demonstrable benefits. A follow-up of such babies into adolescence in Hyderabad, India indicated some benefits of dietary supplementation in pregnancy including less insulin resistance and arterial stiffness(250). In this study, however, there was no programming effect, including in changing muscle mass(245). Other evidence that helps guide us is what happens to South Asians babies born in socio-economically advanced settings, e.g. the UK, where several million South Asians live, with about half of them born there.

The birthweight of South Asian babies born in the UK has been studied in several major studies over about 40 years, and unsurprisingly, it is lower than babies of White UK ethnic groups(240, 248, 249, 251–253). The difference is typically 300–400 g, although in some places like Bradford in the North of England it was 200–300 g (reflecting the lower than average birthweight in the local White British population)(254). Depending on the South Asian population and the location of the study the typical birthweights of South Asian babies in the UK is 2.7–3.0 kg, although sometimes it has been as high as 3.1–3.2 kg. The greatest surprise from these studies, however, is that the birthweight of babies of South Asian mothers who themselves were born in the affluent UK environment are no heavier than those of South Asian immigrants often coming from poor regions. Indeed there is evidence of the opposite, with early studies being contradicted by larger and later ones(249, 252, 254). This shows that the factors affecting birthweight are largely resistant to socio-economic and environmental change.

Insulin is important in determining birthweight and given that insulin tends to be high in both South Asians mothers and their fetuses, this low birthweight is especially surprising. Most studies show high insulin in the cord blood of South Asian newborns(191) but one exception was the study of Indian mothers in New Zealand where their cord insulin was lower than in European or Polynesian babies(255).

The higher birthweight of South Asian babies born in the UK compared with those in India—typically about 200 g—may, at least partly, be a result of the very high prevalence of hyperglycaemia—IGT, IFG, DM_2, and gestational diabetes—of South Asian mothers in the UK(256, 257). If so, it is not likely to be a welcome and healthy change. A small part of the lower birthweight of UK South Asians compared to White British babies is a slightly shorter gestational period—a few days(258).

If, for the purpose of reflection given this is a controversial proposition, we assume the comparatively low birthweight of South Asian babies is innate—perhaps even genetic—we could ponder on why that might be. Well-established hypotheses like the thrifty genotype or thrifty phenotype could be evoked, i.e. the fetus is being prepared for a particular kind of environment(94, 95). Other explanations might relate to body size and shape of parents especially the mother, quite possibly including the pelvic volume, which creates a physical constraint(243, 259). There is, however, a fundamental evolutionary gene–environment explanation that fits with long-established observations on climate and physiognomy, i.e. that the imperatives of heat loss in warm countries place a value on a small size at birth and greater length in relation to weight(160, 188, 260–262). This gives extra surface area for heat loss. The opposite would be needed for heat retention in cold climates. Wells has provided theoretical ideas, a mathematical model, and empirical data from countries across the world to support this idea(188, 261–263).

There is a repeatedly documented association between low birthweight and DM_2 in adulthood(226, 228). The metabolic consequences have also been traced and found to be small in scale compared with the kind of changes occurring in adulthood(264). There are also genetic factors involved, e.g. in one study gene variants associated with DM_2 were also associated with 80 g lower birthweight(265). In discussing this work, Meier et al. also placed emphasis on a reduced beta cell mass in the pancreas as the unifying explanation(266). If there were a reduced production of fetal insulin, which is a growth factor for the fetus, we would expect this to lead to lower birthweight. Reflecting on these observations in the context of South Asians, a lower birthweight could be a result of genetically determined lower beta cell mass and consequently lower fetal insulin. The question is: what evolutionary advantage might there be from this genotype? One possibility, it seems to me, is reduced risk of the fetus being trapped in the pelvic outlet (dystocia) and easier birth, especially given South Asian women's smaller hips and height. The paradox, however, is that South Asian fetuses seem to be exposed to high, not low, levels of insulin.

Table 5.1 provides a brief list of, and commentary on, the main explanations available for the relatively low birthweight, long, and fatty South Asian baby with low muscle mass. There is no agreed explanation for the comparatively low birthweight of South Asians and even whether it is physiological or pathological. Detailed studies in birth cohorts, e.g. Born in Bradford, have not pinpointed the explanation though genetic data have not yet been analysed and integrated with environmental and physiological information(254, 257, 267, 268). We can now interpret the evidence on the thrifty phenotype hypothesis in South Asians, which is considered in the next section.

5.6 The thrifty phenotype and maternal investment hypotheses

The significance of the DOHAD concept for the developing countries, including South Asian ones, was identified early especially as South Asian babies were known to be born with low birth weights, typically 10–15% lower than Northern European ones. One of the turning points in explaining why birthweight might matter was the thrifty phenotype hypothesis (Box 5.1, p 116 and Figure 5.1), a title that echoed the prevailing thrifty genotype hypothesis(95). This placed a mismatch between the environmental conditions during fetal development (later extended to the first two years of life) and those encountered

Table 5.1 Explanations for the small yet, relatively long and fat, South Asian baby

	Explanation	Comment
1.	Genetic factors	Need to be identified specifically but an example is the fetal insulin hypothesis, i.e. genes promote high insulin and that leads to fat deposition.
2.	Parental height	This is clearly important whether via genetic or other mechanisms. Maternal height is especially relevant.
3.	Pre-term birth/shorter gestation	This is true but only by a few days and not enough to explain differences.
4.	Maternal illness, e.g. malaria	This is important but does not explain the differences especially in low-infection environments, e.g. the UK.
5.	Pre-pregnancy weight	South Asian mothers tend to be light, especially in South Asia.
6.	Gestational weight gain	South Asians mothers put on as much weight as others (though they don't take it off easily after birth).
7.	Poverty (through other causes)	Even well-off South Asians have comparatively low birthweight, though higher than poor people
8.	Tobacco including chewing	In South Asian cultures where both smoking and chewing tobacco are taboo,, e.g. Sikhs, birthweights are still comparatively low
9.	Maternal malnutrition	There does not seem to be a protein or calorie deficit
10.	Micronutrients	The evidence on these matter is slim but currently there is active interest in B_{12} in pregnancy, especially in its balance with folic acid (see also Table 5.3)

later, especially in adulthood. Where these are different there is a mismatch, or dysadaptation, this being the factor that promotes diseases. The proposed mismatch is that the low birthweight fetus is programmed for a low nutrition lifestyle but encounters a high nutrition environment. This is what we see with South Asian emigrants to industrialized countries and in urbanized South Asians especially if they have migrated from the rural areas(138, 234, 269).

The potential importance of the hypothesis was recognized but sometimes with scepticism and with alternative explanations. One alternative, for example, is that there are fetal genetic factors influencing birthweight (rather than

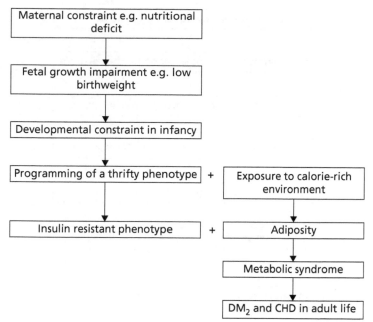

Figure 5.1 Thrifty phenotype hypothesis (also, in essence, and often interchangeably described as the fetal origins, DOHAD, and adaptation–dysadaptation hypotheses)– my simple causal diagram.
Source: data from Hales, CN. et al. The thrifty phenotype hypothesis. British Medical Bulletin. 60(1), 5–20. Copyright © 2001 OUP.

maternal nutrition being the influence), e.g. through insulin, and these are also the causes of adult diseases(265, 270). Several related hypotheses have been proposed including the maternal investment hypothesis of Wells that develops the ideas in the thrifty phenotype hypothesis by providing an evolutionary context (see Box 5.2, p 118, and Figure 5.2)(271). It also fits with the genetic hypotheses we considered in Chapters 2–4 but the ideas are so aligned to the DOHAD hypothesis that I consider it here.

The thrifty phenotype's key explanation is uterine restraint relating to nutritional factors, which might go back a few generations(95). The maternal investment hypothesis, however, sees the effects as being shaped over long timescales. The increasing evidence including, and perhaps especially, in South Asian population is that birthweight is refractory to short-term nutritional factors perhaps inclines us to Wells' standpoint.

There is, however, a slight contradiction and conundrum in these hypotheses and that is adiposity. As we saw (Chapter 3) and will see again in this chapter the South Asians' phenotype is one of brain and adipose tissue sparing. Adipose tissue is a costly resource from a nutritional perspective (9 calories per gram

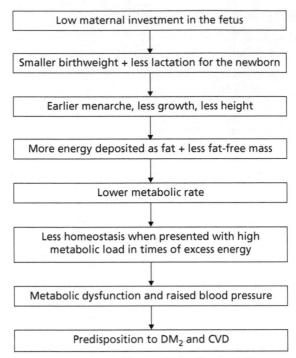

Figure 5.2 Maternal investment hypothesis–my simple causal diagram.
Source: data from Wells, JC. et al. Maternal investment, life-history strategy of the offspring and adult chronic disease risk in South Asian women in the UK. *Evolution, Medicine, & Public Health*. 2016(1),133–45. Copyright © 2016 OUP.

compared to about 3 calories per gram for carbohydrate and about 5 calories per gram for protein). If the South Asian mother is nutritionally constrained or puts in a low investment why is adipose tissue, rather than lean tissue, spared?

5.7 The DOHAD group of hypotheses specifically in South Asians: an examination of the evidence

5.7.1 The focus of the examination

The DOHAD hypothesis is one of the most important research areas with extensive research and scholarship on animals and on humans. The topic has been reviewed on many occasions both by enthusiasts and sceptics and in a range of contexts and populations(226, 228, 272). The hypothesis is pertinent to several animal species and, though possibly less so, also relevant to humans. The question is not so much whether it is relevant in humans, but how important is it in relation to other factors? I will consider this question in relation to South Asians both in the countries of origin and abroad. My primary question is whether DOHAD might largely explain South Asians' propensity to CVD and DM_2. As for about 30 years I have believed this to be the case, it is important that I declare this potential bias.

In this book I generally refer to published articles and reviews and extract illustrative data from them. Unfortunately, for this very important topic, in the only review on ethnic minority groups including South Asians overseas I found, the data were selective and not provided in detail(273). Given the prominence and potential importance of the subject, I have created a table of data on studies directly or indirectly exploring the hypothesis in South Asians (Tables 5.2, 5.3 and 5.4). Before I describe these data, I need to reinforce a few of the epidemiological principles examined in Chapter 1, Section 1.14.

5.7.2 The association between birth and post-birth measures and the effect of adjustment for 'confounders'

In answering the question of whether a difference between ethnic groups, as opposed to humans as a collective, might be explained by a hypothesis, clearly, animal research is not relevant. Human experiments in the DOHAD field are rare and those designed to examine risk factors across ethnic groups rarer still. To my knowledge no experiments in the DOHAD are directly relevant to our central question of South Asians' susceptibility to CVD and DM_2. We are, therefore, reliant on non-experimental, observational data. The key observational study design for our purpose is the cohort study. This produces associations but their interpretation to deduce cause and effect is challenging(27). In Section 1.14 we considered some epidemiological principles and challenges. The biggest challenge in the context of the DOHAD hypothesis is the time between exposure and outcome of CVD and DM_2, which is usually 40 years or more. This puts a reliance on retrospective cohort studies where the exposure data, e.g. birthweight, were collected decades before and outcomes are measured now or in the near future. These can be supplemented by prospective birth cohort studies where the DM_2 and CVD intermediate outcomes are used, e.g. glucose, insulin, or insulin resistance rather than DM_2, or intima media thickness or arterial stiffness rather than CVD itself.

We face other problems in interpreting the role of known causal and probable risk factors beyond the fetal and early life stages, whether in adolescence or in adulthood. For example, is it being relatively adipose at birth, or early life, or in adolescence, or adulthood that matters? All four stages probably matter but the question is by how much and which of them deserves special attention? This knowledge is vital to set up the most effective preventative strategies.

Table 5.2 Birth cohort studies investigating the DOHAD hypothesis in South Asia

Author (first), place, fieldwork dates, publication date	Aims	Sample source	Sample size	Key measurements	Key results	Implications
Kumaran(278) Mysore, India 1934–1954 hospital records; 1993 and 2001 follow-up 2000	To study the association between birth measures and CVD risk factors and glucose metabolism in adulthood.	Survey in 1993 of 7800 households to identify people born in Holdsworth Memorial Hospital where measures had been made since 1934. In 1996–7 further measures were made.	1311 people aged 40 years or older born as singletons were matched to birth records. 536 were matched and 517 participated. Of them 435 participated in the 1996 follow-up.	Weight, length, and head circumference of newborn. Maternal pelvic measurement CVD and DM screen in adulthood. Mixed measures of CHD, e.g. Rose Angina Questionnaire, left ventricular mass, and arterial compliance.	There were few CHD outcomes (n = 52) but the associations were in line with DOHAD. No association with systolic BP, left ventricular mass and arterial compliance. (There were also associations with greater length at birth that remain unexplained.)	The study, overall, provided very limited support for the DOHAD hypothesis. The authors speculate that in India the effects of poor fetal growth may be mediated by insulin resistance.
Stein(276) Mysore, India 1934–1954 1996	To examine the association between dimensions at birth and CHD in adulthood.	Survey in 1993 of 7800 households to identify people born in Holdsworth Memorial Hospital.	Of 1311 people identified 517 men and women had measures taken for this study.	CHD ascertained by questionnaire, ECG, and history of coronary artery surgery. BP and lipids were also measured.	Few people had CHD on ECG (14) and one surgery so most cases (52) were on questionnaire. Most of the latter were women. There was an association with birthweights (inverse) and mothers' weight.	While the results are in the expected direction they lend modest support to DOHAD as the measure of the outcome is not reliable and the number of cases is very small.

Yajnik(100) Pune and Mysore, India Pune 1993 Mysore 1934–1954 2014	To study associations between maternal homocysteine and offspring birthweights, with particular reference to the role of folate and B$_{12}$ metabolism.	See Stein (1996) and Yajnik (2008)	Measures and analysis on 526 mother/baby pairs in Pune and 515 in Mysore.	Mendelian randomization (MR) approach with *MTHFR* gene variant and standard methods using homocysteine measures.	Both MR and standard methods including combining the two cohorts showed high homocysteine was associated with slightly lower birthweights.	This work is important in offering a biochemical basis for a lower birthweight in South Asians that then sets up a susceptibility. Very few people actually had the gene variant (24/1041) so the population-level significance of the finding is unclear. The authors emphasize an imbalance in folate and B$_{12}$ in inducing adiposity.
Bhargava(279) N. Delhi, India 1969–72 with follow-up in 1999—2002 2004	To study which stage of weight gain is related to IGT and DM$_2$ in adulthood.	20,755 women identified in 1969—72 with 8181 live births.	In 1999–2002, 2584 people were located, and 1492 provided outcome data.	Weight and length at birth and regularly until 14–21 years. OGTT with glucose and insulin measurements at 26–32 years of age.	The people developing IGT or DM were, typically, low BMI up to about 7.8 years and high BMI thereafter. However, whatever their birthweight their current BMI was strongly associated with IGT/DM.	There is modest evidence here in favour of the DOHAD hypothesis although the authors emphasize the issue of early adiposity rebound. This is the first of several papers on this topic from this study (see Sachdev and Fall provided below).

(continued)

Table 5.2 Continued

Author (first), place, fieldwork dates, publication date	Aims	Sample source	Sample size	Key measurements	Key results	Implications
Sachdev(211) N. Delhi, India 1969–72 2005	To examine association between birth size, BMI in childhood, and body composition in adulthood.	20,755 women identified in 1969–72, with 8181 live births.	In 1998–2002, 2584 people were retraced. Outcome data on 1526 people.	Weight and length measured at birth then 6-monthly until 14–21 years.	Overweight and obesity were common in adults. Birthweight associated with lean body mass, but not central obesity in adulthood. Also, associated with general obesity in women, not men. BMI gain in later childhood associated with adult obesity.	The findings did not provide strong support for the DOHAD hypothesis, though the findings on lean body mass were noteworthy for insulin resistance and DM_2.
Fall(280) New Delhi, India 1969–1972 2008	To examine the association between birthweight, growth in childhood, and metabolic disorders associated with CVD.	20,755 women identified 1969–72 had 8181 live births	In 1998–2002, 2,584 of birth cohort traced and 1583 participated. Data relevant to outcomes were on 1492 people.	Weight and length measured at birth then 6-monthly till 14–21 years. In 1998 follow-up with detailed data focused on CVD risk factors and glucose metabolism.	Glucose intolerance in adulthood was associated with lower BMI in infancy. Metabolic syndrome in adulthood was associated with rapid weight gain through to adolescence. The association became statistically non-significant after adjusting for adult BMI.	These results pertain to, by Indian standards, an affluent population. These are complex data but, overall, they do not give clear support to the DOHAD hypothesis but throw emphasis on weight gain per se.

Study	Objective	Sample	Measures	Findings	Comments
Lakshmy (281) New Delhi, India 1969–72 2011	To examine association between BMI at birth and childhood and pro-inflammatory, pro-thrombotic factors	20,755 women with 8181 live births	In 1998, 1583 people participated in follow up. Fibrinogen measured in 1492, hs-CRP in 1472 and PAI-1 in 1469 people	Weight and height regularly until 32 years. Fibrinogen hs-CRP, and PAI-I. Adiposity and BMI gain between 2 and 11 years associated with inflammatory and thrombotic factors but BMI at birth was not so associated; in women low BMI at birth and at 2 years was associated with higher fibrinogen.	The evidence for pro-thrombotic/pro-inflammatory effect of low BMI at birth is weak and inconsistent (Table 2 of paper) but it is clear cut in adult life
Raghupathy(282) Vellore, India 1969–73 with follow-up in 1998–2002 2010	To relate CVD risk factors and glucose tolerance to parental size, neonatal size, and childhood growth.	10,670 singleton live births. 2218 participated in 1998–2002 follow up. Rural and urban areas near Vellore, South India. 20,626 married, non-pregnant women were recruited.	Anthropometry at birth, 6–8 years, 10–15 years, and 26–32 years. At the final follow up complete measures available for 1093 of 2218 people. Multiple measures at 26–32 years including an OGTT.	Shorter maternal height associated with higher IGT in offspring. Highest risk of IGT/DM was associated with low childhood and high adult BMI. Insulin resistance associated with rapid weight gain. Birth, infancy, and adolescent weight were not associated with DM_2.	This study has many limitations, e.g. the attrition in the sample size but it is unique. The findings are in line with the DOHAD hypothesis as being thin at birth with accelerated BMI was associated with DM_2. Birthweight was not directly related.

(continued)

Table 5.2 Continued

Author (first), place, fieldwork dates, publication date	Aims	Sample source	Sample size	Key measurements	Key results	Implications
Yajnik(242) Pune, India 1987–9 1995	To determine whether low birthweight is associated with reduced glucose tolerance in Indian children.	A random sample of 404 births at the King Edward Memorial Hospital, plus, 271 babies surviving admission to the special care baby unit with a weight of under 2 kg at birth.	Of the sample of 404 births, 201 participated, of the 271 special babies 178 participated, a total of 379.	Measures at age 4 with an OGTT.	In the sample of 201 birthweight was inversely associated with glucose and insulin, adjusting for current size. In the special care babies only insulin was so associated.	The results are in line with expectations of the DOHAD hypothesis but bias needs to be considered as the association was present with adjustment for current size.
Bavdekar (284) Pune, India 1987–9 1999	To examine the association between birthweight and glucose metabolism at 8 years (Yajnik et al. above reported at 4 years)	As for Yajnik 1985 but an additional sample was taken of 1987–9 births. The special care babies were omitted.	190 of the original sample and 287 additional children gave a total of 477.	Glucose and insulin measures after an OGTT. Anthropometric measures. Total and LDL cholesterol.	All risk factors associated with current weight. After adjustment for current weight birthweight was inversely associated with most factors except index of beta-cell function. Low birthweight and high current fat mass combined were associated with the highest risk profile. Tallness was associated with insulin resistance, especially if parents were short.	There is evidence in favour of DOHAD but the association appears after adjustment for current weight, meaning that it may be a 'change in weight', not birthweight effect.

Study	Aim	Cohort	Measures	Results	Comments
Yajnik(308) Pune, India 1987–9 2015	To see whether insulin resistance in childhood is associated with future CVD risk, i.e. at 21 years.	As for Bavdekar	Of 477 people seen at 8 years, 357 were assessed at 21 years	In addition to OGTT, intima media thickness (IMT) and pulse wave velocity (PWV) were measured. Diet, physical activity, and socio-economic position assessed.	There were some weak associations between measures at 8 and 21 years. In similar analysis with 4 year olds, associations were not statistically significant. Associations between measures at 8 years and IMT and PWV were inconsistent and weak. No association between HOMA-IR or HOMA-B and IMT and PWV.	The authors' claim that prepubertal glucose-insulin metabolism is associated with cardiovascular risk in adulthood is not, in my view, shown on these data. Rather, the glucose-insulin metabolism at 21 years seems more important. The authors' view that low birthweight, insulin resistance and CVD risk are on the same causal pathway is notable.
Kumar(283) Haryana, India 1992–3 2004	To investigate the association of birthweight and BP at 7–8 years of age.	10 villages in Haryana had 339 live births and those to usual residents were followed up. Those born Monday–Saturday had birthweight measured.	214 children were eligible for follow-up—185 enrolled.	Height, weight, BP, and socio-economic circumstances.	No association of importance in birthweight and SBP or DBP in boys or girls or both at 7-8 years.	This small cohort had the advantage of being community based. The results do not support the DOHAD hypothesis.

(continued)

Table 5.2 Continued

Author (first), place, fieldwork dates, publication date	Aims	Sample source	Sample size	Key measurements	Key results	Implications
Yajnik(287) Pune, India 1993 2008	To examine the association between folate, vitamin B_{12} and homocysteine in pregnancy and adiposity and insulin resistance in offspring at 6 years.	Pune Maternal Nutrition Study in six villages near Pune.	700 of 762 live births of whom 653 provided data at 6 years.	Nutritional intake of mothers and B_{12} and other measures at 18 and 28 weeks gestation, and offspring's anthropometry and insulin resistance at 6 years.	Higher folate in mother associated with offspring adiposity and insulin resistance and low B_{12} associated with insulin resistance in offspring.	This work offers a mechanism whereby poor nutrition could lead to metabolic dysfunction, i.e. a low B_{12} in pregnancy especially in association with a high folate.
Rao(288) Pune, India 1993 2009	To study relations between maternal nutrition and fetal growth, with special reference to seasonality.	In 6 villages near Pune with farming population of 770 women delivering babies, 633 babies had data for analysis.	633 full-term normal live births and their mothers.	24 hr recall of foods. Weights of servings recorded the day before. Physical activity by questionnaire. Pre-pregnancy weight and height, and same at 18 and 28 weeks gestation. Baby's birthweight and length.	Food intake of mothers lowest in summer especially at 18 weeks of pregnancy. Birthweights were lower if more exposure to winter during pregnancy.	The study provides unusual evidence that shortage of nutrition and physical activity is contributing to low birthweight in rural Indian babies.

Study	Aim	Population	Sample	Measures	Results	Comments
Winder (289) Mysore, India 1997–1998 2011	To examine whether the size and shape of the placenta predicts BP	1233 eligible women attending the antenatal clinic at Holdsworth Memorial Institute	830 woman took part, 674 delivered at the hospital. Placenta measured in 653 babies. 539 children examined at 9 years. Full data on 171 children	Placental weight and dimensions and anthropometry and BP	In boys no association between BP and birthweight and other measures. In girls BP higher in those with low birth weight. In boys systolic BP was associated with placental dimensions. In girls systolic and diastolic BP associated with placental dimensions	There are some modest yet inconsistent associations as shown by examination of tables 2 and 3 in the paper rather than the selected highlighted results
Hill (312) Mysore, India 1997 2005	To investigate the association of maternal glucose tolerance and fetal growth.	Deliveries at Holdsworth Memorial Hospital, recruited in the antenatal clinic.	Of 1233 eligible women, 830 agreed, and relevant data were available on 674.	3-hr OGTT with a 100 glucose load in mothers. Weight, length and other anthropometry on infants.	6.2% of women developed gestational diabetes. Their babies were 383 g heavier than those of mothers without this. Maternal glucose was associated with birthweight.	Mothers with gestational diabetes were much more adipose than those without. Their babies were heavier, longer and larger in all dimensions than those of mothers without GDM. Birthweight was associated with maternal glucose levels.

Proponents of the DOHAD hypothesis emphasize action even before conception in prospective pregnant women and again early in the life of their offspring. Most public health strategies, however, emphasize risk factors in early adulthood or even once the disease is detected, usually in middle age. This kind of tension needs resolving, starting with scientific analysis of the evidence.

The standard epidemiological approach to analysis is to adjust for other risk factors, to assess the erroneously named independent effect (association actually) of the specific risk factor of interest. So if we are interested in adiposity at birth, 1 year, 7 years, and 21 years and its association with insulin resistance in adult life we might take the 1-year value and adjust for adiposity at 21 years (as a covariate to be treated as a confounder). This kind of analysis has been common practice(274). After such an adjustment procedure, however, the association under study is between the change in adiposity at the two ages and insulin resistance. This is not the same thing as the one we started with, i.e. with adiposity at birth. So we need to examine both unadjusted and adjusted associations to reach an appropriate interpretation.

A general problem that affects all research is publication bias(27). Put simply, researchers, funders, journal referees, and editors are more interested in results that are positive (meaning in this context that they find the association between early life circumstances and health outcomes) than negative or inconclusive. The process of publication is difficult, expensive, and often tedious, involving numerous draft revisions of the manuscript, and also re-analysis of data. It is common for authors to submit to several journals before the paper is accepted. The inconclusive and negative results may never be published causing a misinterpretation of the totality of evidence.

One of the strengths of birth cohort studies is that reverse causation is not possible, i.e. in our example above, insulin resistance at 21 years did not cause adiposity at 1 year. It is quite possible, however, that some factor caused both adiposity at 1 year and insulin resistance at 21 years, e.g. genes controlling insulin action. With these principles in mind we can examine the evidence base.

5.7.3 Evidence for the DOHAD hypothesis in Indians

The studies in Tables 5.2 and 5.3 need to be examined with the principles in Sections 1.14 and 5.7.2 in mind. Table 5.2 summarizes much of the evidence from India, the main source of the data on the DOHAD hypothesis in South Asians. Table 5.3 summarizes some studies outside South Asia. Tables are ordered by the time when the cohorts were established, so reflecting their potential for studying long-term outcomes. This approach also has the merit that different publications from the one cohort study appear together but ordered by date of publication (earlier considered first). The studies are briefly reviewed below.

Table 5.3 Studies investigating the thrifty phenotype and related hypothesis outside South Asia

Author (first), place, fieldwork dates, publication date	Aims	Sample source	Sample size	Key measurements	Key results	Implications
Alvear(294) W. London, UK Unknown 1978	To determine differences in neonatal size in three racial groups	Women giving birth at a hospital in a high immigration area in W. London and their infants.	75 mainly Irish North Europeans, 75 Negroes and 37 Asians of Indian Subcontinent origin. Most of the Asians were non-vegetarian Muslims.	Maternal measures included weight gain in pregnancy. Infant measures were extensive, e.g. anthropometry including three-skinfolds, and mid-arm and calf circumferences.	Maternal BMI was similar across groups but Asian mothers were shorter. Asian infants' birthweight was 2.99 kg, 288 g less than Europeans and they were smaller in every dimension except triceps skinfold. Mothers' triceps skinfold was not correlated with infants' skinfold.	Since maternal weight gain in Asian mothers was similar to Europeans energy intake was judged adequate. Babies' subcutaneous fat reserves indicate intrauterine nourishment was adequate. Limb lengths were similar but lean mass was less. Nutrition does not explain lower birthweight. Micronutrient deficiency and malnutrition in the ancestral line are possible explanations. The authors think the birthweight differences are genetic.
Brooke(295) S.W. London, UK Unknown 1980	To examine growth patterns in British Asians in first year of life.	80 unselected deliveries of 80 Asian infants in St. Georges Hospital, were compared with 243 White infants.	The Asian infants mostly had origins in India (73%) and Pakistani (17%). The Asians were mostly middle class (unlike Alvear's sample).	Maternal height and weight and a range of anthropometric measures on babies.	The mean weight of Asian babies was 3.034 kg (3.363 kg in White babies). Birthweight was not associated with mother's height. Mean length of Asian and White babies was similar. There was accelerated linear growth in first 3 months. At 1 year Asian infants were slightly longer and less heavy than standards.	Catch-up growth in first 3 months suggests intra-uterine growth restriction. However, even in this well-off group of healthy Asian babies weight at 1 year remained lower though length was higher.

(continued)

Table 5.3 Continued

Author (first), place, fieldwork dates, publication date	Aims	Sample source	Sample size	Key measurements	Key results	Implications
West(254) Bradford, UK 2007–2010 2013	To compare birth measures, especially adiposity, in Pakistani and White British infants	13,773 pregnant women attending Bradford Royal Infirmary's maternity service. Of them 8704 were singleton term births to Pakistani or White British mothers	4055 White British babies of whom 612 had leptin measured. 4649 Pakistani babies of whom 775 had leptin measured.	Birthweight, skinfold thicknesses, cord leptin, and multiple co-variables, including blood glucose.	Pakistani babies were lighter and their skinfold thickness was less but not so once adjusted for birthweight. Cord leptin was similar in both groups but was 30% higher once adjusted for birthweight. The findings did not differ by parental/grandparental birthplace.	The lower birthweights (–234 g) of Pakistani babies was affected little by adjustment for many covariates. Skinfold thickness differences were removed by adjustment for birthweight while leptin was higher after this; the only evidence for the 'thin-fat' baby phenotype was leptin levels.
Lawlor(297) Bradford, UK 2007–2010 2014	To examine whether gestational glucose levels explain differences in fat mass reflected in leptin levels between Pakistani and White British infants.	See West (2013). This sub sample was recruited 2008–2009.	Of 1555 eligible infants with cord blood 1415 had provided data (629 White British and 786 Pakistani)	Maternal blood glucose measured by an OGTT at 26–28 weeks. Cord blood leptin levels. Co-variates.	Higher fasting, and post-glucose load, glucose levels were associated with cord insulin and leptin. Pakistani infants had confounder-adjusted 16% higher cord leptin levels, a difference reduced to 5% after adjustment for maternal fasting glucose and cord blood insulin. Similar results were found after excluding mothers with gestational diabetes.	The evidence supports the hypothesis that the relative adiposity of Pakistani infants is a result of high maternal glucose levels (compared with White British mothers). The higher cord insulin in Pakistani infants is also related to maternal glucose levels.

Study	Aim	Methods	Results	Comments
Fairley(299) Bradford, UK 2008–2009 2015(299)	To investigate associations between risk factors for childhood obesity comparing White British and Pakistani children.	See West (2013) for background cohort. This subsample was recruited into a follow-up study (BiB 1000). BMI at 3 years was the outcome with multiple measures of factors potentially related to this. Of 1916 women eligible, 1735 were included and their 1707 singleton births followed up 6-monthly to 3 years.	Pakistani children had lower BMI and a lower percentage with overweight than White British children. Maternal smoking, maternal obesity at booking, and indulgent feeding style were among the few factors associated with BMI, similarly so in White British and Pakistani children. Gestational diabetes was not associated with higher BMI.	Pakistani children were less likely to be overweight and had lower BMI than White British children notwithstanding the higher exposure to maternal gestational diabetes and maternal glucose in-utero (see West and Lawlor above). Risk factors for childhood obesity were not higher in Pakistani children.
Bansal(301) Manchester, UK 2008	To investigate associations between early postnatal growth and BP at 1 year. South Asian infants were hypothesized to be smaller but with greater skinfold thickness than European origin ones.	Women and their infants in a cohort study. Measures include infants' skinfold thickness, weight, and height at birth, 3 months, and in some at 12 months. BP was measured at 12 months. Breast feeding and weaning data were collected. Of 632 women recruited in Manchester, data on 560 infants (189 South Asians and 371 European) were presented. These mothers had uncomplicated pregnancies (no gestational DM or hypertension).	At birth South Asian boys were smaller and shorter with smaller skinfolds; South Asian girls were smaller but their skinfolds were similar to European girls. South Asians grew rapidly. Rapid weight gain but not birth weight, was associated with higher SBP at 12 months but higher birth length and little growth in length was associated with the highest DBP. At 12 months weight, length, BMI, and BP were similar in all groups. A high birth subscapular/triceps skinfold ratio was associated with low BP at 1 year).	The authors emphasize differences in boys and girls, especially in skinfolds (but skinfolds were similar at 1 year by ethnic group–higher in girls than boys). Also they emphasize 'catch up growth' leading to rapid increase in truncal skinfold in South Asian boys especially at 3 months. The authors think these data could explain BP tracking in later life.

The earliest cohort available in India is the South Indian Mysore study known as PARTHENON, based on the birth records at Holdsworth Memorial Hospital(275). These records were discovered by David Barker's team in India led by Caroline Fall. The first paper by Stein et al.—see Table 5.2—examined 517 people who had been born in Holdsworth Memorial Hospital(276). The outcome of interest was CHD. Only 14 people had CHD on ECG, which is a very small number of outcomes for epidemiological studies and results in statistical imprecision of estimated effects. The Rose/WHO angina questionnaire yielded another 52 cases but this is not a reliable outcome especially in cross-cultural settings(277). There was, at best, modest evidence here in favour of the DOHAD hypothesis.

Kumaran et al. reported on the same cohort but also including BP, left ventricular mass, and arterial compliance as intermediate measures of cardiovascular function(278). There were no associations between birthweight and systolic BP, ventricular mass, or arterial compliance. The authors proposed that cardiovascular problems may arise through insulin resistance, the long-held view that we considered in Chapter 1.

A second retrospective cohort study using births between 1969 and 1972 was established in New Delhi also following searches for data by the Barker team. Bhargava et al. reported that of 8181 eligible live births, outcome data were obtained on 1492 people in 1999–2002 (279). Serial anthropometric measures were available in some people up to 21 years. An oral glucose tolerance test (OGTT) was administered at 26–32 years of age. There was no association between birthweight and IGT/DM. The most important and strongest association was between current BMI and IGT/DM. However, people who had a low BMI up to about 8 years and a high BMI thereafter were at the highest risk of IGT/DM$_2$. The concept here was that those who are thin (on BMI) up to two years of age would be at high risk if they became more adipose later in life. In the same cohort Sachdev et al. reported on the association between body composition in early and adult life, with outcome data on 1526 of 8181 eligible live births(211). Birthweight was related to lean body mass but not central obesity in adulthood (though it was associated with general obesity in women). Weight gain later in childhood and adolescence was associated with overweight in adulthood. These two results provided only weak support for the thrifty phenotype/DOHAD hypothesis.

Fall et al. reported on metabolic syndrome and related disorders in adulthood in the New Delhi cohort(280). Glucose intolerance in adulthood was associated with lower BMI in infancy, rapid weight gain in adolescence, and higher weight in adulthood. The association between birthweight and range of outcomes including systolic BP and IGT/DM was weak and statistically not significant. Several of the reported associations with birthweight became statistically significant after adjusting for adult BMI, and as already discussed above this is examining change in BMI rather than birthweight. Overall, this provided little evidence for the thrifty phenotype hypothesis, but as with other papers in this cohort, later weight gain was clearly associated with adverse outcomes.

Also from the New Delhi cohort, Lakshmy et al. examined associations between BMI at birth and through life up to 32 years, with particular reference to pro-thrombotic and pro-inflammatory markers. The associations were extremely clear-cut using measures of BMI in adulthood, but inconsistent and relatively weak in association with BMI at birth(281).

Raghupathy et al. reported results from a prospective cohort study in Vellore, South India, again with involvement of the Barker team(282). The thrifty phenotype concept was an addition to the original aims, with examination of 2218 (of 10,670 eligible) births at 26–32 years with measures including an OGTT. As with the New Delhi cohort rapid weight gain rather than birthweight was the main factor associated with IGT/DM.

Kumar et al. (2004) reported on BP in 185 of 214 eligible 7–8-year-old children whose birthweights had been recorded in rural North India(283). There was no association. This study did not support the thrifty phenotype hypothesis.

Table 5.2 summarizes a series of studies in Pune in Central Eastern India, started in collaboration with Barker's team, under the leadership of Chittaranjan Yajnik. These studies are based on two separate kinds of cohorts, those based on hospital births (1987–9) and those on a rural maternal and child cohort. Unlike the previous studies these were specifically designed to verify and test the fetal origins/ thrifty phenotype hypothesis. As such they deserve special attention so I have additionally summarized the main findings in Box 5.3 (p 120) and Table 5.4.

Yajnik et al. found that low birthweight was associated with higher glucose and insulin at four years of age but this association occurred after adjustment for current size(242). The same conclusion was reported by Bavdekar et al. on the same study group but with a supplemented sample and this time at 8 years of age. At eight years, being tall was, somewhat unexpectedly, associated with insulin resistance(284). In 2015, Yajnik et al. reported on the same sample followed up to 21 years of age, with extra measures of cardiovascular dysfunction, i.e. intima media thickness and pulse wave velocity(285). The associations were weak and inconsistent(285). The associations between birthweight, 4-year measures and 8-year measures and adverse outcomes were relatively weak, compared with the associations with risk factors measured at 21 years.

In 2008, Yajnik et al. reported on 653 of 762 live births in the Pune Maternal Nutrition Study. Maternal nutrition measured at 18 and 28 weeks of pregnancy was related to anthropometry at birth and at 6 years and insulin resistance at 6 years. General nutritional factors were not importantly associated with these

Table 5.4 Key findings of Pune based life-course studies

Author/year of publication	Key finding
Yajnik(242) 1995	Low birthweight children were comparatively insulin resistant at 4 years of age.
Bavdekar 1999(284)	Low birthweight children who had become heavier in childhood had the highest cardiovascular risk profile at 8 years of age.
Rao(309) 2001	Micronutrients were more closely associated with birthweight then macronutrients in Pune Maternal Nutrition Study. There was, relative to other tissue compartments, sparing of subscapular fat and intra-abdominal fat indicating a thin but relative fatty baby. B_{12} deficiency was identified as a prime suspect for low birthweight through the one-carbon metabolism pathway.
Bhate 2008(310)	Maternal B_{12} related to cognitive function of offspring.
Kanade(311) 2008	Micronutrient rich food like fruit and vegetables associated with birthweights.
Yajnik(287) 2008	Maternal B_{12} (low) and folate (high) related to insulin resistance in offspring.
Yajnik(100) 2014	Higher maternal homocysteine linked to lower offspring birthweight by Mendelian randomization study.
Ongoing	A randomized controlled trial of B_{12} and other supplements given pre-conceptually to adolescent boys and girls to examine their offspring's outcomes.

outcomes but green leafy vegetables were, so the investigators focused in subsequent studies on micronutrients, especially folate and B_{12}(286, 287).

Rao et al. (2009) showed an association between fetal growth and season of birth(288). Birthweights were lower in babies exposed to more winter months in pregnancy when food is scarcer. It was proposed that birthweight, and the subsequent association between this and insulin resistance, is a consequence of disturbed 1-carbon metabolism, itself caused by a shortage of vitamin B_{12} together with a high folate level. The hypothesis was tested in collaboration with the Mysore investigators(100). Standard cohort analysis was combined with Mendelian randomization. Very few people had the gene variant associated with low B_{12} (about 2.4%) and the predicted effect on birthweight was very small.

In an international systematic review and meta-analysis of B_{12} deficiency in pregnancy and the association between B_{12} and birthweight Sukumar et al. showed that B_{12} deficiency was common but, except for a few outlier results from India, was not associated with birthweight(110). Rafnsson et al. had earlier reported a systematic review showing little evidence that B_{12} deficiency was associated with CVD(108). This line of enquiry is ongoing.

The concept that birthweight is a marker for other more important changes, e.g. placental function was examined by Winder et al. in Mysore(289). There were some limited associations between placental weight and dimensions and BP but they were inconsistent.

In this set of studies, I found a tendency to construct an interpretation in line with the DOHAD hypothesis, usually by focusing on selected findings. In comparison with the effects of anthropometric indicators in adulthood, the effects of fetal and infant measures were small in scale. Even given some evidence of an interaction between fetal/infant and adult measures the idea that the epidemic of CHD and DM_2 is fundamentally a result of fetal/life rather than adult circumstances is unconvincing. Overall, contrary to my expectations, the evidence for the thrifty phenotype hypothesis in the Indian context was limited and, paradoxically given the low birthweight, not as convincing as that gathered in developed country settings, e.g. the UK where this hypothesis has also been pursued in relation to South Asians as considered in Section 5.7.4.

5.7.4 Evidence for the DOHAD hypothesis in South Asians in the UK

While UK researchers have played a large part in investigating the epidemic of CVD and DM_2 in South Asians(29, 221) and the DOHAD hypothesis(226) empirical research in UK South Asian populations connecting the two areas based on birth cohorts is sparse, though relevant insights are emerging from studies of children and adolescents(290–293). Table 5.3 summarizes the birth cohort data of direct relevance, a body of evidence that is small in comparison with that in India.

Many UK studies have reported birthweights by ethnic group but few have shed insights into the causes or related the differences to the DOHAD hypothesis and its role in CVD and DM_2. Alvear and Brooke examined a small multiethnic group including 37 South Asian mothers and their offspring(294). South Asians were small in all dimensions except skinfold thickness. Mothers' gestational weight gain and infants' fat reserves indicated by skinfold thickness show that maternal nutrition was adequate. Nonetheless, South Asian infants' lean mass was less. The authors drew attention to the possibility of micronutrient deficiency. Brooke and Wood reported that South Asian babies grew fast in the 3 months after birth and by 1 year were slightly longer though less heavy than reference standards(295).

The Born in Bradford Cohort Study is set in a city in the North of England, where about 50% of the births are to the resident Pakistani ethnic group, many of them with origins in Northern Punjab and the state of Mirpur(296). West et al. compared birthweight and other measures, especially related to adiposity, in White British and Pakistani ethnic group babies, with one aim being to see whether the thin-fat phenotype described by Yajnik was observable(254). Leptin, a hormone secreted by adipose tissue, was measured in a subsample. The difference in birthweight of 234 g between the ethnic groups was less than usually reported. The skinfold thicknesses, including the subscapular, were smaller in Pakistani babies but equivalent when adjusted statistically for birthweight. Leptin levels after adjustment for birthweight were higher in Pakistani new-borns, evidence that their bodies have higher fat content than White British babies(254, 267).

The above observation led to the hypothesis that the observed high glucose levels (at the 28 week OGTT) and high prevalence of gestational DM may have led to higher fetal glucose and as a result high fetal insulin. Fetal insulin would promote the deposition of energy as fat. Lawlor et al. provided evidence that was in support of the hypothesis. So, in addition to providing evidence, albeit limited, for a relatively high fat mass, this study also offered an explanation, i.e. higher maternal glucose(297). This result was similar to that reported by Anand et al. in Canada(298).

In this same cohort Fairley et al. studied BMI up to 3 years of age, including a search for factors associated with childhood overweight and obesity. Pakistani children were less likely to be overweight and obese at 3 years despite their increased exposure to higher maternal glucose(299).

These Bradford data, to date, have not provided strong data in support of DOHAD but longer-term follow up is needed. Interim analysis of skinfold thicknesses provide some evidence for the adipose tissue compartment hypothesis with smaller thigh skinfold thickness at 3 years, especially in Pakistani boys(300).

Bansal et al. examined growth in the first year of life showing that South Asian infants were smaller at birth but grew rapidly to catch up with the European origin infants(301). Birthweight was not associated with BP at 1 year but rapid weight gain was.

There is evidence in the UK that South Asian babies are exposed to higher maternal glucose and thereby the fetus (and infant) has higher insulin with adipose tissue sparing as in South Asia. The evidence that this has adverse consequences for CVD and DM_2 is unconvincing. Overall, the UK data concur with South Asia data that South Asian babies are born small and grow fast after birth. The birthweight of South Asian babies in the UK is about 3 kg, a little higher than in South Asia. The low birth weight reflects growth constraint in utero but it does not seem to be a result of macronutrient deficiency. When combined with the evidence from South Asia (Table 5.2) it is not, in my view, a compelling explanation for South Asian adults' susceptibility to CVD and DM_2.

5.8 **Conclusions**

The concepts now integrated into the DOHAD hypothesis, in relation to chronic diseases, have been the most promising avenues for explaining South Asians' tendency to CVD and DM_2 beyond the traditional, established risk factors(234, 273, 302). While capturing both scholarly and public attention, however, they have not greatly altered policy or practice for the prevention of CVD and DM_2, at least in the industrialized and wealthy countries. Nonetheless, these concepts have provided important routes to trying to explain why South Asians are so susceptible to CVD and DM_2. The idea that uterine factors, especially growth restraint related to maternal (and other ancestral) factors, plays a critical role in programming this susceptibility has been compelling. (I am one of many scholars and researchers who have pinned their hopes on this hypothesis.) The evidence in Tables 5.2 and 5.3, however, provides little support for it.

In the process of seeking uterine and early life risk factors, the research puts the spotlight on adult risk factors, and at most, on the change between early life and later life risk factors. In their systematic review of birthweight and obesity Yu et al. concluded that high birthweight was associated with higher prevalence of obesity in later life and low birthweight with a lower obesity(303). So it is a move from this trajectory that may cause the problems of adult diseases, not the birthweight (or the factors birthweight is a proxy for) itself. Weight in early life is associated with weight gain in later childhood and adulthood(304). In trying to increase birthweight, the logical goal of this set of hypotheses, we may be increasing adiposity in South Asian babies and setting a lifelong increased tendency to adiposity and obesity. Caution is required.

I conclude that even though the story recounted here has hardly begun, and many surprises surely await us as more research with longer term outcomes occurs(305), it is unlikely that the dominating, root causes of the CVD and DM_2 epidemics in urbanized South Asians lie in their uterine and early life circumstances. This verdict acknowledges that the DOHAD hypothesis has a part to play but it is not, in my (new) view, the critical one. There is still much to learn in this area including preconceptional circumstances(306).

We will return to this in Chapter 9. We now turn to mainstream factors that have been the mainstay of CVD and DM_2 causal thinking for the last 50 years, i.e. socio-economic and psychosocial factors (Chapter 6) and the traditional risk factors (Chapter 7).

Box 5.1 The thrifty phenotype hypothesis

Type 2 (non-insulin dependent) diabetes mellitus: the thrifty phenotype hypothesis. Hales CN, Barker DJP. Diabetologia 1992;35:595–601 *and* updated in British Medical Bulletin 2001;60:5–20(95).

My introductory remarks

The ideas in this hypothesis were not developed with South Asian populations in mind but they were quickly recognized as being important for them, because the South Asian baby is born relatively small. Important studies examining the hypothesis are ongoing in India (see sections 5.7.3 and 5. 7.4 and Yajnik 2008 in Table 5.2). The account below starts with the original exposition and then considers the 2001 update. I have summarized the hypothesis in Figure 5.1, a simple causal diagram.

The original paper

The paper opens with the hypothesis that poor fetal and early post-natal nutrition induces nutritional thrift with consequences, including poor development of the pancreas, that increase susceptibility to DM_2. The paper then reviews insulin deficiency and insulin resistance in the path to DM_2, noting that in the Ely study in the UK people with IGT were shorter than controls.

The paper also introduces the fetal origins hypothesis for CVD, i.e. that impaired growth and development lead to permanent changes in structure or function (programming) that increase risk in later life. Early evidence for this came from observing the correlation between neonatal mortality and CVD deaths in England 70 years later, subsequently corroborated with observations on the Hertfordshire birth cohort. Low birthweight, associated with high placental weight, and low weight at 1 year in boys was linked to raised BP and plasma fibrinogen in adult life. Poor maternal nutrition was thought to be the underlying factor. A study was done to see whether glucose tolerance might also be related similarly. This was demonstrated in the Hertfordshire cohort. Adult obesity added to the effects of low weight at 1 year. The hypothesis was identified as compatible with the high prevalence of diabetes in the developing world.

The effects, whether on glucose or hypertension or other outcomes, were postulated to depend on the timing of the growth impairment. From conception to birth there are 42 cell divisions compared with about 5 after birth so the potential importance of the early period was clear. By birth nearly

Box 5.1 The thrifty phenotype hypothesis (*continued*)

all neurons and renal glomeruli are present, and by 1 year about half of the pancreatic beta cells are. The latter are vulnerable in early life, and damage to them is the proposed route to DM_2 later. The effect on beta cells is seen as both direct (numbers) and indirect (structure, innervation, and blood supply). The authors then pose and answer six key questions. One of the questions is about which nutritional factors are involved, and amino acids are picked out as especially important. A shortage of amino acids would be sensed by the beta cells and less insulin produced and as insulin is a key growth regulator, fetal growth would be reduced. In looking for genes relevant to DM_2 therefore, those for fetal growth and development could be important.

The authors then contrast their interpretation with Neel's thrifty genotype hypothesis to formulate the thrifty phenotype hypothesis. Undernourishment implies less need for insulin. If, however, good nutrition arises later in life the body is unprepared, and DM_2 could result. Change in circumstances is judged as critical. They predict that as maternal (and hence fetal) nutrition improves across the generations DM_2 will decline.

Update paper in 2001 (British Medical Bulletin)

The update summarizes the original paper, and informs us that the association between birthweight, length, and thinness has been replicated widely. The point is emphasized that we need to understand what is programmed. Poor growth is closely linked to insulin resistance rather than insulin secretion. The growth trajectory in childhood, and not just in utero and in infancy, is now highlighted as important. Accelerated childhood weight gain is pinpointed as a problem. The results from studies of the Leningrad and Dutch famines are considered as generally supportive and insightful for understanding and underpinning the hypothesis. The evidence on the relative roles of genes and environment is interpreted as remaining unclear. The concept that different nutritional influences, and the timing of influences, will alter outcomes is emphasized.

Some experiments in rats, where the thrifty phenotype is induced by a low protein maternal diet, are cited as showing the importance of nutrition in early life in setting appetite. The differences in males and females, alluded to in 1992, are now accepted as correct. Interestingly, the adaptation to nutrition is aligned by the authors with similar cross-generational adaptations to environmental temperature.

Box 5.1 The thrifty phenotype hypothesis (*continued*)

New, speculative features include the effects of maternal hyperglycaemia, and there is increased emphasis on vasculature, and involvement of the hypothalamic–pituitary––adrenal axis and sympathetic nervous system.

The authors conclude the hypothesis has been strengthened, and ready for intervention studies and incorporation into policy.

My concluding remarks

This hypothesis has been widely influential, including in India, from where prospective and retrospective cohort studies have provided corroborative data and additional understanding including on mechanisms. It is intuitively appealing. The way I see it is this: if you build something with the finest materials it will be strong, functional, and lasting (like a Rolls Royce) but if it is built from meagre materials you cannot expect the same. There is a nuance here. The object, whether car, or body, or organ, will work better and longer if it is used in the ways it was prepared for. A car designed for the road will not last or function well off-road. In essence, on this hypothesis South Asians are not well built for the environment they are now encountering and this underlies their susceptibility to CVD and DM_2. No matter how appealing the hypothesis is it needs to be examined critically, which I do in Section 5.5. At present, I do not find the evidence stands up to the promise.

Box 5.2 Maternal investment hypothesis

Wells J et al. Maternal investment, life-history strategy of the offspring and adult chronic disease risk in South Asian women in the UK. Evolution, Medicine and Public Health 2016;1:133–45 (271).

My introductory remarks

This hypothesis further develops the ideas in the thrifty phenotype concept. The paper is unusual in that it both articulates a hypothesis and tests it out in a sample of South Asians. I have summarized the hypothesis in a simple causal diagram as Figure 5.2.

The paper

The DOHAD hypothesis proposes that low birthweight and rapid weight gain after infancy are key mediators of obesity and adult cardiometabolic

Box 5.2 Maternal investment hypothesis (*continued***)**

diseases. The authors build on these mediators in their capacity load model. Metabolic capacity, in the model, is related to early life growth and governs the potential to maintain homeostasis in the face of metabolic load in later life, which is increased by risk factors including obesity (high load).

Energy is allocated for maintenance of the body, growth, reproduction, and immune function. Evolution, however, prioritizes reproduction. A concept of slow and fast life histories is introduced. The latter are favoured when mortality risk is high.

The metabolic capacity of the offspring is related to maternal investment during pregnancy and lactation, and low investment is said to predict shorter lifespan, a shorter reproductive career, and a fast life history. Low metabolic capacity, together with high metabolic load, is predicted to increase CVD risk.

The authors studied UK adult South Asian women. The women provided information on their own birthweight, breast feeding, and menarche by recall (with help from their mothers). Key physical measurements were made including resting metabolic rates. Birthweight and breast feeding duration were the indicators of maternal investment. Only 58 of 210 respondents provided the full data for the analysis.

Higher birthweight was associated with later menarche and greater height. Lower birthweight was associated with more fat mass. Indices of fat mass were associated with BP. The resting metabolic rate of those born overseas was lower than those born in the UK.

The authors conclude that the findings support the hypothesis, i.e. that less maternal investment indicated by low birthweight was associated with earlier menarche, reduced height, more adiposity, and higher BP. This state induces CVD in the presence of an elevated metabolic load, especially excess energy deposited as central fat.

My concluding remarks

The hypothesis could explain why South Asian ethnic groups exposed to low energy, high pathogen environments have high CVD risk after migration to affluent countries. Surplus energy in the new environment may lead to rapid maturation and reproduction (and not growth and maintenance) with a mismatch of high metabolic load and low metabolic capacity. The empirical evidence is somewhat sparse though intriguing.

Box 5.3 The Pune Maternal Nutrition Study

D'Angelo S, Yajnik CS, Kumaran K, Joglekar C, Lubree H, Crozier SR, et al. Body size and body composition: a comparison of children in India and the UK through infancy and early childhood. Journal of Epidemiology & Community Health. 2015;69(12):1147–53 (182).

Katre PYC. Pune Experience: Influence of early life environment on risk of non-communicable diseases (NCDs) in Indians. Sight and Life. 2015;29(1):91–7 (307).

My introduction to the study

Pune is a major Indian city in the state of Maharashtra in Western India, lying about 100 miles east of Mumbai. Inspired by the developmental origins of adult disease hypothesis (and David Barker), and under the leadership of Chittaranjan Yajnik, a series of investigations have taken place that have established the relevance of the hypothesis in India and have led to new avenues of investigation including micronutrients in fetal life. For this box the focus is a birth cohort study.

Pune Maternal Nutrition Study

In six villages near Pune, health status including anthropometry was measured in over 800 pregnant women who were identified and enrolled before conception. Data were collected on these woman before they became pregnant, an unusual feature and strength as most birth cohort studies recruit women once their pregnancy is established. Among the measurements were health behaviours with a focus on food intake and physical activity, and fetal growth with ultrasound. Detailed measurements were also made on the newborn babies.

The mothers were small and thin even by the standards of Indian rural people with a mean weight of 42 kg, mean height of 1.52m, and a BMI of only 18 kg/m^2. Their babies had a mean birthweight of 2.65 kg. The ponderal index (weight/length^3) was 24.5 g/cm^3. This birthweight was at the lower end of the range of birthweights reported in Indian babies. These babies were compared with babies born in Southampton, UK. The Southampton babies had a mean birthweight of 3.45 kg and a ponderal index of 27.3 g/cm^3. This is not untypical in Northern Europe though, again, it is at the upper end of the range in reported studies. The key observation, however, came from comparing anatomy, particularly adipose tissue reflected in skinfold thickness. The differences between Indian babies in Pune and British babies in Southampton were greatest for abdominal and mid arm circumference (both much bigger

Box 5.3 The Pune Maternal Nutrition Study (*continued*)

in Southampton), and least for length and subscapular skinfold (Pune babies were only slightly smaller). To emphasize, even the subscapular skinfold was smaller in Pune babies than in Southampton-born babies but only marginally so while the other measures were much smaller. So, the issue here is not about actual levels of adiposity but adiposity relative to other tissues.

Yajnik had already coined the paradoxical phrase 'thin and fat Indian' and this work had shown something similar in Indian newborns, i.e. low birthweight, thin, long baby with low muscle and abdominal tissue, but as reflected best in the subscapular skinfold, a well-developed torsal, subcutaneous fat compartment.

The aspects of maternal diet associated with a higher birthweight in this cohort were dairy products, green leafy vegetables, and fruits.

Maternal body size before pregnancy was associated with the baby's weight. The skinfold thicknesses in the babies were associated with short stature and high body fat cohort in the mothers.

Authors' interpretation and new lines of work

The authors named the pattern they discovered the 'Indian thrifty phenotype' and interpreted it as a consequence of the well-established biological phenomenon whereby priority is given to brain growth and development. Insulin resistance and other changes allow diversion of nutrients to the brain at the expense of some other tissues (except, evidently, central fat). These mechanisms may serve the fetus well but may programme changes that have adverse consequences in later life. The authors also invoke air pollution and infections as characteristics of urban Indian life that may exacerbate the cardiometabolic consequences.

Three new lines of work were developed as a result of this: follow up of these babies; the study of micronutrients, especially vitamin B_{12} and its relationship with folic acid; air pollution and its cardiometabolic effects (Pune is a highly polluted city).

My concluding remarks

The interpretation of the significance of the Pune studies is work in progress. It is interesting that the brain, as reflected in head circumference, and torsal fat, as reflected in subscapular skinfold, are relatively unaffected by a comparatively much lower birthweight. Brain sparing is always perceived as a virtue but torsal fat sparing is not. We need to reflect on this arbitrary, and possibly erroneous, distinction.

Socio-economic development and the demographic and epidemiological transitions: effects on psychosocial circumstances and lifestyles

6.1 Chapter 6 objectives are to:

1. Describe the relationship between socio-economic development, accompanying changes in psychosocial status and lifestyles, and the rise of chronic disorders (the demographic and epidemiological transitions).
2. Evaluate whether the above changes can explain the susceptibility of South Asians' to diabetes, stroke, and CHD.

6.2 Chapter summary

Diabetes mellitus, CHD, and ischaemic, but not haemorrhagic, stroke are closely linked to rising affluence and the accompanying changes in life expectancy and in lifestyles. These changes take place in the context of the demographic and epidemiological transitions. These phenomena could be a sound explanation for the rise in diabetes, CHD, and stroke in populations including South Asians but cannot, alone, explain why the rates of these diseases exceed those in populations who are already at an even more advanced stage in these transitions. Changes in psychosocial status and lifestyle accompanying these transitions have been especially rapid in the South Asian diaspora. The recent high heat cooking hypothesis, which proposes South Asians' cooking styles produce atherogenic substances including advanced glycation products (AGEs) and trans-fatty acids, illustrates how affluence and behaviours might influence disease. These explanations are considered in relation to the genetic and developmental origins hypotheses to look for points in common. Together, these general explanations set the stage to examine specific risk factors.

6.3 **Introduction**

The chronic diseases, especially CHD, DM$_2$, and cancers such as those of the breast and colon, are commonly described as diseases of modernization, civilization, industrialization, affluence, and other similar words. This is only true, and only partially so, at the level of populations and not of individuals. At the individual level all these and other chronic diseases are ancient. Paradoxically, it is some infectious diseases that tend to be modern, e.g. HIV/AIDS, caused by microorganisms that previously did not cause human diseases. Certainly, DM$_2$ was well known and described by Indian and other physicians writing about 2000 years ago(84). Atherosclerosis can be seen in imaging studies of Egyptian mummies, and angina, CHD, and stroke would certainly have been an outcome of this pathology then as now. The labelling and diagnosis of CVD outcomes is relatively new and has reflected increased understanding of the pathology. These chronic disease were not common causes of death and disability until the 20th century. Some indirect insights on circumstances in ancient times are provided by modern day examination of contemporary hunter-gatherers and traditional farming communities. Atherosclerosis is rare and so is hyperglycaemia, although this changes rapidly with modernization(313–316). This is true in South Asia too. Nonetheless, the potential to develop CVD and DM$_2$ was present in ancient times and these outcomes develop rapidly even now when hunter-gatherers and subsistence farmers change their lifestyles.

Understanding the forces that have led to these diseases in epidemic form elsewhere is important to South Asians as they are not an exception but are following an established trend. Lawson has pointed out that liberalism and globalization of markets has led to, amongst many other outcomes, cheaper food, higher incomes, and greater freedom of choice (including in foods)(317). These changes occur in the context of many others including longer life expectancy. It is in this kind of broad context that we need to examine the case of South Asians.

The scope of this chapter is potentially vast so the focus is on whether there are any specific factors in South Asians populations that might explain why they get more CVD and DM$_2$ than other populations that are at a more advanced stage of the demographic and epidemiological transitions.

6.3.1 **The demographic and epidemiological transitions**

In Chapter 1 I considered the idea of competing causes of disease. CVD and DM$_2$ are diseases that take decades to occur, and mostly the first symptoms are delayed until about the fourth decade and usually much later. Atherosclerosis and hyperglycaemia have probably been present for years in most such people but without any noticeable problems. For most of human history life span was short because most people died from diseases of childbirth and infancy, infections, nutritional deficiency, accidents, and war. Only the few people surviving till middle age would have been at risk of overt CVD and DM_2.

As socio-economic advances occur, and nutrition and housing improve, more people live into middle and old age and beyond to get overt CVD and DM_2. This is clear in South Asian people living abroad where life expectancy is high, on a par and sometimes higher than in the majority populations of these countries(318), even although more of life might be spent in ill health (319). This demographic shift is also clear in the metropolitan, urban, and semi-urban areas of South Asia(24, 103). Some rural areas have not been greatly affected by socio-economic development and these have, relatively, been spared from the rapid rise of CVD and DM_2 (24). The clearest indicator of this change is in the prevalence of obesity which rises rapidly after rural-to-urban migration(320, 321).

It is not the geography that matters most, however, but the lifestyle change. The same kind of lifestyle changes have already reached many South Asian villages and this trend is likely to accelerate. As people live longer they succumb to the diseases of older ages, i.e. chronic diseases, which is the epidemiological transition, itself a consequence of the demographic transition with the age structure of the population shifting towards an ageing society(23). This transition also leads to a preponderance of women over men as fewer women die in childbirth, and their longer life span is expressed. The change in disease patterns that ensues from a combination of aging, socio-economic, and environmental change, and lifestyle change is called the epidemiological transition.

If the CVD and DM_2 epidemics were solely a result of the demographic transition it would be a matter for celebration. Unfortunately, the epidemiological transition is also affected by numerous additional changes in society that accelerate the processes leading to CVD and DM_2. The most obvious, detrimental accompanying changes include eating more than is needed and a reduction in physical activity increasing the risk of obesity, and other behaviours such as cigarette smoking. Such changes increase CVD and DM_2. The demographic transition also leads to changes in the way societies are organized and in the environment, e.g. in overcrowding and air pollution(322, 323). These changes, in turn, catalyse the epidemiological transition in ways considered in Section 6.4.

6.4 The spread of the epidemic of CVD and DM_2 globally: implications for the epidemic in South Asians

There is now detailed documentation of the way CVD and DM_2 change their incidence as societies change. The trend is usually uncontroversial but the underlying reasons are still being debated(324–326). There is sufficient knowledge, however, to shed light on both the current situation in South Asia and to forecast the likely future(24, 327).

The description here applies to atherosclerotic CVD and DM$_2$. It is worth noting, however, that haemorrhagic stroke generally declines with socioeconomic development. This implies that the causes of haemorrhagic and atherosclerotic stroke are somewhat different, even although raised BP is a risk factor they have in common, including in South Asia(328).

Distinguished physicians of the 19th century who studied diseases such as CHD, including Sir William Osler, noted they were rare, and it was in the early decades of the 20th century that MI and angina were separated and ways of making the diagnoses described(329). By then, CHD was becoming common, quite possibly because of the rapid rise in smoking cigarettes and changing diets. The rapid rise in CHD rates was identified as a serious problem in the post-first world war era, most especially in the US. These concerns were an impetus for large-scale research to understand the causes, e.g. the Framingham Heart Study, which started in 1948(330). At that time the pathology of atherosclerosis was already well described and a common clinical view was that it was a natural, degenerative consequence of ageing. Nonetheless, ideas on the factors that promoted atherosclerosis were being formed and debated. A hundred years earlier the pathologist Rudolf Virchow had already written that atherosclerosis was a result of the combination of thrombosis and deposition of lipid material(331). What was not clear was why this combination occurred and why the consequence, CHD, was becoming commoner.

The substantial rise in a disease beyond its baseline or background incidence rate is by definition an epidemic(27). The first step in its control is recognition that the epidemic is a reality. The second step is to set up surveillance systems to track the epidemic over time, geographical places, and the kind of people most affected. The easiest and perhaps most important measure of outcome is the mortality rate. In the US CHD mortality rates in the middle of the 20th century were highest on the West Coast, were rising fast, and affected men more than women. The rates rose rapidly till the mid-1960s when they started to decline and are still declining(332).

In the UK the same pattern was observed but about 10 years later than in the US, with the decline starting in the mid-1970s, also about 10 years later, with ethnic differences becoming increasingly evident(333). The UK pattern was also seen in much of Northern Europe, Canada, Australia, and New Zealand. The two advanced, industrialized nations that were largely spared were France and Japan(334, 335). The reasons for this sparing are unclear but are much debated. There are predictions that the epidemics in these countries are merely delayed, but if so the delay has been so prolonged that this explanation is unlikely to be true.

The general view is that the epidemic affected the wealthy groups first. These were also the first groups to see a decline in rates. The poorer sections of society in these countries subsequently had much more CVD than the wealthy groups. The causes of the rise and fall of CHD has been studied and debated carefully, given it was the commonest cause of death in the latter 40 years of the 20th century. As the spread across the world was from an apparent focal point in the western part of the US, the idea that it was an infection has been considered but discarded. Rather, it seems to be a behavior-related epidemic. With socio-economic development a set of behaviours became common, of which the most important was the rise of tobacco use, especially as cigarettes(336). The difference in tobacco use in men and women explains much of the difference in disease rates. Further, we saw a rise in the consumption of processed, energy-dense foods, a decline in physical activity levels, and many other changes that are discussed in Chapter 7 as the classical cardiovascular risk factors. The rapid rise in the prevalence of obesity and DM_2 actually happened mainly after CHD rates started to decline in the 1970s, and even more recently in South Asia(324, 337, 338).

New technologies, especially powerful medications to reduce BP and cholesterol, but also health care facilities, added greatly to the decline in CHD mortality that was started with behaviour change such as smoking cessation(339). The trend for atherosclerotic stroke over the same timescale is less well studied but in many respects the picture is similar to that described for CHD, although in countries such as the UK blood pressures have been declining for more than a hundred years, with a concomitant decline in stroke.

The question arising for South Asian countries and populations is which path are they likely to follow in the face of socio-economic development? Twenty or thirty years ago South Asia might have hoped to emulate the surprising and favourable French or Japanese pattern but the experience of the South Asian diaspora was already signalling that the US or UK pattern was more likely. Now it is clear that an epidemic of CHD is accompanying socio-economic development in South Asia, despite a relatively low prevalence of cigarette smoking in women and vegetarianism in many subgroups of the population(24). While this might seem an inescapable price to be paid for socio-economic advance we should look to the global experience to put in place mitigating actions.

Being overweight and, especially, obese was uncommon in most countries until about the 1980s. Historically, obesity was associated with high privilege, wealth, and status. Nonetheless, obesity was commonly associated with stigma. Now, in wealthy societies such as the US and UK more than 50% of the population is overweight or obese. The prevalence of overweight and obesity is even high in young children and there is a steady increase with age, and this problem is increasingly recognized in South Asians (46, 340). This remarkable change in only about 40 years was not predicted. Indeed, as our understanding about healthy living, and the causes of chronic diseases rose, the importance of remaining normal weight was increasingly emphasized over these decades. This epidemic in weight gain has spread internationally, hitting middle-income countries and urbanized areas of low-income countries. The contrast between the decline in some risk behaviours, e.g. smoking, and the rise of others, e.g. exercising insufficiently and eating enough to gain weight, is noteworthy. The consequence of the rise in overweight and obesity has not been seen in a rise of CVD, presumably because the trends in other risk factors with stronger causal effects have outweighed the adverse effects of weight gain.

As with CVD, obesity affects the wealthy countries and groups first and then the less wealthy. Improvements also occur in the wealthy first. This general trend is presently clear in South Asia—obesity prevalence, and its attendant adverse effects on dyslipidaemia, are much higher in the wealthy compared to the poor(341). In a review of the association of risk factors for non-communicable diseases and socio-economic status Allen et al. examined 75 low- and middle-income countries(342). Their results typify what is also seen in South Asian countries as most of the studies were from India. The lower socio-economic status groups used more tobacco and alcohol, and consumed less fruit, vegetable, fish, and fibre. By contrast the higher socio-economic groups undertook less physical activity and had more fats, salt, and processed foods in the diet. From the experience of the economically advanced nations, we can predict that the other groups will catch up, and then even overtake the wealthy ones, who will have begun to reverse this trend.

The single most obvious effect of the rise in obesity has been the rapid increase in DM$_2$. While the obesity epidemic is a complex matter, ultimately, energy intake has exceeded needs(343). The availability of food supplies has increased at the same time as mechanization has reduced expenditure of energy in physical activity. The story is, however, complex with many nuances beyond the scope of this book. Obesity will be discussed further in Chapter 7, especially in its role as a CVD and DM$_2$ risk factor in South Asians.

The migration process, whether from rural to urban areas or from South Asia to industrialized, wealthy countries in Europe or North America, accelerates the obesogenic and diabetogenic processes(344, 345). Unsurprisingly, the adverse change in CVD risk factors from rural to urban environments in one country, such as India(344, 346) seems to be much smaller than in a move from India to the UK(60, 61). In Hermandez et al.'s review, rural-to-urban migrants tended to be intermediate in their risk factor patterns compared to those settled in urban areas(347). Migration and social change are a source of psychosocial stress, considered in Section 6.4.1.

6.4.1 Psychosocial factors: mental health, stresses of migration, and racism

When the epidemic of CHD first came to widespread notice in the 1940s or so it affected, particularly, well-off men. Among the ideas that were sparked off by this observation two are particularly relevant here, i.e. that CHD was a result of the kind of pressured life of high ranking (executive) roles and/or of a personality type characterized by a pressured life. A series of psychosocial risk factors have been examined over the years(348, 349). Many of these ideas, especially personality type, were not upheld by research but it is worth noting that in the later epidemic of the CHD and DM_2 in South Asians we have seen the same pattern, i.e. the highest rates of disease in the populations with higher social and economic status.

Psychosocial factors are a composite of mental health problems such as anxiety and depression, personality traits such as type A or type B, and stressors such as strain in the workplace, discrimination possibly based on race or ethnic group, and the difficulties of migration and resettlement in a new country(348, 350, 351). This is a complex matter that is hard to study especially in relation to physical health problems such as CVD and DM_2.

In popular culture and lay language, the above psychosocial factors might be labelled as stress. Stress of this kind is a difficult matter to define, measure, and study as a cause of disease. Stressors activate production of the hormones cortisol and adrenaline/noradrenaline. Over a short time and in response to environmental threats such stress is necessary, but over a long period there is a failure of normal function. The concepts of homeostasis and allostasis are relevant here. In homeostasis the body maintains stability of its functions even in the presence of environmental stimuli for change (e.g. core body temperature doesn't change in hot environments). Allostasis allows a resetting of the values around which homeostasis occurs, e.g. clearly BP is re-set in some circumstances and becomes higher for prolonged periods and even permanently(352).

Recent research has linked stress to activity in the amygdala of the brain and thereby to vascular inflammation, postulating a path that fits the pathology(353). Stress has been taken seriously by researchers as a cause of both CVD and DM_2, not usually as a single factor but as one or more of the psychosocial factors mentioned in the opening sentence above. These factors have mostly been studied in descriptive epidemiology with few interventional studies as trials, although some trials have been done on intermediate outcomes, usually BP levels using stress reducing activities such as yoga, often with breathing exercises, as the intervention(354–356). This is relevant as this kind of activity is popular and respected in South Asia.

The importance of psychosocial factors is undeniable, especially as they also affect the risk factors we consider causal, e.g. smoking cigarettes, BP, diet quality, and obesity(349). See figure 6.1 (p 134) for my simple causal diagram for such factors. The two questions of particular importance for this book are: 1) whether these factors have direct effects that are not through the known causal factors and 2) whether the pattern of psychosocial risk factors might explain the high risk of CVD and DM$_2$ in South Asians, especially in comparison with White European origin populations.

Of the many psychosocial factors studied depression, low control and strain at work, the stresses of poverty, and discrimination (most clearly racial but probably other kinds) are strong candidates as causal factors for CVD for either exerting their effects through other risk factors or independently(348, 349). The mechanisms of action for independent effects are most likely through the endocrine systems controlling corticosteroids released by the adrenal gland and the autonomic nervous system releasing adrenaline and noradrenaline. In turn, these systems might affect atherosclerosis through inflammatory processes and lipid metabolism or affect heart rhythms or function(357, 358).

Migration itself, whether rural-to-urban, or international, is undoubtedly a stressor as well as a powerful cause of changes in an array of lifestyles and life choices relevant to CVD and DM$_2$. Migration is also related to other psychosocial factors such as depression and work strain. It would probably be impossible to isolate the direct effect of migration independent of these other changes.

Might the susceptibility of South Asians to CVD and DM$_2$ be attributable in an important way to the kind of psychosocial factors above? In South Asian countries now, as in the US and Europe in the 1930s and 1940s, CHD and DM$_2$ are affecting the well off more than the poor, although already there is some evidence to the contrary. (The situation for stroke is more complex as most data do not separate atherosclerotic and haemorrhagic stroke, so we will set it aside for the present.) The kinds of explanation based on executive stress and the self-driven type A personality did not hold in US and European settings and are unlikely to be relevant to South Asians either.

We have no reason to think South Asians are especially prone to depression in comparison with, say White Europeans. By contrast, a high proportion of South Asians living in urbanized settings are working in jobs where autonomy and self-control are low, incomes are low, and strain and job demands are high. This also applies to many emigrant South Asian populations, especially when emigrants are not gaining work opportunities and status commensurate with their qualifications and abilities, e.g. the common anecdote of the Pakistani taxi driver who has a university degree from Karachi that is not recognized in the UK or the US. The results of the empirical studies on this matter have not been clear cut, and in some places South Asians are in self-employment where job control is high unlike many other jobs(359, 360). There is a great deal of discrimination of various kinds both in South Asian countries themselves and in the countries of emigration(350). In South Asian countries, however, the most susceptible groups for CVD and DM_2, the relatively wealthy, are not, at least not yet, the ones most discriminated against; these being the poor, the lower castes, and religious minorities. Racial discrimination is, potentially, an important explanation in countries such as the UK, and we will look at the situation in Section 6.4.2, focusing on UK as most studies of psychosocial risk factors in South Asian populations have been done there.

6.4.2 Psychosocial factors in UK South Asians

A recent unpublished systematic review for the Master of Public Health degree by my postgraduate colleague Debjani Mukhopadhyay of psychosocial factors related to CHD in South Asians in Europe and North America only found eight papers from four studies that reported comparisons with a reference population, and all were in the UK. Some of these publications subdivided the population by religious subgroup or country of origin but mostly they were combined as South Asians(350, 359–365).

About 4 million people of South Asian ethnicities (Indian, Pakistani, Bangladeshi, etc) live in the UK and the population is rising. South Asians there comprise a mix of regional and national origins, social and economic status, and occupations. More than half of them were born in the UK. Many South Asians enjoy high economic status and work in the professions and in business. Overall, however, most work in lower status occupations and generally their occupational status is lower than that expected from their educational qualifications. Despite excellent anti-discrimination laws and policies there remains, as in all societies, racial and cultural prejudice in the UK, which is readily admitted by the public in surveys(366).

The immigrants had the stresses and strains associated with resettlement in a new country. Their children had the stresses of combining and reconciling their South Asian and British cultures. In trying to understand the very high rates of CVD and DM_2 in UK South Asians researchers have tried to examine the role of psychosocial factors. The evidence base is small but can be summarized as follows:

- South Asians, especially women, may have more depressive disorders than the majority White populations, and these disorders may not be treated early and thus lead to disproportionately more hospitalization(350, 367).

- Work-related strain and lack of control may be greater in employed South Asians, though this may not be true overall, as a high proportion of South Asians are self-employed when job strain and lack of control are not such problems(359, 360).

- Perceived and reported racial discrimination is a problem for a surprisingly small proportion of the South Asian population(366). People, however, may not always recognize the presence of racial discrimination, which is commonly reported by the White majority population in the UK(366). Either way, the evidence linking this to either CVD or DM_2 is negligible, even though it has been linked clearly to mental health outcomes(368).

- The disruption of social networks through migration especially (whether abroad or to the city from a village), can lead to loneliness(350, 361, 362, 369).

- Stress and migration issues are perceived as important by South Asians in relation to CVD and DM_2. The effects might be subtle and lie in disrupted social networks and reduced opportunities for social interaction especially for women(369–371).

One way of judging the potential importance of such psychosocial factors is to compare UK South Asians with UK Chinese, whose migration history and life circumstances are similar. UK South Asians have about 2–3 times the CHD rate and about 50% more stroke and DM_2 than the UK Chinese(4, 58). Although not conclusive, this kind of observation veers us towards other explanations.

Overall, without denying the importance of psychosocial factors, especially in influencing the pattern of the recognized causal factors, the evidence that they are especially important in South Asians is weak. The explanation for the South Asians' susceptibility to CVD and DM_2 is unlikely to reside, at least directly, in psychosocial factors.

People with severe psychosocial distress are more likely to be prone to poverty and vice versa and the role of poverty in CHD and DM_2 is examined in Section 6.5.

6.5 **Poverty as a cause of CVD and DM$_2$, especially in South Asians**

Poverty is a dominant influence on health and disease, and with few exceptions, the effects are adverse. Yet, socio-economic advancement is accompanied by the rise of chronic diseases including CVD and DM$_2$. Traditional farming and hunter-gatherer societies tend to be free of these diseases but they arise quickly when they adopt the customs and behaviours of urbanized or semi-urbanized life(313–315, 372). It might be thought, therefore, that poverty is protective against CVD and DM$_2$. This is doubtful, There has been a study showing extensive atherosclerosis in both poor and not poor South Asians, and others indicating poverty does not protect against atheroma(373, 374). In countries such as the UK, CHD, and DM$_2$ are now, though not in the early stages of the epidemic, more common in poor people than in well-off people.

Clearly, the role of poverty is complex. It is not poverty or wealth, per se, that leads to CVD or DM$_2$ or protects us from these diseases, but how they affect the way we lead our lives. We have already considered the role of socio-economic development in creating the demographic and epidemiological transitions. These occur not because of money per se but the changes in our environment, especially our homes, workplaces, technologies including birth control, and a wide range of health-related behaviours.

With an escape from poverty, a quest that is one of the driving forces in human life, come new opportunities, including a move from hunger, whether intermittent or chronic, to satiety. We see a move from goods such as televisions and fridges being unattainable or luxuries to being everyday acquisitions and experiences. I would like to share an anecdote that will chime with hundreds of millions of South Asians and one that is central to the epidemic under scrutiny. My grandparents were typical South Asians living in Punjab, India, at the end of the 19th and beginning of the 20th centuries who had to work long hours to maintain their households. Luxuries were few and reserved for special occasions. Among these luxuries were ghur (sugar molasses), and much less frequently, a jalebi or a pakora. Meat was not eaten, and milk and ghee were in short supply. By my parent's time both being born in 1925 in India, and after migration to Scotland in 1955, there was a modest improvement. Meat was eaten once or twice a week while Indian sweets, milk, and ghee were quite commonly consumed, though they were still seen as luxuries. By my generation's time, none of these food items was a luxury and there was no impediment to fried savouries and sweets such as jalebi as they were not only plentiful but cheap in relation to income. Many other changes occurred including access to mechanization which reduced the requirements for physical activity on a day-to-day basis. It is perhaps no surprise that average adult waist sizes rose about 20–25 cm (12 inches) across these three generations.

We will examine behaviours that are fundamental to understanding CVD and DM_2 in Chapters 7 and 8. Dietary change has been a focal point for research in this field for 50 years or so. The research has produced contradictory conclusions and uncertainties. Along with dietary change, however, we have had two phenomena that have received insufficient attention: 1) the processing of foods using chemicals and 2) the way food is cooked. As an example of how the move from poverty to wealth might, inadvertently, influence disease I would like to discuss in Section 6.6 the recently proposed high heat cooking hypothesis, as summarized in Box 6.1 (p 137)(107).

6.6 The influence of wealth: the example of cooking practices

Traditional societies, especially hunter-gatherers, but also subsistence farmers, ate a great deal of raw or lightly cooked food. However, cooking food has major benefits, including the following. If the temperature is high throughout the food, the heat will sterilize it and decrease the risk of infection. The food is easier to chew and digest and more energy is extracted from it. The flavours are changed, adding to enjoyment. Most human societies mastered and retained fire, using it for many purposes including heating, keeping predators at bay, and cooking. Cooking consumes a lot of fuel, and is expensive, if not in money, then in time to collect, e.g. as firewood. Firewood is very difficult to collect in many parts of South Asia now. Cooking fuel has had to be used sparingly in much of South Asia until recently.

As societies become wealthy, fuel becomes readily available and the technologies to use it for cooking are highly developed. Technologies such as the tandoor oven can achieve temperatures of 400–500°C which is remarkable (and some open flame grills go even higher).

High heat cooking is known to destroy some vitamins, e.g. vitamin C. Heating food has another effect and one that has had little study in health research and practice, although it is well understood in food science—altering its chemical composition. In Box 6.1 (p 137) I summarize a paper that I initiated on some of the potential effects of high heat cooking on the chemical composition of foods and, in turn, on CVD and DM_2 especially in South Asians. I see this paper as a beginning of a new chapter on the possible causes of South Asians' propensity to CVD and DM_2. I chose this as an example of how economic advance might, alongside the benefits, have unpredicted and unexpected side-effects, here the production of newly formed (neo-formed) chemical products, with adverse effects that might initiate or compound the processes that lead to CVD and DM_2. The hypothesis is summarized as a simple causal model in Figure 6.3. I will return to this hypothesis in Chapter 9.

6.7 Conclusions on socio-economic and psychosocial factors

We have covered, albeit lightly, vast topics that are undoubtedly of central importance in the evolving epidemic of CVD and DM_2 in South Asians. I have summarized the ideas in simple causal models as Figures 6.1, 6.2 and 6.3. The themes of socio-economic development, the demographic and epidemiological transitions, and psychosocial stress and strain are universal ones, and it is likely that the consequences already seen in countries such as the US and the UK will

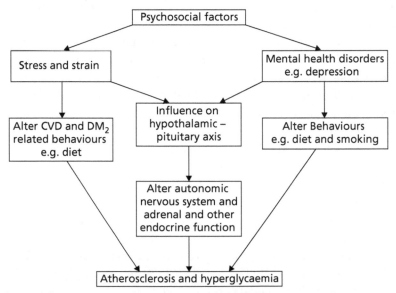

Figure 6.1 A simple causal diagram linking psychosocial factors to CVD and DM_2.

be similar in South Asia. Obviously, this has practical consequences, i.e. South Asian countries are forewarned and, therefore, can prepare, although in the major cities the consequences are already plain.

Is there anything specific to South Asians in this account? There may be a particular convergence of potentially interacting forces: the continuing presence of high rates of infection and sub-nutrition combined with particularly rapid modernization, with its attendant pollution and overcrowding. Razum and colleagues have pointed out that immigrants to Europe from developing countries may undergo an especially rapid epidemiological transition(375). The same may be true for urban South Asia, where the pace of change from agricultural to industrial lifestyles has occurred within a generation or two, at least in some places, where it was spread out over a century or more in Europe and the US(24).

The biological effects of the psychosocial and socio-economic forces are likely to be through the established cardiovascular risk factors as discussed in Chapter 7.

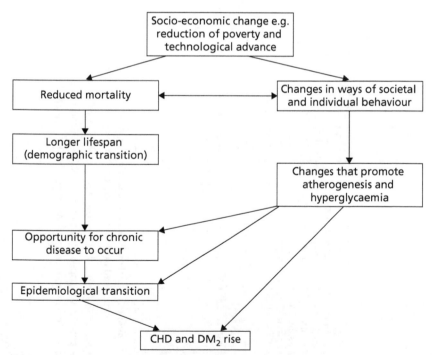

Figure 6.2 A simple causal diagram linking psychosocial factors to CVD and DM_2.

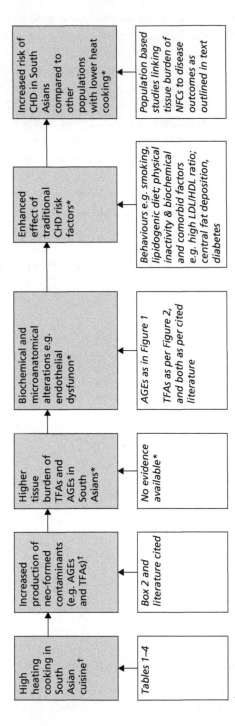

The figure contains the following boxes and annotations (reading left to right):

High heating cooking in South Asian cuisine†

Increased production of neo-formed contaminants (e.g. AGEs and TFAs)†

Higher tissue burden of TFAs and AGEs in South Asians*

Biochemical and microanatomical alterations e.g. endothelial dysfunon*

Enhanced effect of traditional CHD risk factors*

Increased risk of CHD in South Asians compared to other populations with lower heat cooking*

Tables 1–4

Box 2 and literature cited

No evidence available*

AGEs as in Figure 1

TFAs as per Figure 2, and both as per cited literature

Behaviours e.g. smoking, lipidogenic diet; physical inactivity & biochemical and comorbid factors e.g. high LDL/HDL ratio; central fat deposition, diabetes

Population based studies linking tissue burden of NFCs to disease outcomes as outlined in text

†Statement based on literature and evidence in paper
*statements need further basic and epidemiological research

Figure 6.3 A summary of the high heat cooking hypothesis in relation to South Asians' risk of coronary heart disease in relation to the evidence presented in the paper. *Source:* data from Kakde S, Bhopal RS, Bhardwaj S, Misra A. Urbanized South Asians' susceptibility to coronary heart disease: The high-heat food preparation hypothesis. *Nutrition.* 33:216–24. Copyright © 2007 Elsevier.

Box 6.1 High heat cooking hypothesis

Kakde S, Bhopal RS, Bhardwaj S, Misra A. Urbanized South Asians' susceptibility to coronary heart disease: The high-heat food preparation hypothesis. Nutrition. 2017;33:216–24 (107).

My introductory remarks

Since the 1980s I have wondered whether there is a shared dietary toxic
factor in South Asian groups across the world. One shared culinary habit
I observed was the prolonged frying of onions, often with garlic, ginger,
and spices as the starting point of cooking. I recently examined a book of
recipes of South Asian foods. Nearly every recipe included oil, usually fried,
even those for rice and breads(376). The investigation of this possibility
(by Smitha Kakde working with me) quickly led to an understanding that
this process led to neo-formed contaminants (NFCs) of which there are
many, but that the critical factor was heat, not simply the medium in which
the cooking took place or the specific foods cooked. Our focus turned to
oils, frying and heat independently and together. Given the special interests
and expertise of co-authors Bhardwaj and Misra in trans fatty acids (TFAs)
(377), we decided to focus on two kinds of NFCs i.e. AGEs and (TFAs) as
examples.

The paper

The paper opens with the observation that the high susceptibility of urbanized South Asians to CHD is incompletely explained by either general hypotheses or specific risk factors. Diet seems to be important but in ways that
remain opaque. The hypothesis is introduced as moving in a new direction
from evolutionary concepts to cultural ones, i.e. that high-heat cooking promotes NFCs, such as AGEs and TFAs, that lead to endothelial and other
dysfunctions that enhance the effects of traditional risk factors to increase
the risk of CHD in South Asians. The paper is primarily based on literature
review and discussions with experts, though empirical data are presented on
the effects of heating oils on the production of trans fats. The simple causal
models in the paper for AGEs and TFAs are summarised in Figure 6.3 and
more detailed ones are in the paper.

Evidence is presented that high-heat cooking, especially at temperatures
above 150°c, rapidly accelerates the production of NFCs, including AGEs
and TFAs. Reheating further accelerates production of TFAs. Animal and

Box 6.1 High heat cooking hypothesis (*continued*)

human evidence showed these kinds of NFCs were damaging through several mechanisms including oxidative stress, inflammation, lipid metabolism, endothelial dysfunction, and ultimately atherosclerosis. They also promote insulin resistance. We found evidence of clinical effects of high NFCs and clinical benefits of low NFC diets. We found no direct evidence to guide us on whether South Asians had a higher tissue burden of NFCs or whether such a burden had a clinically important effect on their CHD risk.

We, therefore, examined the issue indirectly by comparing Indian and Chinese cuisine by literature review and discussions with informed people. The Indian cuisine made more use of high-heat cooking methods, e.g. the tandoor oven and less use of low heat cooking, e.g. boiling and steaming, than the Chinese cuisine. We showed that the foods cooked at high temperature had higher AGEs than foods cooked at low temperatures. We presented evidence that Indian snacks had far more TFAs (sometimes hundreds of times more) than Chinese snacks. We concluded that there was sufficient evidence to warrant further research on this hypothesis, and set out a research strategy.

My concluding remarks

This hypothesis is a simple one compared with all the others presented in this book and is relatively easily testable. Furthermore, it could lead to rapid change if there is more evidence for it. However, cooking techniques are deeply ingrained and should not be disturbed lightly. There are benefits of high-heat cooking, e.g. hygiene and digestibility is increased. So, we need more evidence before advocating change at a public health level.

Chapter 7

Established CVD and DM$_2$ risk factors: reappraisal in relation to South Asians

7.1 Chapter 7 objectives are to:

1. Reconsider the role of the established CVD and DM$_2$ risk factors (introduced in Tables 1.4 and 1.5), particularly their importance in South Asians

2. Reconsider the view that the explanation for South Asians' susceptibility to CVD and DM$_2$ cannot be ascribed to established risk factors.

7.2 Chapter summary

The causal basis of the established risk factors rests mainly on cohort studies (often backed by case-control studies) sometimes with supplementary data from trials, Mendelian randomization studies and experiments in animals. As the findings have been replicated in many countries there is general acceptance of their global generalizability.

In South Asian populations, specifically, the direct evidence is limited as most of the research to date is from case series or cross-sectional studies. There are a few case-control and cohort studies that confirm the associations are as expected. This chapter re-examines the common claim, including in this book, that these established risk factors do not explain the pattern of disease in South Asians. This claim is clearly true for DM$_2$, but can usually also be substantiated for CHD and stroke.

The lifestyle-related risk factors can be grouped into those where an excess is a problem (e.g. diets leading to adiposity or a high glycaemic load) and those where a deficit is a problem (e.g. insufficient physical activity). These kinds of risk factors, particularly in the context of adverse socio-economic circumstances, provide an excellent basis for causal thinking. So far, even combined with a wide range of biochemical and physiological risk factors, however, such factors are insufficient, though necessary, parts of a convincing explanation for the excess of DM$_2$ and CVD in South Asians. Future research may need to put more emphasis on insufficient physical activity, change in lifestyles as a risk factor in itself, and cultural explanations.

7.3 **Introduction**

Strong evidence on the causes of CVD was provided by the pioneering Framingham Study(330). Framingham is a small town on the West coast of the US that was attractive to the investigators because it had a stable population, allowing people in the study to be followed-up easily. The study started in 1948 and is still going on. More than 1200 scientific papers have been published from the original study and its offshoots. The pivotal contribution was the demonstration that several of the potential causes identified from the experience of clinicians were demonstrated to be associated with CVD outcomes in the long term. The phrase 'risk factor' was coined by the Framingham investigators. The phrase is used variably. I use it to mean a factor where the evidence is sufficient for it to be a serious candidate for consideration of causal status. When causality is agreed, it would be logical to simply say causal factor(27). Custom and practice, and perhaps caution (if not humility) often inhibits writers from taking this step.

Table 1.3 sets out nine causes of CHD, and Table 1.4 five causes of DM_2, for which there is evidence-based consensus. There are many other associated factors, some of which are considered in Chapter 8. Tables 1.3 and 1.4 have, in common, adiposity and obesity, physical inactivity and tobacco but surprisingly genetic and developmental factors still do not always feature in agreed lists of CVD risk factors. Much of the empirical data underpinning Table 1.3 first came from the Framingham study. The study also established the primacy of epidemiology in human population health research on CVD. The results from Framingham were corroborated internationally in numerous other cohort studies, and generally, found to be widely applicable. So, for example, the associations between high levels of cholesterol, high BP, and MI have been widely demonstrated and through careful analysis accepted as causal factors.

Most of the larger-scale, cohort studies were done in wealthy, industrialized countries with strong traditions of epidemiology with little such work, if any, in low-income countries. Within these countries there has been relatively little work on ethnic minority populations including South Asians(98). There were doubts about whether the established risk factors would also apply in countries including in South Asia, e.g. Bangladesh and Pakistan. Was it really true that evidence from Framingham would apply in Dhaka, Bangladesh's capital city and in other such places? The answer, perhaps surprisingly, is yes. In addition to local studies, this principle has been confirmed by international collaborative research on a grand scale, e.g. the case–control study INTERHEART and the even more ambitious cohort equivalent, i.e. PURE(85, 323, 378).

With some nuances, the risk factors have turned out to have similar associations with disease outcomes internationally, including in South Asian countries. Differences tend to be refinements not radical departures. For example, tobacco products increase the risk of CVD across the world but in South Asia these may be used orally and in leaf based products (e.g. bidis) and not just in commercial cigarettes. Tobacco in these forms is unquestionably harmful but the estimates of associated risk are not so precisely known as for cigarettes and many South Asian populations see them as beneficial rather than harmful(379, 380). The association between BMI as a measure of overweight and obesity and hence as a risk for CVD has been a focus of attention, with contradictory evidence on whether it needs to be replaced by other measures, e.g. waist, and this controversy is usually centred on South Asians. INTERHEART found waist/hip ratio was a measure more clearly associated with CHD than BMI(85). These are the kind of modest exceptions that have proven the rule.

In this chapter, I examine each of the major risk factors to: 1) give a broad indication of how common the risk factor is, 2) to highlight some important subpopulation differences, and 3) consider whether the factor might explain the CVD and DM_2 epidemic in South Asians, particularly in comparison with White European populations. For a fuller exposition on each risk factor, I refer readers to relevant articles. I have provided simple causal diagrams on how the risk factors might, together, lead to CVD and DM_2 in Figures 7.1 and 7.2. I then re-examine the currently accepted view that the high susceptibility of South Asians to CVD and DM_2 cannot be explained by the pattern of traditional risk factors. If this is true then studies that have examined these factors as a package, not singly, should support this(1, 18, 381). This kind of examination requires modelling a number of variables (risk factors, confounding factors, mediating factors, interacting factors, and outcomes) using multiple regression or other statistical methods(27). I review these studies carefully, both to extract what we do know and what we still have to learn. One of these studies is examined in Box 7.1(p 171) to provide familiarity with the methods and the quantitative data given in Table 7.1(1).

7.4 **High arterial blood pressure**

The heart pumps the blood into the arteries at considerable pressure. The pressure is, by tradition, measured in millimetres of mercury (mmHg). The typical BP in an artery is 120 mmHg. This is about 1600 mm water, i.e. about 160 cm. If a major artery is cut the blood will rise 160 cm into the air, perhaps hitting the

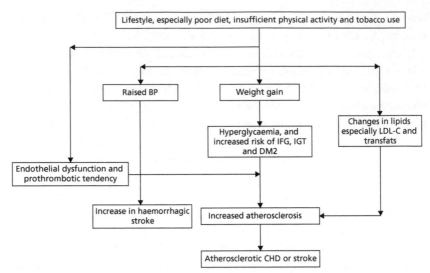

Figure 7.1 A simple conceptual causal diagram on how the classical risk factors might cause CVD.

ceiling. This pressure is needed to ensure circulation of the blood throughout the body. The circulatory tree has to cope with this pressure. It is not surprising that even at normal pressures blood vessels rupture, sometimes causing devastating internal bleeding. BP rises with age, a process that in most populations continues into old age, although there are some traditional societies where this does not occur or is very slow, a benefit that is lost with migration to urban environments(372, 382). In some people BP becomes very high, even above 200 mmHg systolic. The risk of a blood vessel rupturing, especially with a major stroke, then becomes very high.

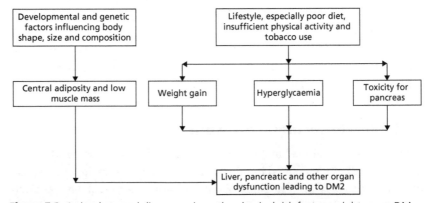

Figure 7.2 A simple causal diagram – how the classical risk factors might cause DM₂.

Table 7.1 Forouhi et al.'s study examining a package of traditional risk factors to explore why South Asians are at relatively high risk of CVD compared to White European populations (1)

Author, year of fieldwork, publication, date, location	Aim of study	Populations studied/ assessment of ethnicity	Number of study participants	Selection of participants	Analytical method	Variables included in analysis	Age and fully adjusted (95% CI) measure of risk	Interpretation
Forouhi 1988–1991 2006 London, UK	To measure the CHD mortality rate in European and S. Asians. To assess whether the baseline risk factors account for differences in mortality	Men of European and South Asian ethnic groups, assessed on several variables.	1787 Europeans 1420 South Asians.	77% were from general practices. 23% were from factories.	Mortality rates from CHD (any mention on death certificate) using person-years at risk, adjusted for relevant variables, using survival time analysis and Cox regression. Tests for interactions between ethnic group and risk factors.	Anthropometry (including waist) BP ECG Glucose Insulin Lipids (total cholesterol and HDL-C and triglyceride) Smoking Physical activity score Medical history Socio-economic status Metabolic syndrome Diabetes Insulin resistance (HOMA and HOMA-IR)	Age adjusted hazard ratio 1.64 (1.24, 2.16) Fully adjusted hazard ratio 2.20 (1.54, 3.14)	Despite several different models with various adjustments the higher risk of CHD in South Asians could not be accounted for statistically.

Source: data from Forouhi, NG. et al. Do known risk factors explain the higher coronary heart disease mortality in South Asian compared with European men? Prospective follow-up of the Southall and Brent studies, UK. *Diabetologia* 2006;49:2580–8. Copyright © Springer.

CHD and especially stroke risk is exquisitely sensitive to changes in BP—a 2 mmHg rise in systolic BP increases stroke by about 6%, and South Asians seem to be particularly sensitive, possibly as a result of accompanying hyperglycaemia(383). Yet, after migration from a rural to an urban environment BP typically rises by 10–20 mmHg, and even more following international migration, e.g. from the rural Punjab to Southhall, London(60, 61). This is, in turn, closely related to rises in salt intake and weight gain.

The additional insights from cohort studies such as the Framingham Study include that there is a graded relationship between rising BP and higher CVD risk, i.e. 100 mmHg confers less risk than 110 mmHg etc, and this less than 120 mmHg etc(384). This graded effect starts at less than what we consider to be normal BP. When I was a medical student in the 1970s the cut-off for high BP was 160 mmHg and now it is 140 mmHg generally and 130 mmHg in those with DM_2, with some people advocating even lower cut-off points, which are currently under discussion(385). BPs of 100mmHg systolic and 70mmHg diastolic or lower are common in thin South Asian people, especially in rural areas, although hypertension is undoubtedly common in many places across South Asia.

The association between rising BP and increased risk of CHD and stroke has been established internationally, including in South Asian populations(384, 386). It is a major cardiovascular risk factor—perhaps even the single most important one(62, 387). It is certainly the most important one for stroke and one of the most important for CHD.

South Asians have exceptionally high risk of stroke and moderately high risk of CHD compared to UK White Europeans(5, 383, 388). We would predict that they would have comparatively high BP. Is this prediction correct? The answer has been elusive because of the heterogeneity of South Asian populations, and no doubt because of rapidly changing lifestyles and socio-economic circumstances that lead to changing population level BPs. Rises occur in BP with urbanization, in association with weight gain and reduced physical activity, and probably through changes in diet, especially salt intake. South Asians are, indeed, prone to a high prevalence of hypertension. Studies across the world, however, show South Asians' BP and prevalence of hypertension tends to be similar to European origin populations, but lower than urbanized African origin (including African American) populations(389–392). There are big differences between Indians, Pakistani, and Bangladeshi populations, with a gradient of reducing BP in that order(392). Despite their lower BPs urbanized Bangladeshis tend to have the highest rates of stroke, CHD, and DM_2 among the South Asian populations(58). This can be observed both in South Asia and in South Asian populations living in the UK and elsewhere abroad. There are also big differences in the pattern of systolic BP by sex between adult Indians (about 7 mmHg higher in men), Pakistani (about 4 mmHg), and Bangladeshi (about 3 mmHg) and virtually no difference in diastolic.

There is emerging evidence in the UK that the differences in BP in different subgroups of South Asian adults, e.g. Bangladeshi and Indian, are not echoed in children and adolescents(393). Battu et al. have confirmed the heterogeneity in BP in Indian, Pakistani, and Bangladeshi adults, but the similarity in BP in children from the three South Asian groups(728). Most likely this indicates that the homogenization of lifestyles and environmental circumstances, and growth patterns, is leading to convergence of BP. The alternative explanation is less likely in my judgement, i.e. that BP diverges not in childhood but at a later age, although we have shown exactly this latter pattern in African origin populations in the UK(394).

Young et al. have hypothesized that the propensity to develop high BP in environments where there is abundant salt, calories, and cool climates is a result of evolutionary adaptation to heat(395). They have summarized genetic and other evidence in support of this hypothesis, including data on body shape. If correct, then South Asians, at least those from the hot regions, would be susceptible to rapid increase in BP after migration to cool climates (possibly including their exposure to air-conditioned homes and workplaces).

BP is important in the causation of CVD in all South Asians but it is not sufficiently commoner to explain the comparatively high risk of CVD. Especially compelling is the finding that Bangladeshi adults have high CVD despite comparatively low BP(396). Explanations for this paradox include that South Asians are more than usually sensitive to the adverse effects of high BP possibly because of hyperglycaemia(397), that the hazards occur at a lower BP, and that it is the pressure in a particular part of the arterial tree (e.g. the aorta and other central arteries) that matter(396). South Asians tend to have higher arterial stiffness and pulse rate, both of which raise central BP(398–400). The possibility that squatting might also raise central BP in South Asians and hence contribute to high rates of stroke has been proposed(396, 401–406). The possibility that BP interacts with other risk factors, e.g. diabetes, particularly strongly in South Asians, thus creating additional risk and that central BP matters greatly will be examined in Chapter 9.

7.5 Lipids including LDL-C and Lp(a)

Rudolf Virchow, the 19th century pathologist, had noted the potential role of blood lipids in atherosclerosis(331). However, it was only after the epidemic of CHD was causing alarm in the 1930s and 1940s that work accelerated on this possibility. The challenge is formidable because lipid biochemistry is complex, and this is compounded by complexity in the lipid composition of the human diet. Additionally, there is individual and population-level variability in lipid metabolism, which may be both induced and programmed, possibly by early exposure to different kinds of lipids.

Blood lipids have been a central focus of research on atherosclerosis for over 70 years, but remain a controversial topic(407, 408). It seems logical that if a fatty material is accumulating in the artery (atherosclerosis), it is coming from the blood. This causal pathway is accepted as, in essence, correct. The question is which circumstances promote this process. The obvious answer is high levels of blood lipids do so and many kinds of research showed this is, in principle, true though the story continues to be refined(409). In the genetic condition familial hypercholesterolaemia patients have extremely high levels of cholesterol and CVD risk, which can be reduced by reducing blood cholesterol levels(115).

The picture that has emerged, however, is a nuanced one. Blood lipids have many functions including in inflammation, control of inflammation, and wound healing. These lipids may alter their functions after undergoing biochemical change, for example, LDL-C can be oxidized, acetylated, and glycated, and the atherogenic effects are different, and probably greater, than unaltered LDL-C(410). The tendency to glycation is likely to be greater in South Asians because of greater hyperglycaemia and possibly because of high heat cooking as considered in Chapter 6 and 8.

Some lipids are neutral or potentially beneficial for CVD, the best example being HDL-C, which is a part of total cholesterol(411). The focus, therefore, turned to LDL-C and VLDL-C. It is accepted that LDL-C is on the causal path for atherosclerosis. There are subtleties that need consideration, e.g. whether the size of the LDL-C particle matters. Small, dense LDL-C particles may be more atherogenic than larger, less dense ones, and are present in larger numbers in South Asians(412). The role of triglycerides is less clear than LDL-C though evidence suggests this lipid is also a cause of CVD, which is particularly important as it is linked to metabolic syndrome and hyperglycaemia, both common in South Asians(413).

South Asian adults in urban setting have a characteristic lipid profile that differs from White Europeans. Their HDL-C is comparatively low, LDL-C is similar, and triglyceride level is high compared with European origin populations. This is seen in adults and children alike(414, 415). This picture is partly linked to insulin resistance (see Section 7.7). In a paper from Uganda in 1959, Shaper et al. showed Asians (meaning South Asians) had higher cholesterol than Africans, and vegetarians had higher levels than non-vegetarians(416). Until recently, when the causal role of HDL-C has been questioned(411), the low HDL-C of South Asians was considered a good explanation for their higher CVD risk, but this now seems unlikely, although the story is still incomplete(409, 417). The similar and sometimes slightly lower LDL-C level is not surprising given typical South Asian diets, but it probably closes off on another explanatory avenue. South Asians do have smaller and denser LDL-C particles, a feature of DM_2 and its precursor states. This, however, has been shown not to be the explanatory factor for their high susceptibility to CVD(1).

Attention has been given to other lipids, mostly notably lipoprotein(a) (Lp(a)). Enas Enas's writing have given special emphasis to this lipid fraction in South Asians(418, 419). Several studies(419, 420), but not all (421–423), have shown Lp(a) levels are relatively high in South Asians, and systematic reviews demonstrate Lp(a) is a causal risk factor for CVD(424). This lipid fraction is under strong genetic control. The (a) part of the name refers to a highly glycosylated protein, itself attached to LDL. Lp(a) has a role in inflammation and attracts inflammatory cells much more than other lipoproteins(425). It may be that South Asians have higher Lp(a) as part of an evolutionary strategy to combat infections. Although the spotlight has been on Lp(a) for many years it is still unclear what its true significance is, including in the issue of South Asians' susceptibility. The lipoprotein is much higher in African origin Black populations than in South Asians but they do not have the same susceptibility to CVD as South Asians.

There are strong advocates of Lp(a) as the key factor behind South Asians' risk of CVD. At present, the evidence to support this advocacy is not strong. Misra et al. found little support for a special role for Lp(a)(421). In their study of CHD, Ramachandran et al. found an association with a range of risk factors including lipids and oxidized LDL-cholesterol, but not with Lp(a)(378). Even if it was a key factor it is not easy to lower Lp(a) levels with effective, well-tolerated medications or other methods. Nicotinic acid (niacin), the main treatment, has side-effects and while it does work it is not easily tolerated(424).

Mostly, researchers have measured cholesterol and its sub-fractions rather than the proteins that carry the cholesterol, e.g. apolipoprotein B (mainly LDL-C). Our causal understanding of South Asians' tendency to CVD is unlikely to alter greatly by measuring the lipoproteins although clinical care might improve(426). In the Newcastle Heart Project lipoprotein levels were similar in Indian, Pakistani, Bangladeshi, and European origin populations even though HDL was low(9). However, in theory, as borne out by INTERHEART, measuring lipoprotein particles could be important in South Asians given their similar LDL-C levels are disguising their larger number of small, dense lipoprotein particles(426).

A form of lipid whether in the diet or in the blood that is frequently considered but could be especially important in South Asians is discussed separately to give it more prominence—trans fatty acids.

7.5.1 Trans fatty acids

Trans fatty acids (TFAs), also known as trans fats, as a cause of CVD are seldom mentioned especially in the literature on CVD in South Asians. TFAs in the blood are rarely measured in individuals or reported in epidemiological studies. It may be that the role of TFAs was accepted so quickly and policy action was taken so fast that the causal link is taken for granted and hence sometimes ignored(427–430). The epidemiological evidence that TFAs are atherogenic and associated with CVD has been reviewed recently and found to be strong(427, 428). Nonetheless, we need a note of caution. In a recent trial, Radtke et al., fed volunteers, aged 45–49, 2% of their nutrients as dairy TFAs or industrial TFAs(431). After 4 weeks there was a rise in cholesterol but no effect on endothelial dysfunction and other intermediate outcomes. So, it is unclear how they have their effects if not through cholesterol. The story is still incomplete especially on the effects of different kinds of trans fat.

In the countries that pushed for this change, including the US and the UK, trans fat content of the diet is now negligible but this is not true in many other parts of the world including South Asia, where the topic still needs careful consideration. Stender et al. measured industrial trans fats in food purchased from supermarkets and ethnic shops meaning those catering for ethnic minority groups(432). Mostly, the levels were <2% as recommended but in 83 products from ethnic food shops, often supplying South Asian populations, the content was 12%.

Trans fatty acids (TFAs) are fatty acids that have a particular chemical structure (one or more non-conjugated double bonds in the trans-configuration). When oil is heated in manufacturing in the presence of a catalyst and hydrogen, some of the unsaturated fatty acids are converted into this structure. When vegetable oils are hydrogenated, a process that converts liquid oils into semi-solids fats, or are refined in other ways, TFAs are created. When oils are heated in the home or catering establishments, TFAs are also created, and increased further with each re-heating(107, 377, 429, 433).

Kakde et al. have recently reviewed the role of TFAs with particular reference to South Asians(107). We found animal and human evidence points to a role for TFAs in biochemical processes that are pertinent to the causation of both CVD and DM₂. These oils are vegetable, and cholesterol-free, but they pose a risk for CVD and DM₂. Five grams of TFAs per day are associated with a 23% increase in CHD risk(427, 428).

Kakde et al. found no data measuring TFAs in South Asian populations or examining their role directly. We know, however, that Vanaspati oil is popular in India (it is often called ghee but it is not) and is hydrogenated vegetable oil, e.g. from palm oil, and is high in TFAs(433, 434). However, it was clear that South Asian foods and cooking methods promote consumption of TFAs(107).

Consensus dietary guidelines for Indians recommend that less than 1% of daily energy come from TFAs. Kakde et al.'s review of South Asian foods, especially snacks, was informative(107). The estimated trans fat content of jalebi, a popular sweet often bought from street vendors and made of sugar and flour and deep fried in oil, was 17.7 g/100 g; and in chat, a popular savoury dish, it was 16.4 g/100 g. By contrast, TFAs were close to zero in equivalent Chinese snacks. Chinese people have far less CHD, and a little less DM_2, than Indians and other South Asians. This work on TFAs was set in the context of the high-heat cooking hypothesis with attention also given to other chemicals produced during cooking, especially advanced glycation end-products. The hypothesis was summarized in Chapter 6, Section 6.6 and in Box 6.1(p 137). We noted earlier the potential added harm from glycated LDL-C(410).

There have been many twists and turns in the quest to understand South Asians' susceptibility to CVD and DM_2 so drawing attention to one relatively new explanation would invite a repeat of previous experiences of false trails. Nonetheless, I think trans fat consumption in South Asians merits much more, detailed empirical investigation.

As we considered in Chapter 1 and will discuss in Chapter 9 a change, or perhaps more accurately, a disturbance of lipid biochemistry remains at the heart of credible explanations for the epidemic of CVD in South Asians, quite possibly in conjunction with diets that potentiate the risk, whether as fats or other compounds. It is extremely worrying that all pointers in South Asia suggest rising levels of both consumption of fats and blood lipids(327, 433).

7.6 **Tobacco**

Tobacco products are agreed as causing CVD in all populations(379). Most of the evidence comes from studies of cigarette smoking, and to a lesser extent pipe and sheesha (waterpipe) smoking(435). The risk comes, primarily, from inhalation. Pipe smokers tend not to inhale and sheesha habits are variable. The non-smoking people who inhale others' tobacco smoke are also at raised risk. The limited work on the effects of bidis which are like a self-rolled cigarette except that a leaf is used instead of paper indicates that the risks are no less than with cigarettes(436). Even one cigarette per day is enough to raise the risk of CVD substantially(437).

Tobacco is a complex substance (4500 chemicals have been identified) and the exact mechanisms and components that lead to CVD and possible DM_2 are not clear. As summarized in Table 1.4 the absorbed products of tobacco promote endothelial dysfunction, thrombosis, and atherosclerosis. The key ingredient in inducing biological, tobacco addiction is nicotine, and this applies to smoking and all other ways of using tobacco, including chewing(438). This substance is of increasing and singular importance because it is used as a tobacco-cessation aid, e.g. in nicotine patches and as the active ingredient in so-called e-cigarettes, which are not harmless(439). In itself, however, nicotine is not considered an important cause of CVD although it has effects on cardiovascular physiology(440).

The use of tobacco products is surprisingly variable across South Asia because cultural forces are strong. There are also major differences by social and economic status and urban/rural life. There are strong social taboos against smoking tobacco in nearly all groups of South Asian women and in surveys few report it, although its use is highly variable across social classes and places(441). Clearly, there is a tendency not to admit to smoking because of social stigma. This has been checked using objective measures of tobacco use such as carbon monoxide in the breath and the tobacco metabolic product cotinine in the saliva. These tests confirm the prevalence of smoking tobacco in South Asian women, for example in the UK, is low(9, 10). Remarkably, this is often also true in daughters of South Asian women living overseas and even across many generations, e.g. Surinamese people living in the Netherlands who left the Indian subcontinent about 100 years ago or more (442, 443). Even although the proportion of people smoking rises across the generations, it remains much lower in South Asian women than in men and also lower than in women in the countries of settlement. Sikhism, for example, forbids the use of tobacco (by decree on 13/4/1699), and in both Sikh men and women smoking is rare, and this behaviour is being retained across generations(444).

Tobacco is a major risk factor for CVD so the low prevalence of this risk factor, alone, would be expected to show in a comparatively lower CVD rate and to less extent lower DM_2 rate, which we don't see either in South Asian women or Sikh men and women in the UK, for example(1, 10). This is one of the paradoxes that need explaining.

In South Asian men the smoking of tobacco varies hugely by religion, region, urban-rural location, socio-economic position, and other factors. Generally, smoking tobacco is commonest in Muslim men, especially Bangladeshis, particularly in the poorer, rural populations(9, 445). Smoking in men is less common in Hindu and Sikh populations than in Muslims in the same country, which is very clear in the UK(446, 447). On this basis we might expect Muslims in the UK and probably South Asia to have higher rates of CVD than Hindus but that is not obviously so in South Asia, though this might be occurring overseas(4, 58, 448). It is true that Bangladeshi men in the UK are at especially high risk of CVD and this might be partly related to smoking tobacco(9, 58).

Tobacco is also used orally, either chewed as a cud or as part of a package of products, e.g. as paan, a product that is widely available not only in South Asia but also overseas in countries such as the UK(449). Chewing paan is common in men and women and even in children in South Asia. It is interesting that social taboos against smoking do not always extend to oral tobacco(380, 450). Paan may be perceived as a smoking cessation aid, which is unfortunate as less harmful, and more effective alternatives are available(451). The role of these products in causing oro-pharyngeal cancers is well established but they have not been considered as potent as cardiovascular risk factors as smoking tobacco. This may be because the mode of delivery or mode of processing of tobacco is important in the causation of cardiovascular disease or it may be related to the amount of the noxious agents that enter the bloodstream. Gupta provided data on smokeless tobacco users in Mumbai: an association was seen with mortality(436). Heavy use of oral tobacco, might be an important risk factor in South Asians(379, 452).

Overall, in relation to tobacco we can conclude that it is vitally important in the causation of CVD in South Asians but with the possible exception of some groups of Muslim men, especially Bangladeshis, the high risk in comparison with White European groups is not attributable to tobacco. The greater mystery is why nearly all South Asian women and Sikh men and women in particular, do not have comparatively low CVD given their low, sometimes even reportedly zero, tobacco consumption.

Tobacco products are also associated with the causation of DM_2(453, 454). The evidence base for a causal effect is less firm than with CVD. Even assuming a causal effect, it is not possible to attribute the comparatively high prevalence of DM_2 to tobacco. DM_2 in South Asian subgroups does not reflect the huge variation in tobacco use, e.g. Sikh men and woman rarely consume tobacco but DM_2 is very common. Once again, the possible effects of tobacco in explaining some of the high risk of DM_2 in male Bangladeshis needs to be considered.

Tobacco can also be used in other ways, e.g. snuff, but the principles above are sufficient to discount these usages as part of an explanation for South Asians' comparatively high risk of CVD and DM_2.

The babies of mothers who smoke are born smaller, by about 100g, than babies of non-smokers. This could, potentially, be of importance in individuals given the developmental origins of adult disease. As most South Asian women do not smoke it is not, however, an important explanation for the CVD and DM$_2$ epidemic in South Asians. Nonetheless, the significance of this in relation to CVD and DM$_2$ in South Asians is unclear.

It is important not to demote tobacco as a primary target in our efforts to control CVD and DM$_2$ in South Asians. This said, tobacco is not, in itself, the reason why South Asians are particularly susceptible to CVD and DM$_2$.

7.7 **Food, diet, and nutrition**

There is a widespread perception, and one that seems correct, that food has an especially prominent place in South Asian cultures(48, 455–458). There is un-doubtedly truth in this as food is more than nourishment. It has a central place in health, well-being, family and social unity, social status, and celebration. The traditional maternal role revolves around food. Recent qualitative research in Edinburgh and London has given insights into how children (including adult children) are expected to eat the family meals, irrespective of whether they have already eaten elsewhere as the external meals are not considered proper food(345, 459). In the Bangladeshi community in London, children were having five eating events a day plus two calorie-laden beverages, with rice with meat or fish being seen as essential to good health(345).

Unquestionably, diet is the most controversial issue in the causation of CVD and DM$_2$ with much still to learn(407, 408, 460–462). There have been numerous twists and turns and even reversals of direction in mainstream thinking. Yet, notwithstanding the difficulties of studying the causal role of diet and nutrition in CVD and DM$_2$, it is important, though there are still deep disagreements on what aspects of diet are important and how.

The role of dietary fats, particularly saturated fats from dairy products, eggs, and fresh meat in the causation of CVD is being revisited(433, 460, 463, 464). Saturated fat has been a central plank of the dietary hypothesis on CVD for most of the last 50 years. Similar controversies have simmered for decades on the health risks of sugars such as, sucrose, glucose, and fructose, and of salt(463, 465). The important principle that emerges from these controversies is that in thinking about the role of diet and nutrition in the epidemic of CVD and DM$_2$ in South Asians, it would be wise to be circumspect, especially as much of the evidence has not come specifically from these populations. Yet, there are a multiplicity of emphatic opinions enunciated by influential members of the public, medical professionals, and research teams. Some advocate abandoning milk (as an ostensibly unnatural food for adult mammals), ghee, sweets of all kinds, salt, and even all flesh. In the next section I consider whether there are dietary or nutritional factors that might explain the epidemic of CVD and DM$_2$

especially in urbanized South Asians. First, we will start with what the evidence agrees on.

7.7.1 Diet, CVD, and DM$_2$: the evidence and its implications for South Asians

Fruits, vegetables, nuts, seeds, and whole grain, and high fibre carbohydrates have withstood careful scrutiny as protective, or at worst neutral, in relation to CVD and probably also for DM$_2$, though an excess of even these foods would lead to weight gain and increased risk(466–470). It has not been possible to extract the specific active ingredient from these foods so that we can take it as a food supplement or a pill, e.g. the antioxidant properties of fruits and vegetables cannot be mimicked by taking antioxidant pills.

Fish, white meats such as chicken and fresh red meat (this in small quantities) are not likely to increase or decrease CVD or DM$_2$ risk in any important way(463, 471). The same applies to dairy foods and eggs, certainly in the context of a balanced diet(463, 464, 472). If dairy foods, eggs, and meat are consumed in large amounts, blood cholesterol levels including LDL-C rise and that is not desirable. Processed meats, especially red meat in large amounts and regularly, may be harmful(473, 474) but this is not typical of eating patterns of South Asians.

Mono-unsaturated and polyunsaturated fats and oils may have cardioprotective properties(407, 475, 476). Saturated fats are associated with raising LDL-C and are unlikely to be beneficial even if they are not unquestionably harmful as previously thought, and some researchers deny any benefits from reducing dietary fat(407, 408, 427, 460). It is critical to note that fats are complex and different versions have different effects. Many saturated fats are probably fine when consumed in small quantities. Hydrogenated TFAs are harmful as discussed in Section 7.5.1.

The complex and controversial story on dietary fats is unfinished but at this point we can summarize it as follows: TFAs should be avoided and where zero consumption is not possible, they should comprise less than 2% of daily calories: saturated fats should be controlled to prevent LDL-cholesterol rising, and the widely agreed upper limit of 20% of daily calories is still holding; mono-unsaturated fats such as olive oil and polyunsaturated fats such as sunflower oil can be used and can supplement, or even supplant, saturated fats. If fat consumption is reduced, it should not be replaced by simple carbohydrates but by complex ones. These are the kind of guidelines that have held over five decades(477).

Alcoholic drinks in small amounts (one or two drinks a few times per week) are neutral or possibly even cardioprotective but are harmful for cardio-metabolic health when consumed in large quantities, especially on one occasion as in binge drinking(62, 478, 479). Alcohol reduces potentially harmful postprandial glucose levels(480, 481). Given its other health disadvantages, such as cancers, accidents, and social disorders, starting to drink alcohol is not recommended in the prevention of CVD and DM$_2$.

Salt raises BP and hence increases risks of CVD, so in normal circumstances, less than 6 g per day is advised though 3 g is mostly sufficient(463, 482). This guidance may need relaxing when salt loss is excessive, e.g. through sweating vigorously in hot environments.

Many micronutrients have been linked to CVD, including antioxidant vitamins, folic acid, and vitamins B$_{12}$ and D(463). There is no clear causal evidence on these substances, and not enough to justify supplements to prevent CVD and DM$_2$. The trials that have been done indicate no benefit and sometimes harm. (Vitamins are discussed in more detail in Chapter 8).

Micronutrients have been under scrutiny in the maternal diet in relation to the health of the newborn especially from the perspective of the DOHAD hypothesis(110, 234). Human studies of micronutrients have been equivocal on benefits in relation to DM$_2$ and CVD (some are considered in Chapter 8) but there are clear-cut benefits of folic acid for congenital abnormalities. Similarly, the effects of micronutrient excess, deficiencies, or imbalances in the pregnant mother on CVD and DM$_2$ in the offspring are unclear in humans. In Chapter 5 I referred to experimental evidence in mice on the role of diet in altering mitochondrial function across the generation (Section 5.4) as a proof of concept. Clearly, we have much to learn on this topic.

The way food is processed and cooked may be more important than the core, nutritional ingredients themselves, although highly processed foods tend to have high levels of sugar, fat, and salt(107, 433, 483–485). Processed meat, for example, confers a greater risk for CVD (and cancers) than fresh meat(474). Processing fats raises the level of TFAs(377). Some oils are likely to start with a high level of TFAs and these will increase with heating and reheating(377).

Frying is commonly associated with cardiovascular risk but it is a complex matter(486). The effects will depend on the oil and the heat. Frying with olive oil, for example, is not harmful and may even be beneficial(475). Nigam et al. intervened by counselling on lifestyle and changing the cooking oil in Indian people with fatty liver(487). People cooking with olive oil showed a marked change including 5 kg of weight loss compared to the soybean/safflower oil group.

The high heat cooking hypothesis (Chapter 6, Section 6.6) proposes that the chemical reactions in the mix of sugars, proteins, and fats occurring especially at temperatures above 170°C, produce many new substances including TFAs and advanced glycation end-products (AGEs) that promote atherosclerosis and other adverse outcomes that may promote hyperglycaemia(107). A low AGEs diet has been shown to have benefits in animal and human experiments(488–490). Open flame and high heat cooking methods for meat have been associated with DM_2 in cohort studies(491).

Can diet and nutrition explain the epidemic of CVD and DM_2 in South Asians? The diet of South Asians is extremely varied, and yet most South Asian populations are at high risk. This observation, alone, moves us away from a focus on specific ingredients.

In most respects, the traditional South Asian cuisines, especially in the balance of ingredients in rural settings, are healthy from the perspective of CVD, though possibly less so for DM_2 given their high carbohydrate content, although even this probably does not matter in agrarian settings, with other changes required to induce disease(492, 493). the idea that high carbohydrate diets lead to high levels of insulin, thereby leading to adiposity seems over-simplistic, even in the context of South Asians' propensity to insulin resistance(494, 495). Traditionally, the cuisine consists of a variety of grain breads such as chapatti, or rice (sometimes both), pulses eaten as dhaals, and vegetables usually braised as a curry, or in a form of soup (sambhar)(107). These staples would be supplemented by fresh vegetables such as onion, tomato, chilli, lemon, and lime. Other fruits such as melon, papaya, and mangoes would be seasonal and comparatively expensive so would be eaten in moderation. Yoghurt and similar products are also popular but in small amounts. Flesh is expensive and would be eaten in moderation, and the same was true of desserts, especially those made of dairy foods (called *mathiae*). This traditional diet is not especially atherogenic and in truly rural places where it is consumed CHD and DM_2 are very rare(53). In a recent remarkable observation (but unremarked by the authors) in rural Maharashtra not one of 149 men aged 30–50 years had DM_2 on an OGTT. Their average BMI was 20.1 kg/m². The traditional diet of such rural people is clearly not a problem for DM_2 prevention in traditional settings(53).

The forms of vegetarianism widely practiced in South Asian countries with highly refined carbohydrate and oils are, evidently, not cardio-protective or protective against DM_2, although we might have expected them to be, though modest benefits are sometimes found(470, 496, 497). For example, Gujerati Hindus are mostly vegetarian but they have amongst the highest rates of CVD and DM_2 amongst South Asian groups. Clearly, these diets are very different from vegan types of vegetarianism which is associated with lower weight and cardiovascular/DM_2 protection.

Modernization, wealth creation, and urbanization has occurred very fast in South Asian countries and this can happen in weeks or months in emigrant

South Asians(48, 321, 346). Experimental volunteer studies in relevant populations (though not in South Asians) show that the change in biochemical
profile in the face of such rapid urbanization, or the opposite, a return to a
traditional lifestyle on cardiometabolic health is dramatic. In Tarahumara
Indians, for example, plasma cholesterol rose by 31% after only 5 weeks (from
3.13 to 4.11 mmol/l) on a high fat, high calorie diet leading to 3.6 kg weight
gain. The adverse changes were observable in the first week(498). This is the
kind of change we see in rural to urban living in India(499). These kind of foods
cause oxidative stress and inflammation. It is in these urbanized environments
(including agricultural regions where urbanized lifestyles have arrived) that
South Asians' risk of CVD and DM$_2$ is most evident. (24) What is it about these
environments that might be causal? What might be the explanatory factors in
common in these dispersed and disparate populations of South Asians?

The first obvious change is eating the same or more food whilst reducing
physical activity(321, 346). This is clear from a typical rise in weight of about
10–20 kg a few years after emigrating from a South Asian country to one in
Europe or the US(61, 500, 501). Similar though not such extreme changes are
seen after rural-to-urban migration in South Asia(320). This kind of weight
change is highly explanatory of increased risk of DM$_2$ and is in line with the
adaptation–dysadaptation hypothesis in that South Asians programmed to be
slim (BMI typically 19–21) put on weight (BMI 24–27). This would not explain
the high risk of CHD as the relationship between weight and weight gain of this
magnitude and CHD risk is not strong enough as we consider in Section 7.9.

The second change is the increased consumption of fats and processed foods
made possible by these hitherto expensive and highly desired items becoming
affordable(433). A remarkably quick rise in fat consumption has taken place
in urban South Asia, especially in richer people, as methods of processing oils
have led to cheaper products(433, 434). We have already, observed, however,
that not all fats raise CVD risk. It depends on the fat. It is clear that the consumption of hydrogenated fats, including TFAs, has risen. Hydrogenated vegetable oils such as the kinds known as Vanaspati, replacing ghee made from milk,
are widely used and are heated and reheated. We know, however, that Vanaspati
oil is high in TFA(433, 434). South Asians are consuming TFAs and probably
other harmful substances through this kind of cuisine. As already stated TFAs
are very high in typical South Asian sweets such as jalebis. Such sweets are also
high in cholesterol oxide(502).

In the Health Survey for England 1999, dietary patterns were examined by
ethnic group including Indians, Pakistanis, Bangladeshis, and Chinese(503).
Bangladeshis had the highest intake of red meat (Indians had the least) and
fat and least for fruit. Indians and Chinese had the lowest fat intake. It is hard

to interpret the role of such patterns when there is so much variation. Using a 5-day weight inventory method, Miller et al. showed that Indians (38.4%) had much the same fat intake as Europeans (38.2%) but low marine oil consumption(504). Several such UK studies indicate that fat comprises about 40% of the calories in South Asians' diets. In India, fat consumption is rising fast but is closer to 30% than 40% of calories, but it is likely to reach that(505). In the INTERHEART study, including South Asian countries, diet was associated with MI(506). Fried foods were associated with MI but not in a linear fashion, the association being clearest for the highest level of consumption(506).

The other common factor is the widespread use of high heat when cooking as considered in Chapter 6, Section 6.6(107). The possibility that this kind of cooking produces substances that also increase cardiovascular and DM_2 risk needs careful study. Chinese people are much less prone to CVD than Indians and there are many potential reasons for this but one is that their cuisine and cooking techniques are less atherogenic, including using lower cooking temperatures and consuming less TFAs(107).

It is not possible to come to a clear conclusion on the role of the composition of the diet in the epidemic of CVD and DM_2 we see in South Asians. Nonetheless, it is important even if only through the weight gain that accompanies increasing affluence. There may be additional subtle reasons such as the balance of ingredients. Studies in the UK, however, show that diets of South Asians are either similar or more in line with healthy eating guidelines than those of comparable White Europeans and yet their risk of CVD and DM_2 is higher(507–509). While the fat content of their diet tends to be high (about 40% of calories) much of this is mono- or polyunsaturated. The possibility that South Asian cuisines may generate or contain some toxic ingredients needs to be considered as in, for example, the high heat cooking hypothesis. Might there be some essential ingredient missing from the typical South Asian diet, e.g. vitamin B_{12} or Vitamin D? We will consider this possibility in Chapter 8.

7.8 **Hyperglycaemia and its consequences**

Diabetes mellitus (DM), both type 1 caused by a deficit of insulin and type 2 that results from defects in insulin function and is the primary concern of this book, are unquestionably major causes of CVD, including in South Asian populations(510–512). The causes of DM_2 generally (Chapter 1, Section 1.8) apply to South Asians. In studies on Europeans and Asians, people with DM_2 typically have 50—100% more CVD than those without(513). Some of this excess results from associated risk factors, e.g. BP is also commonly high in DM_2. The evidence suggests similar associations in South Asians.

DM is defined as a disorder of glucose metabolism. Classically, the definition has been based on a plasma glucose level of 11.1 mmol/l or more, measured on more than one occasion or with typical clinical symptoms and signs(514, 515). This is the level of glucose that is linked to microvascular diseases such as retinopathy. Gerstein has proposed that many of the complications of diabetes may be a result of microvascular problems with ischaemia at the capillary level(70). South Asians are highly prone to such micro-vascular complications at least partly because of the difficulties in controlling blood glucose even in trial settings(516, 517). It is possible that microvascular complications in South Asians occur well below the cut-off of 11.1 mmol per litre.

Currently, there are several ways of biochemically measuring whether glucose levels are high and several definitions of DM_2 although the WHO's approach remains fundamental (514). The details of all the definitions available are not important here except to note that South Asians are, relative to other comparable populations, hyperglycaemic on several different measures, e.g. fasting glucose, glucose after eating, glucose as measured with a glucose tolerance test, and other measures of long-term exposure(9, 518–520). One of these long-term measures, with a strong graded relationship to cardiovascular outcomes, is glycosylated haemoglobin usually measured by HbA1c(510, 521). The point to note is that many proteins, lipids, and other molecules are glycosylated, not just haemoglobin. HbA1c is not only raised by hyperglycaemia but also by blood disorders called haemoglobinopathies which are commoner in South Asians than Europeans. HbA1c in South Asians tends to rise and this trend is highly resistant to interventions to prevent or reverse it. In South India, Dilley et al. reported that a higher HbA1c was associated with CVD risk factors even in normoglycaemic populations(520). Insulin, glucose, and HbA1c are raised in South Asian children too(291, 522).

It would be logical to presume that hyperglycaemia is the main reason why DM_2 is a cause of CVD(523). The evidence on this, however, is not clear. An association between IGT and CHD has been shown though the strength of the relation is quite weak with a relative risk of about 1.5, or even lower especially after adjustment for other cardiovascular risk factors(519, 524). An association with IFG is usually demonstrable though weaker still. When glucose is studied as a continuous variable, often using HbAIc, without using clinically relevant cut-offs for IFG, IGT, and DM_2 there is a relationship with CVD. If this were a causal relationship then we might expect that interventions that reduce glucose would reduce CVD. That expectation has not been unequivocally verified by some relevant interventions, although in sub-group analyses some small benefits can be seen, usually done on people with DM_2(70, 525, 526). An exception is the Da Qing diabetes prevention trial that reported reduced CHD in Chinese men some two decades after the intervention which was on people with IGT(527). I doubt this result can be attributed to a reduction of glucose by a life-style intervention on glucose levels 20 years earlier. Until it is replicated some caution on its interpretation is needed.

South Asians have comparatively high fasting and postprandial glucose levels, reflected in a high prevalence of IFG, IGT, and DM_2(528, 529). DM_2 has, however, remained uncommon in South Asia until about the last 40–50 years though it was noted as a problem of well-off people in India in the 1880s(84). Amongst the causes identified in the early decades of the 20th century were lack of outdoor exercise and starchy food (including Indian sweets). It was not until the 1980s that serious, large-scale research got underway, establishing that DM_2 was about four times as prevalent in urbanized South Asians as in White Europeans(35). It is remarkable that, according to Arnold(84), in 1928 Scott also estimated but without a study, that diabetes mellitus was 4–6 times com-moner in Indians than Europeans. He identified being in the 'better class', fes-tive sweets, and indolence as related factors. In 1966 the World Congress on Diabetes in the tropics took place in Bombay. While it was justified on the basis that there was a special type of diabetes mellitus there, it turned out to be the same disease and disease process as elsewhere(84).

South Asians also have high insulin, at least partly as a response to hyper-glycaemia, that persists because of peripheral muscle insulin resistance and might also reflect high-carbohydrate diets(456, 530–532). The reasons for raised insulin resistance have not been pinpointed but probably relate to adipose tissue which secretes molecules, including free fatty acids, that pro-mote it. McKeigue was amongst the major contributors to testing the hypoth-esis that insulin resistance underlay South Asians' tendency to CVD(221). He proposed this was either a direct action of insulin or an indirect result of insulin's effects in promoting upper body adiposity and altering lipids, e.g. in promoting triglyceride-rich lipoproteins(14, 221). Evidence of a direct effect of insulin on cardiovascular health is limited and conflicting, and overall, the current view is that it is not a causal risk factor in itself. The hyperglycaemia/hyperinsulinaemia/insulin resistance hypothesis has not withstood scrutiny as the key explanation for South Asians' tendency to DM_2(1). So, how do we explain the paradox whereby we accept DM_2 as a major cause of CVD but not so readily its precursor hyperglycaemic states, including insulin resistance? The answer is that DM_2 is a complicated dis-ease with multiple metabolic consequences, particularly, but not solely, re-lated to glucose but also, for example, relating to lipids and hypertension. It may be that a complex of abnormalities promote atherosclerosis rather than hyperglycaemia alone(533).

There is an alternative explanation, i.e. that CVD and DM_2 share common causes, e.g. obesity, high BP, and physical inactivity. It may be, therefore, that the effects of DM_2 on CVD are not direct. This is partially true but even thin, active people with DM_2 or DM_1 are at greater risk of CVD than their counterparts without DM.

While hyperglycaemia and its related states, especially DM_2, are very important in raising risk of CVD they are not strong candidates to wholly or largely to explain the enhanced susceptibility of South Asians at the population level. Likhari et al. showed that 36 South Asians (Sikhs) had similar glucose levels but higher HbA1c than 103 White people, indicating greater protein glycosylation at any level of glucose; they also demonstrated this in people with IGT(521). Perhaps lifelong exposure to slightly higher glucose and other glycating agents, with glycation of many proteins contributing to arterial stiffness, may be important. We will consider this matter of arterial stiffening in Chapter 8 and again in an integrated way in Chapter 9.

7.9 Obesity, adiposity, and central adiposity

I have partially considered the role of adipose tissue and its distribution, especially in Chapter 3, noting that several hypotheses are centred on it. Obesity and overweight are terms that are defined by the WHO using the BMI, which is simply the weight in kilogrammes divided by the height in metres squared (weight ÷ height²). A BMI of ≥ 30 kg/m² is obesity and of ≥ 25 kg/m² is overweight by the WHO definition. At this obesity cut-point, in Europeans 25% of the body's composition in males is fat, with 35% in females(534). In South Asians body fat is much higher at this BMI (535–537). The equivalent BMI for the same fat composition of the body in South Asians could be as low as 22 or up to 25, but much lower than 30(176, 538). Females have higher fat levels and South Asians females are prone to developing obesity, more so than South Asian men, especially as they escape from poverty. Above these low cut-offs adverse health consequences are demonstrable for hyperglycaemia and DM_2 (539–541) but not for mortality, including CVD(154–156, 158, 542).

Most of the controversy about obesity, until recently, was on whether its adverse effects on CVD were direct, i.e. related to adipose tissue, or indirect via other risk factors, e.g. raising BP, and lipids. In other words, if BP and lipids did not change (or were controlled) would obesity still raise risk? The current understanding is that there are both direct and indirect effects of overweight and obesity. The direct association with CVD and mortality, however, is weak or non-existent in South Asians but it is very strong for DM_2. A second controversy is even more recent, i.e. whether the WHO cut-offs are appropriate or whether adverse effects also occur at lower BMIs. The answer for DM_2 seems to be yes, they do, albeit the effects are smaller. The third addition to our understanding is the observation that the measurements of BMI, alone, is insufficient as both the relative amount of adipose and other tissues (especially muscle) and the distribution of adipose tissue is important(543). We considered such points earlier, particularly in Chapter 3, but they are worth re-emphasizing as they are especially important in South Asians.

South Asian adults, especially men, mostly have lower BMIs than comparison populations such as White Europeans(9, 415). There is a comparatively low BMI for children too as shown in an international systematic review but rapid change is underway as the obesity epidemic slows in industrialized countries and accelerates in developing ones(48, 324, 544). The comparatively low BMI is seen especially in men but is also true in most studies of women, with some exceptions, mostly abroad or in wealthy populations in South Asia(441, 500). This generally lower BMI (despite some exceptions) does not fit with their higher CVD and DM_2 risk. The plausible explanation is that they have much less muscle mass and that South Asians have relatively more fat at any BMI than White Europeans(138, 157, 204). Furthermore, as we noted in Chapter 3, a higher proportion of this fat is central and less of it is in peripheral depots, especially the lower limbs(101). The reason for the centralization of fat are not clear. In Chapter 3 I discussed two evolutionary hypotheses (Sections 3.6 and 3.7). There may be other reasons relating to more immediate factors such as diet or exercise patterns(545, 546).

Chandalia et al. have reported South Asians have larger adipocytes than a European origin reference group(177). The implications of this are unclear, though such cells are more active than small cells(547). The potential importance of central adiposity, ectopic fat, and large adipocytes in South Asians has been emphasized by, among others, Misra and Khurana(548). Contrary to expectation, however, Johannsen et al. found people with small adipocytes were more likely to become insulin resistant on overfeeding than those with large cells(549). The role of ectopic fat needs more study before we can reach clear-cut conclusions. For example, it would be premature to assume ectopic fat around the arteries and heart is necessarily harmful, even although it sounds compelling, and there is cross-sectional evidence of an association with atherosclerosis(550). In a recent review mostly based on studies on mice Kiefer et al. observed that perivascular fat is associated with less vasoconstriction (a good thing)(551). Some ectopic fat depots act like brown fat and are activated by cold. It is possible that ectopic fat in some locations is harmful for cardiometabolic health but in other locations it is beneficial. If the observations on mice apply to humans it might help explain, amongst other reasons, why weight loss helps prevent DM$_2$ but not CVD(552). Garg et al. showed that in a sample of South Asians compared to four ethnic groups in the Multi Ethnic Study of Atherosclerosis, South Asians had the most hepatic fat but least pericardial fat(553). Some of this central fat, which is intraperitoneal, is linked to the liver as the blood from its veins, and hence the hormonal and inflammatory products, enter the liver's (portal) circulation. This is one possible explanation for its special importance in metabolic disorders. This is, obviously, not so for other central fat compartments, i.e. skinfold fat.

The argument has been made (and largely convincingly, although there is not a consensus(554)) that the BMI cut-off points for overweight and obesity need to be much lower in South Asians, the guidance mostly settling on a BMI of 23 for overweight and either 25 or 27.5 for obesity(86). The additional argument is that measures of central obesity (in practice waist or a ratio of waist to height) are needed and also that the waist cut-offs should be lower(85, 478, 555). Indeed, the IDF guidelines are that a waist of 90 cm, about 35 inches, is indicative of central obesity in South Asian men compared with 95 cm in other men (the recommended cut-off is 80 cm—about 32 inches—for all women)(556). This argument for lowered cut-off points seems sound for DM$_2$ but its consequences for other important health outcomes, e.g. all-cause mortality(154, 156, 158), infections, maternal outcomes(256), and possibly even CVD is unclear. There is also no agreement on the implications for children, so there is still much to do. This said, South Asian children do have similar BMI and sometimes more adiposity than comparison European children(179, 557).

The effects of obesity (and by inference adiposity even without obesity) are cumulative over the life-course. South Asians are born with relatively high fat levels especially centrally as discussed in Chapter 3 (but not in total amount). The reasons for, and the implications of, this are under investigation. Lifelong adiposity may have different, probably more adverse, results from adipose tissue merely acquired in later life(558).

I discussed in Section 7.3 that when a factor is agreed as causal it is usually universally so. Given smoking cigarettes increases mortality and lung cancer in British doctors, we expect it to do this in all populations, as it does. Given obesity increases mortality, CVD, and diabetes in the European origin and Eastern Asian populations(158, 166, 167, 559) we would expect it to do so globally, including in South Asians(46). It might seem unnecessary to question this assumption and request empirical evidence. Nonetheless, and, fortunately, researchers have sought to verify that overweight and obesity are harmful to South Asians. Three large cohort studies have, contrarily, failed to demonstrate this is so for the most important outcome—mortality(154–156). The evidence of an adverse effect of overweight/obesity on mortality, CHD, and stroke in

South Asians is also limited and contrary(542). The role of overweight/obesity in DM_2 is, however, clear using a range of measures(560). It is unclear why overweight/obesity is not associated with raised mortality and CVD in South Asians. Possibly, the people who are overweight/obese are better off and better nourished and therefore have lower mortality. This unexpected finding therefore, could be a result of confounding. There may, however, be benefits of a larger adipose tissue mass especially where infections are common(165). Adipose tissue is complex and has many functions and is a major contributor to immunity and appetite control. These and other explanations need investigation.

These contrary, complex and sometimes unexpected observations have led to an emphasis on measures of centralized and ectopic fat such as waist : hip ratio in studies of South Asians(561, 562). While a large waist size is strongly indicative of central obesity a large waist/hip ratio may reflect a small hip size, itself indicative of either low muscle mass or a small lower limb fat compartment. A large waist/hip ratio is, therefore, hard to interpret. However, both waist and waist/hip ratio are associated with insulin resistance and similar outcomes in South Asians(221).

Presently, it is not possible to attribute the relatively high risks in comparison with White European populations of either CVD or, even more surprisingly, DM_2 to obesity, overweight or even distribution of adipose tissue. Indeed, recent research indicates these factors do not explain the high prevalence of diabetes in South Asians(2). This does not undermine the importance to health of obesity in South Asian populations. It merely says that overweight and obesity do not seem to be the explanation for the particularly high susceptibility we see in comparison with other populations.

There is one alternative but closely related explanation that may be important and that is that change in weight has a strong effect on outcomes, and this is likely to apply to South Asians (558, 563, 564). The association between weight gain and insulin resistance is stronger in South Asian children and adults than in Europeans(565, 566). In truly rural South Asia, typically the BMI is about 20(567). If this rose to 23 (about 7 kg extra), might that be especially hazardous and more so than having a BMI of 23 all your life? If so, why? One possibility is that at earlier ages an increase in adiposity is accompanied by an increase in other tissues, including muscle. At older ages this might not be so. This explanation goes against work indicating that it is the lifetime exposure to being overweight that matters, i.e. the effects are cumulative(558, 568, 569). In Norway about half of Pakistanis migrating into the country gained 16 kg or more after migration(501, 570). This is not untypical on emigration of South Asians to wealthy industrialized countries. However, it is far more weight gain than in settled communities. Mutsert et al. found in US health professionals that between 21 years and 60–65 years weight gain was 4.5 kg(571). Both weight at 21 years and weight gain raised disease risk.

The change in weight hypothesis has been tested in several general cohort studies that have not been on South Asians and the results have not corroborated a view that change, rather than actual weight, is a special problem(106). There is an additional nuance with weight change. The intra-abdominal fat compartment is the most active and reduces and enlarges rapidly. Subcutaneous fat is lost and replaced less readily. If weight is lost and regained there is a tendency for preferential gain of intra-abdominal fat relative to subcutaneous fat. As we have considered, intra-abdominal fat is most strongly associated with cardiometabolic disorders, including insulin resistance. It is also associated with an atherosclerotic pattern of lipid particles, e.g. small LDL-C particles.

There is an additional important and puzzling observation that warns us to take care before making strong recommendations on overweight and obesity in South Asians: in large studies of BMI and all-cause mortality, there is a strong association with underweight but not with overweight and obesity(154, 156, 158, 572). The priority problem in much of South Asia is underweight. Nonetheless, especially in the context of the developmental origins of adult disease hypothesis, these ideas about adiposity in relation to muscle across the life-course need investigating in South Asian populations.

Overall, however, I conclude that despite the focus on it, the relatively high susceptibility of South Asians to CVD cannot be explained satisfactorily by the amount or distribution of adipose tissue. It is important in DM_2 in South Asians but there are other equally, perhaps more important, factors.

7.10 Physical activity

Humans have evolved as a highly active species which expends much time and energy by foraging and hunting its food, collecting water, exploring, and wandering, as well as leisure-time activities such as singing and dancing(573). This activity, together with traditional cuisines, mean that people were physically fit and lean. This is normal physiology, and inactivity is abnormal(574). Physical activity leads to the metabolism of free fatty acids, i.e. lipids, so it is not simply using calories but specifically calories from fat. By contrast, the brain primarily metabolizes glucose (574). Brain work and stress, by contrast, both promote a positive energy balance(574). Typically the average BMI in people living in traditional ways is around 19–21 kg/m^2(313). South Asians in either tribal, hunter gatherer societies or in traditional, agricultural settings without mechanization even now have BMIs in this range. Studies of such populations show a virtual absence of DM_2(53).

Physical activity at home and in work is deeply ingrained into normal, traditional, rural South Asian life, whether this is pumping and carrying water from a well to the home or ploughing the land. In 1997 I visited my sister in Moga, a large town/small city in Punjab, where I was born. She was in that context a person of moderate wealth living in her own home. Her water came from a well in the courtyard and I learned through experience that it was hard work to draw it. This was, until recently, normal life. Maintaining physical health by means such as yoga, massage, or the exercise regimens of warriors are also part of South Asian life. In some accounts of the modern phenomenon of sedentary South Asian populations it has been stated that there is no concept of exercise in Indian languages. That is incorrect, e.g. the word 'vurgish' in Punjabi/Hindi captures the concept of exercise perfectly and is widely used. Physical activity is extolled, if not commonly practised, as a key to good health.

Given this background it is surprising, and yet on reflection understandable, why in modern, mechanized, urbanized environments, generally in all populations, there is a serious, virtually global problem of insufficient physical activity, and especially in South Asians both abroad and in urbanized environments in South Asia(62, 575–577). In modern environments much of the physical activity of day-to-day life has been reduced by the motorized vehicle, household appliances, and elevators and escalators. The effort needed to acquire, prepare, and cook food, and to gather fuel for this, has diminished too. Home and personal entertainment devices encourage a sedentary lifestyle, e.g. the average time spent watching television alone exceeds 20 hours per week in many communities. When computing, tablet, and mobile phone time is added there is not much time left—and lack of time is the main reason people give for not taking exercise(578–583).

In long-industrialized, advanced economies such as the UK and US a new culture of leisure-time physical activity has emerged that is a substitute for day-to-day activity, e.g. jogging, running long distances, and going to the gym. This only partially compensates for the reduction in physical activity of everyday living. The understanding of the effects of such activities is evolving (584). Currently, about 5 × 30 minutes of moderate bouts of such activity per week is recommended. The 30-minute period may be broken up into chunks of 10 minutes. There is evidence that South Asians may need much more, including more muscle-building anaerobic exercise, to achieve the same benefits as White Europeans(217, 585). There are also CVD and DM_2 related benefits of short bouts (1–3 minutes) of high intensity exercise and of anaerobic exercises such as lifting weights, though these have been less well studied(218).

These new physical activity cultures are not embedded as normal, especially in urbanized South Asians, and a minority of the population participate in them. Most of the studies of the health benefits of physical activity have centred on leisure-time activity. The evidence that this kind of activity aids in the prevention and control of CVD and DM_2 is strong and this is accepted as a causal relationship(586–588). The benefits of other kinds of activity, e.g. housework or in the workplace have been less well studied, but the principles are likely to be similar(584). The details may, however, differ as often leisure time exercise is outdoors while housework is mostly indoors. There may be benefits of being outdoors, e.g. sun exposure. The benefits of physical activity relate to time spent and are short lived, e.g. the biochemical changes such as reduced insulin resistance that follow exercise last days, not months, as shown in a trial in UK South Asians(589).

As South Asians have urbanized, the level of daily, normal physical activity has plummeted and a new culture of organized leisure-time physical activity has emerged, albeit slowly and in a small proportion of the population. Many studies in different countries have shown that leisure-time physical activity is comparatively low in South Asians populations . Extensive data have been collected in the UK, perhaps unusually, in virtually all age groups. These show that in children and adults alike, and possibly even in infants, South Asians have less self-reported and objectively measured physical activity than comparable White British counterparts, with some favourable changes occurring across the generations(576, 590–592). Females have less physical activity than males (576, 590). This difference is reflected in South Asians being less fit than Europeans as measured objectively by maximum oxygen uptake methods during vigorous exercise, a finding that applies to children as well as adults (224, 585, 593). Females are less fit than males. Given this, South Asians have reduced capacity to utilize fatty acids, an activity that takes place in mitochondria especially in the muscle(212, 585). Exercise changes and improves skeletal muscle mitochondrial function. In Konopka's study a 12-week exercise programme restored such function in obese women with polycystic ovary syndrome(594).

The greatest surprise, and one that needs confirmation, is a recent finding that to enjoy the same cardiometabolic benefits of exercise, South Asians need to do about twice the amount of physical activity as White Europeans(585).

A great deal that is known about attitudes to physical activity in South Asians, especially but not only in the UK, and many of the findings seem to be generalizable across South Asian populations. The most helpful insights come from qualitative studies of South Asians' beliefs, perceptions, and attitudes to physical activity in relation to health(578–583, 595-600). Such studies have explored barriers to, and promotors of, physical activity. These studies have shown no surprises. People partially understand the health benefits of physical activity and have positive attitudes and intentions, though these are insufficiently converted to actions. Barriers to action are usually lack of time, other responsibilities, feeling tired, and lack of money or facilities. There are, however, cultural reasons reported that are especially relevant to South Asians, and especially women. One of these is modesty and codes of behaviour. Exercising in the presence of the opposite sex is not acceptable to some men and many women

Physical activity that requires clothing that highlights body shape or exposes the skin is not acceptable in some South Asian cultures, especially, but not only, in women. There are also issues of priority and propriety. There is a social attitude that there are other matters, e.g. looking after the family, education, work, and socializing that take priority, and that it is improper and indulgent to spend time, especially alone, in leisure-time physical activity. Concerns are also reported about personal safety in taking exercise outdoors. There are difficulties in exercising while fasting, e.g. at Ramadan. Nonetheless, in a small study of Muslims in the UK weight lost while fasting was quickly regained(601). The older South Asians who are now getting CVD and DM_2 were raised when transport was limited and life was physically tough and exercise was unavoidable. The freedom from such burdens is usually perceived as a boon. Much of South Asia is hot for most of the year and it is not attractive to take exercise outdoors. Air-conditioned indoor premises such as gyms are expensive to visit. In countries such as the UK, South Asian people report that the cold, windy, and wet weather especially through much of the winter inhibits their outdoor physical activity. Ramadan and other festivals, and lengthy trips abroad can disrupt habits that may be difficult to re-establish. Leisure-time physical activity is, however, theoretically valued for its health and social benefits

Clearly aerobic physical activity is important in the prevention, control, and rehabilitation of CVD. It is almost certainly even more vital for both prevention and management of DM_2. For DM_2, in addition to aerobic activity, muscle tone and bulk are important. This requires additional anaerobic exercises, most probably using weights or other means of working muscles against resistance(218). The observation that South Asians need a great deal more of such exercise than Northern Europeans (perhaps 1 hour per day compared with 30 minutes), if verified as it probably will be, elevates the challenges, especially given the cultural matters that we considered(585). In guidelines published in 2012, Misra et al. recommended 60 minutes of exercise daily in Indians (this can be generalized to South Asians)(217). In adults they recommend 15 minutes of muscle resistance exercises and 15 minutes at the workplace, the remainder as leisure-time activity. This is much more than in most guidelines in Europe, and US, where 30 minutes of moderate exercise is recommended 5 days/week.

Over the last 50 years the comparatively low level of leisure-time physical activity in South Asians has not been promoted as a dominant explanation for their epidemic of CVD and DM$_2$. This contrasts with the attention given to insulin resistance and obesity/distribution of adiposity. I think that this risk factor's role has, hitherto, been underestimated. We will consider the practical implications in Chapter 10.

7.11 Salt in the diet

The role of salt as a cause of CVD has provoked controversy even though a high intake undoubtedly raises BP, which is a major cause of CVD, especially stroke(463). The current controversy is about how much salt people should have. The current consensus is converging at about 6 g daily meaning 3 g of sodium, substantially lower than is typical in South Asia(602). Obviously, this will vary depending on climate, occupation and other factors etc. Typically, in wealthy, modern urban societies the average salt intake has been about 9–12 g per day although this is dropping quite fast. Much of the salt is invisible and in processed foods, and a high level of salt, sugar, and fat in combinations is typically why foods are tasty and hence popular(434). South Asian cuisines, e.g. Gujarati, routinely combine these substances on the plate even in home cooking. As South Asia has urbanized and as South Asians abroad adopt local dietary customs, including eating much more of processed foods, the salt intake of South Asians seems to be rising. Given these background observations is it possible that South Asians' susceptibility to CVD, and especially stroke, is a result of their salt consumption?

We have already observed in Section 7.4 that average BP in South Asian populations is either comparatively low (Bangladeshis and Pakistanis) or similar (Indians) to reference populations so it doesn't seem likely that the excess CVD risk is simply a consequence of raised BP or salt consumption.

Direct measurements of salt intake in South Asian populations in community settings have rarely been published but salt consumption was high in northern India(602). I conclude that while the role of salt is important, in itself it is not a good candidate for explaining South Asians' particular susceptibility to CVD.

7.12 Explaining the susceptibility of South Asians to CVD and DM$_2$ using classical risk factors

Many cross-sectional studies across the world have examined the pattern of the classical risk factors in South Asians, often comparing them with White Europeans, but sometimes others including Chinese, Malay, and African origin groups(9, 176, 416, 603, 604). The picture that emerges is fairly consistent: there is no obvious reason why South Asians have high rates of these diseases given the pattern of classical risk factors. One exception to this rule was the Newcastle Heart Project that studied an unusually broad range of factors and which concluded that in Bangladeshis in particular, but less so in Pakistanis, and not in Indians, the overall pattern of risk factors for CVD was adverse in comparison with White Europeans(9). The pattern we find across a large number of studies, many of which we have considered already above, can be summarized as follows:

◆ BP is similar or lower

◆ Tobacco use is much lower in all women and Sikh men and often lower in other men, with the main exception of Bangladeshi and Pakistani men

◆ Diet quality is mixed with, in affluent South Asians, high fat but also more fruit, vegetables, and fibre

◆ Physical activity is less (as is fitness)

◆ Overweight and obesity is less on WHO definitions while adiposity is similar though high in relative terms, and the waist-to-hip ratio is high

◆ Hyperglycaemia and DM$_2$ are greater

◆ LDL-C levels are either similar or lower (data on TFAs in blood are not available but they are probably high)

◆ Data on psychosocial factors are inconclusive, with suggestive evidence of adverse patterns.

The only risk factor that is accurately measured, commonly available, and invariably greater is hyperglycaemia/DM$_2$ and this explains why it has gained so much attention. However, an accumulation of recent data place leisure-time physical activity into the same category. These adverse influences are balanced by favourable ones, e.g. in tobacco use.

Similar analyses of risk factor patterns have been done for DM$_2$ and other than relative adiposity and relatively centralized distribution of adipose tissue there are no strikingly adverse patterns of risk factors. Overall obesity and overweight (on WHO definitions) tends to be comparatively low. Accordingly, we see a greater focus on alternative explanations for DM$_2$ than CVD in South Asians, especially those relating to genetics and the DOHAD hypothesis.

The examination of each risk factor separately has been augmented by their study as a package. These studies have come to the same conclusion—on the basis of the classical risk factors neither South Asians' extra risk of CVD nor of DM$_2$ can be explained. Box 7.1 and Table 7.1 summarize an important study in this arena on CVD, the follow-up of the Brent and Southall cross-sectional studies originally led by McKeigue(1, 18, 99, 221). Similar work has been reported on metabolic syndrome and its association with CVD and DM$_2$(605). The study focused on insulin resistance and the related upper body fat hypotheses but the results were not in line with the hypotheses(1, 18). In extensive analyses with different sets of variables the differences in populations in either CHD or stroke could not be explained. This work puts a brake on some 30 years of focus on insulin resistance, requiring new explorations(221, 456). The PURE international cohort study is currently examining the broader physical, socio-economic, and psychosocial environment especially in the transition to urbanization(323).

7.13 Conclusions

The established CVD and DM$_2$ risk factors cause CVD and/or DM$_2$ in South Asians as they do in all populations and Figures 7.1 and 7.2 are simple diagrams to illustrate this. Even where the data are either sparse or inconsistent, e.g. on the relationship between overweight, obesity, and CVD, the likely explanation is that the associations have been influenced by socio-economic factors and will, in time, emerge. Currently, in much of South Asia overweight and obesity are more common in the well-off groups who may have lifestyles that counteract the adverse effects of overweight/obesity, e.g. a better quality diet. The key point, however, is that the population level patterns of these classical risk factors do not help us understand South Asians' particular susceptibility to CVD and DM$_2$.

In Chapter 1 I stated the explanation was either:

1. South Asians have more of the risk factors, or,
2. Are affected more by such risk factors at any given level (i.e. there is an effect modification that can be demonstrated by study of statistical interaction), or
3. There are other, yet uncovered, factors that either affect disease outcomes directly or through the known risk factors.

The current evidence is unsupportive of either the first or second of the above explanations, so, we must look to the third. We will do this in two ways. First, we will examine other possible causes of CVD and DM$_2$ in South Asians in Chapter 8. Then, in Chapter 9, we will integrate the hypotheses in Chapter 2–5 with the standard epidemiological work on associations in Chapters 6–8.

Box 7.1 Examining the ethnic difference in CHD using cohort data on a package of risk factors and modelling outcomes

Forouhi NG, Sattar N, Tillin T, McKeigue PM, Chaturvedi N. Do known risk factors explain the higher CHD mortality in South Asian compared with European men? Prospective follow-up of the Southall and Brent studies, UK. Diabetologia. 2006;49:2580–8 (1).

My introductory remarks

If a risk factor, say X, was the explanation for the higher risk of CHD in South Asians than Europeans, then we would expect it would be more prevalent in South Asians. Risk factors may have varying relative prevalence with some being more, and others being less, common. Judging their overall effect is difficult but statistical modelling could help. This study is one of the most important of this genre and cemented the long-standing view that known, established risk factors do not explain the higher risk of CHD in UK South Asians compared to UK European origin men.

The paper

The paper opens with important statements including that insulin resistance might underlie the high risk of CHD in South Asians and that data from prospective tests of this and other hypotheses are very limited.

This study comprises a long-term follow of the samples in the cross-sectional Southall and Brent multi-ethnic studies done in 1988–1991 in West London. The 3207 South Asians and European men in these studies were analysed here. They were 40–69 years at baseline.

Details about the study are in Table 7.1 including the variables adjusted for. The noteworthy features in data collection included these: reliable assessment of ethnicity (name, country of birth, appearance, and if necessary direct enquiry); the use of an overnight fast to collect glucose, lipids, and to do a 75-g fasting OGTT; and a physical activity score including work, leisure, sports, and travel time.

Metabolic syndrome was defined using IDF guidelines. Mortality data came from death certificates all completed by a doctor, as is compulsory in the UK, and coded using the WHO's International Classification of Diseases. The statistical methods were standard ones and performed following accepted principles. Nearly everyone (99.4%) of the sample had data to allow

Box 7.1 Examining the ethnic difference in CHD (*continued*)

a person-time denominator calculation. Tests for interaction were included which means that if the effects of risks factors varied by ethnic group, this would be captured in the analysis.

The risk factor distributions were as expected, i.e. features associated with insulin resistance were much commoner in South Asians than Europeans with considerable variability in other variables—some higher (low HDL-C), many similar, and some lower (smoking). There were 202 CHD deaths, 94 in Europeans, 108 in South Asians. The relationships between risk factors and outcomes were similar to those expected, with some exceptions, perhaps the most important of these being no association of note between BMI or waist circumference and CHD in either Europeans or South Asians.

As expected, age-adjusted CHD mortality was about 60% higher in South Asians than Europeans. This jumped to a 114% higher risk after adjustment for smoking. No other adjustments brought the level of risk near to that of Europeans. There were no statistically significant interactions, indicating risk factor–outcome relations were similar in South Asians and Europeans. The authors emphasized their study was small and not designed to study interactions.

The authors wondered whether they captured the risk factors fully, e.g. duration of diabetes was not available. Then they considered the potential role of novel risk factors that they did not measure, e.g. CRP, adipokines, or Lp(a).

The authors concluded that the traditional risk factors are very important in the genesis of CHD in South Asians and Europeans alike but these, including insulin resistance, do not account for the between-ethnic group variation in CHD mortality. Adjustment for co-morbidity or social class and education did not alter this conclusion.

Concluding remarks

This paper, essentially, showed that the package of established risk factors, including a range of indicators of insulin resistance (as well as metabolic syndrome and diabetes as co-morbidities), does not explain the higher CHD mortality of South Asians compared to White Europeans in the UK. The special significance of this paper is that one of the authors, Paul McKeigue (now my colleague in The University of Edinburgh), was a leading proponent of the insulin resistance hypothesis with much of the argument resting on the baseline cross-sectional phase of this study.

Chapter 8

Other risk factors and explanations

8.1 Chapter 8 objectives are to:

1. Consider, in outline, some of the many specific explanations that have been proposed but not established, not been studied in depth, or are under active consideration including:

   - Inflammation and infection
   - Thyroid dysfunction
   - Renal function
   - Cardiovascular system anatomy and physiology
   - Lactose intolerance
   - Vitamin B_{12} deficiency
   - Folic acid and vitamin D deficiency.

2. Evaluate whether any of these ideas need upgrading as serious contenders for future scholarship and research.

8.2 Chapter summary

As is usual with medical and scientific puzzles, there have been numerous creative ideas to explain South Asians' susceptibility to diabetes, CHD and stroke that have not been developed into either fully articulated hypotheses or have rarely or never been included in hypothesis testing or evaluation studies. These include thyroid dysfunction, lactose intolerance, vitamin B_{12} and folate deficiency, infection, and chronic inflammation. Vitamin D deficiency has been studied intensively recently in relation to chronic disease including some work on South Asians. Cardiovascular anatomy and physiology has been explored in observational work. These explanations have little theoretical foundation but they need some consideration. The relations between the ideas here and those in Chapters 2–7 are emphasized.

8.3 **Introduction**

The risk factors in Chapter 7 are acknowledged as important to the causation of CVD and DM_2, though there are periodic controversies about one or other of them. Currently there is controversy about the causal role of saturated fats, lipids, and even LDL-C in CVD. As a package they are, nonetheless, widely agreed to account for most CVD and DM_2 at the population level in populations worldwide(85). The estimates of the risk accounted for range from as low as 60% to as high as 90%. The higher numbers are usually in analysis that adjusts for mismeasurement and biases. Despite this level of success there is a sense that there are, in all populations, important undiscovered aspects of the pathology of CVD and DM_2.

The search for factors that cause, or accurately predict, CVD and DM_2 has been intense. This seemingly endless quest partly reflects that there is no coherent, theoretical foundation for the empirical evidence to rest on. Another driver of this restless research is the number of anomalies. We can't satisfactorily explain differences between population subgroups, e.g. men and women, rich and poor, and the focus here, ethnic groups. The search for the so-called emerging risk factors entails grand-scale research databases on a multiplicity of measures, especially biochemical, and increasingly in the study of metabolites by tracing the formation and function of gene products (named the 'omics' revolution)(606, 607). The search beyond the classical risk factors has not added materially to the predictive power of models, but it has added to our understanding of biological mechanisms, though not particularly to understanding South Asians' susceptibility(121, 608). Trying to explain South Asians' susceptibility to CVD and DM_2 has provoked new ideas including some not explored in the mainstream of the emerging risk factors field.

In this chapter I consider factors that have been seen as especially relevant to South Asians. The evidence, however, tends to be sparse so evaluation of their importance is difficult. It may be that some of them are worth detailed study. This chapter does not enter the 'omics' type of research as, in my view, it is too early in its evolution to assess its value in relation to CVD and DM_2 in South Asians. I have listed the explanations in this chapter in Table 8.1.

8.4 **Vitamin D**

Vitamin D is mostly obtained from precursor molecules formed in the skin that are produced by exposure to ultraviolet B (UVB) radiation which is in some (not all) sunlight. Glass filters the UVB from sunlight as does the atmosphere in winter in high latitude countries. Fog and cloud also block this radiation. Small

Table 8.1 Other non-traditional risk factors as explanations for the high susceptibility of South Asians to CVD and DM_2

Section	Factor	Brief comment
8.4	Vitamin D deficiency	A compelling case can be made theoretically but the empirical evidence is largely unsupportive.
8.5	Vitamin B_{12}, folic acid, and hyperhomocysteinaemia	As for vitamin D
8.6	The pro-inflammatory state	It is unclear whether the pro-inflammatory state simply reflects greater centralized active adipose tissues or other paths.
8.7	Pro-coagulant state	There is contradictory evidence on this and an important role is unlikely.
8.8	Infections and microbiota	A compelling theoretical case can be made but the empirical evidence is limited. DM_2 and TB are associated but it may be DM_2 causes increased TB, not vice versa.
8.9	Renal function impairment	Renal function is impaired by CVD and vice versa. This is important at individual level but unlikely to explain population level differences.
8.10	Thyroid function being low	A good example of a postulate that has not been tested out.
8.11	Lactose intolerance/milk drinking	A good example of an idea that enters popular discourse and even earns professional approval but without evidence.
8.12	Anatomy and physiology of the circulatory system e.g. narrower, stiffer arteries	This needs more study (see also Chapter 9).
8.13	Miscellaneous	
8.13.1	◆ Other co-morbidities	These are causally important but unlikely to explain population level differences.
8.13.2	◆ Other genetic factors	Potentially important but evidence is needed. Unlikely to be important explanation.
8.13.3	◆ Other lifestyles	This needs more thorough investigation.
8.13.4	◆ Other biochemical disturbances	This needs more thorough investigation.
8.13.5	◆ Toxins	This needs more thorough investigation.
8.13.6	◆ Breast-feeding	South Asians tend to have relatively high exposure to breast-feeding, normally associated with good health. Evidence on cardiovascular benefits and harms is limited.
8.13.7	◆ Cortisol	No evidence of importance.
8.13.8	◆ Alcohol	Requires more investigation.
8.13.9	◆ Consanguinity	Unlikely to be important explanation.

amounts of vitamin D come from diet. Vitamin D is essential for the prevention of the bone disease osteomalacia, which is caused by a shortage of calcium, but it is also important in many other physiological and biochemical functions including inflammation, cell growth, and insulin secretion(609).

The potential role of vitamin D in the development of chronic diseases including cancers, CVD, and DM_2 has been studied intensively and consistent associations have been shown in cohort studies between low vitamin D and high levels of these diseases(610, 611). The evidence has stimulated clinical trials, some of which are in progress. To date, the evidence from trials that vitamin D is important in the causation of CVD and DM_2 is weak and most associations in cohort studies may be as a result of confounding(612–618).

The reason this issue is important for South Asians is that they have comparatively low levels of vitamin as usually measured in the form of 25-hydroxy vitamin D in serum, not just in cloudy climates overseas as in the UK, but also in South Asia itself(619–622). Some studies in the UK show very low and even undetectable levels in a substantial number of South Asians(619). Vitamin D deficiency in children leads to the disease called rickets, which has been a problem in the relatively affluent South Asian population in Scotland(622). South Asian children, especially emigrants living in areas of sparse sunshine, are known to be at comparatively high risk of rickets, and South Asian women, more than men, to osteomalacia. Given its prevalence, and its association with chronic diseases(463, 611, 623), vitamin D deficiency is a contender as an explanation for urbanized South Asians' high risk of CVD and DM_2 as diverse South Asian populations manifest vitamin D deficiency.

The reasons for the low vitamin D in South Asians are fairly well understood. A dark skin requires longer exposure time to manufacture vitamin D than a light skin(118, 624). The skin needs to be exposed and not hidden by clothes and South Asian women, especially, often cover up for modesty. Urbanized life is lived indoors and behind glass. Glass absorbs UVB and the exposure to sun needs to be direct. Chemicals such as phytates in South Asians' diet, e.g. in chapatis, may block absorption of calcium from the intestine, compounding bone problems(621, 625). Unsurprisingly South Asians in Northern Europe have low vitamin D levels but even in the Indian Subcontinent the levels can be low even in people exposed to much sun. The research evidence from trials is quite sparse, inconsistent, and unconvincing.

Nagpal et al. gave 100 Indian men large doses of vitamin D in a trial and reported no important cardio-metabolic changes, except that those with central obesity and lowest vitamin D levels had some increased insulin sensitivity(626). A trial by Madar et al. in immigrants to Norway showed no beneficial effects of vitamin D supplementation on metabolic function(627). In New Zealand, a trial of vitamin D supplementation in South Asians had only small effects on metabolic dysfunction(628). The evidence from trials across the world showing little such effect in other populations supports this conclusion(612, 617, 627). There is a mismatch between the evidence from cohort studies and trials. The likely reason is that chronic diseases cause vitamin D deficiency (called reverse causality) rather than vitamin D causing chronic diseases; and that the kind of people who have vitamin deficiency also have other risk factors that are the true causes, e.g. low outdoor physical activity that both causes CVD and DM$_2$ and low vitamin D for lack of exposure to outdoor sunshine. People with large fat stores have lower vitamin D, which is fat soluble and so may be stored there, and they are also prone to CVD and DM$_2$.

It is premature to rule out a role for vitamin D deficiency in the CVD/DM$_2$ epidemic in South Asians but presently the evidence base for this is weak. It is premature to advocate a supplementation programme to prevent CVD and DM$_2$ (though there is such a case for bone health).

8.5 Vitamin B$_{12}$, folic acid, and hyperhomocysteinaemia

People with genetic disorders of metabolism that lead to high levels of the molecule homocysteine in the blood (hyperhomocysteinaemia) have high risk of CVD (629). Hyperhomocysteinaemia can occur for non-genetic reasons that are very common, the most important being shortage of vitamin B$_{12}$ or of folic acid (vitamin B$_9$). These vitamins have diverse functions particularly in cellular regulation. They are fundamental to carbon metabolism (the process of 1-carbon metabolism)(630). Recent observational studies, including in South Asians, show a small reduction in birthweight in offspring of mothers associated with high homocysteine levels(100). This means that, if causal, the effects on CVD and DM$_2$ could be over the life-course as in the DOHAD hypothesis as well as from hyperhomocysteinaemia directly in adulthood. Several studies have shown high levels of homocysteine in the blood in South Asian adults, including in comparisons with European populations(97, 631). This difference is related to deficiency of B$_{12}$ and folate, the former being particularly common in vegetarians(632, 633).

Vitamin B$_{12}$ is provided only by microbial metabolism and is mainly obtained by humans from a narrow range of foods, mostly animal products, and in lesser amounts in foods such as pulses. In South Asians generally, and in vegetarians especially, vitamin B$_{12}$ levels are comparatively low, and this is the case during pregnancy. Foods typically consumed by South Asians are low in vitamin B$_{12}$(634). Unsurprisingly, this is more of a problem for Hindus, many of whom are vegetarian, and less so for Muslims, who are generally not vegetarians.

Extremely low B_{12} leads to macrocytic anaemia and neurological disorders but the effects of low, not deficient, levels are unclear except through a rise in homocysteine levels.

Folic acid is mostly obtained from vegetables, especially green leafy ones, but is also present in many other foods. Folic acid deficiency leads to many disorders including macrocytic anaemia, just one marker of how this vitamin and B_{12} are involved in the same kind of biochemistry, including in the metabolic path leading to high homocysteine(629). Although South Asians eat fruits and vegetables, generally their homocysteine levels tend to be comparatively high, whether living in South Asia or not(97, 631, 635). A third B vitamin called pyridoxine or more commonly vitamin B_6 also raises homocysteine levels(629). This vitamin is less often discussed but it would be reasonable to presume the principles in relation to B_{12} and folic acid would apply to B_6.

The reasonable question, therefore, is whether either a shortage of these vitamins, or an imbalance in their relative amounts, might explain South Asians' susceptibility to CVD and DM_2. Trial-based evidence is not available on this question, though fortification of food and food supplements do reduce homocysteine(636). The cohort studies relating B_{12} and CVD were not on South Asians but they do not show important links between B_{12} levels and CVD outcomes(108). Case–control studies in India and Pakistan examining the association between CVD outcomes and homocysteine levels provide some evidence in favour of this explanation, but it is hard to interpret the causal validity of the evidence(637, 638). Chambers et al.'s case–control study showed 8% higher fasting homocysteine level in both Europeans and Indian Asians with CHD than controls without (B_{12} and folate were lower in Indian Asians than Europeans)(97). So, direct effects of B_{12} or folic acid (including through homocysteine) are not, at least yet, evidence based candidates for explaining South Asian population' susceptibility to CVD and DM_2.

The effects of B_{12} and folic acid on South Asians' risk of CVD and DM_2 through fetal development and reflected in low birthweight are of interest. The evidence base is slim. In a recent meta-analysis of low B_{12} in pregnancy and low birthweight the association was seen only in Indian studies and not internationally and was somewhat implausibly strong there(110). Conclusions on indirect effects via fetal development are premature but are under study as we have considered in Chapter 5(246, 287, 630, 639–641). Overall, the evidence that deficiencies or imbalances of these vitamins or excess of homocysteine underlies South Asians' susceptibility to CVD and DM_2 is not compelling.

8.6 **The pro-inflammatory state**

Inflammation is vital to tissue repair and healing. There is always inflammation as part of the wear, tear, and repair system required for normal life, including ensuring that the microorganisms that live in/on our bodies do not become pathogenic (which some do when the immune system weakens). Infection is considered more in Section 8.8.

South Asians, compared with White Europeans, often have biochemical evidence of a higher level of inflammatory activity(208, 642). Markers that show this include the molecules immunoglobulin G and CRP(643–645). This might be a consequence of ongoing atherosclerosis or of high levels of oxidized LDL-C which both promote inflammation; the latter being associated with ghee and other South Asian foods(410, 646, 647). If the former it would be consequence and not cause of atherosclerosis. It is possible that a reinforcing cycle is created, e.g. atherosclerosis stimulates inflammation which in turn promotes atherosclerosis.

There are other possibilities that are potentially important for causal understanding. As we discussed earlier (especially Chapter 3 and 7), South Asians have a higher proportion of their body weight as fat especially in the most active, central depots. Fat is an immune function tissue and produces pro-inflammatory molecules including leptin and IL-6(208). For this reason alone, we could expect South Asians to have higher levels of inflammation, and indeed they do. High levels of adipose tissue are agreed as likely to be part of the causal pathway to CHD and DM_2. This may occur through pro-inflammatory or other functions of fat cells. Low grade inflammation of this kind could induce insulin resistance, endothelial dysfunction, and enhanced coagulation. The higher level of inflammation could also be non-causal either because of reverse causality, confounding, chance, or co-existence of two phenomena. Overall the evidence points to a non-causal role for CRP and other markers for inflammation.

The high susceptibility of South Asians to CVD and DM_2, especially in relation to White Europeans, is not likely to be explained directly by their pro-inflammatory state. In the UK, several studies have examined inflammatory markers in South Asians compared to White populations, especially CRP levels(10, 208, 642, 648–654).

Overall, the results have been inconsistent, though compatible with the view that CRP is higher in South Asians, a difference probably attributable to greater adiposity, especially centrally. Probably CRP and other inflammatory markers seem to be good predictors of CVD but are not direct causes, a view recently supported by Mendelian randomization studies(655). Nonetheless, the possibility that a pro-inflammatory state might be producing a pro-coagulant state needs examining.

8.7 Pro-coagulant state: a tendency to blood clotting (thrombosis)

When a blood vessel is damaged, especially when there is bleeding, one of the crucial methods of repair is through the clotting of the blood which is called thrombosis. The blood clot plugs the tear of the blood vessel. The same process occurs with minor vessel wall damage, e.g. an erosion on the arterial wall which is more likely where there is an atherosclerotic plaque. The blood clot, the thrombus, could impede or even stop the blood flow through the vessel thereby causing angina, MI, and stroke depending on the location and extent of the blockage.

Normally, the blood clot adheres to the damaged surface but it can break free of the artery or break up into pieces, which may block smaller branching arteries downstream. Such a travelling clot fragment is an embolus and is particularly important as a cause of stroke although it can lodge anywhere in the arterial tree with severe consequences. As atherosclerosis and its precursor conditions, including endothelial dysfunction of the arteries, increase so does the likelihood of blood clotting on the arterial wall (and subsequent embolism). We can see the two processes are interdependent. Atherosclerosis, however, is in this case the cause and clotting/embolism the effect. It is not easy to distinguish cause and effect in case–control studies illustrating an association between cardiovascular outcomes and clotting factors(637). The blood clot will be resolved and eventually removed though an inflammatory process that may leave some scar tissue and calcification that can be the focus for subsequent atherosclerosis and can narrow the artery permanently.

If a person (or a population) has a tendency to blood clotting that increases CVD risk. Inflammation of the arterial wall can enhance clot formation at that site. A clotting tendency, for example, as reflected in high levels of the clotting molecule fibrinogen increases CVD risk. Nonetheless, this is not one of the major CVD risk factors, even although some evidence of associations is available(656).

Does the high risk of CVD in South Asians relate to a procoagulant state? One of the key markers of coagulation is fibrinogen which is easily measured in plasma so it is a common measure of a pro-coagulant state. A Mendelian randomization study of fibrinogen did not show evidence of a causal association with CHD(657). Studies in South Asians, many of them done in the UK, have shown a mixed picture. The Health Survey for England showed fibrinogen levels were similar across a range of ethnic groups including in South Asians(10, 503). The Newcastle Heart Project also showed no higher fibrinogen in South Asians compared to Europeans(9). Studies by a research group in Leeds, England, have, however, shown higher fibrinogen in South Asians than in White controls(658).

Thrombosis is, however, a complex phenomenon with many other factors including platelets and other molecules involved in a cascade of chemical reactions(656). In addition, there are mechanisms to prevent thrombosis (plasminogen) and molecules involved in the removal of thrombus (fibrinolysis), and there are associations between them and insulin resistance(658). Their actions may reduce the stability of atherogenic plaques, increasing the risk of plaque rupture and MI.

Some of these molecules, including fibrinogen, are related to insulin resistance and possibly also to the extra cardiovascular risk associated with DM$_2$. It may be that some of the adverse effects of insulin resistance and DM$_2$ occur through enhancing thrombosis(659).

I do not think that the state of knowledge encourages us to give priority to these factors as a primary reason for South Asians' susceptibility to CVD and it is more likely they are providing mechanisms for the effect of one or more of the primary causes. As such, they are more likely to be a consequence of other causes or a mechanism through which other causes have, at least partially, their effects.

8.8 Infections, microbiota, CVD, and DM$_2$

Atherosclerosis activates the immune system with the production of inflammatory molecules and local increases in the number and action of phagocytes and other immune system cells. Inflammation for other reasons promotes atherosclerosis too, possibly through causing changes in the delicate single-cell layer lining of the arteries, the endothelium(660). We discussed the importance of endothelial dysfunction in Chapter 1.

Infections provoke inflammation and create a pro-inflammatory state. Sometimes infections are generalized, with transportation of the microbes through the arteries and the production of inflammation throughout the body. Even localized infections, e.g. an abscess of the gum or the disease gingivitis create generalized inflammation. In animal experiments atherosclerosis can be accelerated by exposure to infections. The theoretical basis of infection as a cause of atherosclerosis is strong. Many microbial species are present in atheroma plaques but whether they are harmless bystanders called commensals, consequences, or causes has been very difficult to resolve(661–663).

Table 8.2 Some specific infections and microbial processes associated with CVD

Helicobacter pylori
Chlamydia pneumoniae
Mycoplasma pneumoniae
Herpes simplex virus 1 and 2
Cytomegalovirus (CMV)
Epstein Barr virus
Hepatitis C
Hepatitis A
Gut microbiota
Gingivitis (periodontal disease)

It is important to consider the role of infections in the genesis of CVD generally and, given the high exposure to infections in much of South Asia both currently and historically, specifically so in South Asians. The research base is now substantial, and both specific infections and generalized infective states (burden of infection over a lifetime) have been examined. Some of the infections studied are listed in Table 8.2. Remarkably, exposure to some microbes is extremely common, e.g. antibody to chlamydia is present in about half of the population or more, including in Sri Lanka(664). It is possible that some infective agents invade the arterial wall and create local inflammation, but indirect effects are more likely. Despite many promising leads with evidence of weak or moderate associations between several specific infections and CVD, none of these have achieved causal status as a primary cause of atherosclerosis leading to CVD. There is good evidence that there is a raised risk of heart attack during and shortly after an acute infective illness such as influenza(662). These kind of acute effects, however, are not credible candidates for explaining ethnic variations in CVD or more specifically South Asians' susceptibility to CVD. These kind of acute infections seem to bring forward cardiovascular events in those with previous atherosclerosis.

Much of South Asia is currently in the epidemiological transition whereby the traditional problems of infections and diseases of malnutrition are still common even as the modern problems of over-nutrition and chronic diseases are rising. The research shedding light on the possible link between infections and CVD in South Asians(644, 664, 665) has not, overall, provided much evidence to favour this pathway(643–645). Nonetheless, the possibility remains that one or more infections, perhaps in early life, prime the body towards atherosclerosis in later life. This is a continuing area for research, even although generally it has not lived up to its early promise, especially with the failure of trials of antibiotics to help treat atherosclerotic diseases(646). New avenues that may be especially relevant to South Asian populations include oral health, especially periodontal (gum) disease. Causal effects are, however, more likely to be through a general pro-inflammatory state (Section 8.6) than the result of specific actions of microbes.

Type 1 diabetes mellitus is considered to be a result of immune dysfunction triggered by viral infections usually in childhood. The exact viruses and mechanisms are yet to be established. The effect is a destruction of the pancreatic beta-cells such that insulin cannot be produced in the required quantities. Unsurprisingly, there is a question of whether DM$_2$ might also be caused, at least partly, by infection. In DM$_2$, as with CVD, there is a link between markers of inflammation such as CRP and IL-6 and disease. These markers may be consequences of DM$_2$ or the association may be a result of a common cause, i.e. confounding. There is a strong link between tuberculosis and DM$_2$, but the immunity of people with DM$_2$ is compromised and their exposure to the tubercle bacillus is more likely to lead to clinical tuberculosis(529). It is less plausible, though possible, that exposure to the bacillus leads to pancreatic dysfunction or insulin resistance.

The possible role of infections in evolutionary timescales to shape the distribution of adipose tissue (e.g. central deposition in South Asians) was discussed in Chapter 3(207).

Overall, despite its simplicity and attractiveness there is insufficient evidence to support the hypothesis that the pattern of exposure to infections explains South Asians' tendency to CVD and DM$_2$(643). Stefler et al. systematically reviewed studies that compared infection patterns (and non-specific indicators of infection) in South Asians and European origin White populations in developed countries to help establish lines of investigation. Up to 2011 only 21 studies were found, with data on 17 specific infections(643). South Asians had higher infection exposure to *E. coli* and the tubercle bacillus but lower exposure to herpes simplex, hepatitis C, HIV, and varicella zoster. For other infections, including periodontal pathogens and *Chlamydia pneumoniae* there were inconsistent differences. Markers of infection and pro-inflammatory states, such as IgG and endotoxin, were higher in South Asians. In general populations, the evidence was once compelling enough to justify trials of antibiotics in the treatment of MI but the strategy has been abandoned for lack of evidence.

There is now a resurgence of interest in the role of gut microbiota in explaining chronic diseases. Animal experiments show microbiota are extremely important to health, e.g. germ free mice are thin(666, 667). The gut microbiota affect the energy harvested from food, fatty acid metabolism, the composition of adipose tissue, and many other relevant matters(667). It is difficult to envisage how specific infections and microbiota would affect South Asians so widely—South Asians in South Asia, emigrants to other countries, and the descendants of migrants. Also, why would these factors affect South Asians, but not the Chinese, in comparison with Europeans? There may be explanations relating to local environments, diet, antibiotic use in animal husbandry, and human health, etc. At present, however, we cannot pinpoint a role in explaining ethnic variations.

Given that South Asians brought up, even born in, developed countries show susceptibility to CVD and DM2, infection is not looking like a strong candidate explanation. Some early life infective event might prime later susceptibility to CVD and DM_2, but there is no clear evidence for it.

8.9 **Renal function**

Kidney diseases cause a multiplicity of different kinds of adverse CVD outcomes including MI, heart failure, and stroke(668). The kidney is, of course, also severely affected by atherosclerotic diseases, so it tends to be a cyclical adverse process. The kidney is vitally important in regulation of BP and some of the adverse CVD effects of renal dysfunction may arise via hypertension. South Asians have much more renal failure than White Europeans, perhaps even seven times as much, a problem long-related to DM_2(669, 670). Renal failure is, fortunately, quite rare and is not itself a cause of the general epidemic of CVD and DM_2. Indeed, it is more likely that the susceptibility to atherosclerosis and DM_2, and these diseases, lead to much of the renal failure, which then leads to more CVD, thus creating a vicious circle(668).

The causes of the South Asians' tendency to renal failure are outside the scope of this book, but they almost certainly overlap closely with the causes of CVD and DM_2 that we are discussing. One point of interest is that in being born small, South Asians are born with relatively small kidneys with fewer nephrons than comparable White European babies(671). Whether this, in itself, matters is unclear given that one normal kidney is enough.

Renal failure is preceded by a long period with signs that there is a problem, e.g. there is more protein in the urine than we expect. This is usually detected by measuring albumin in urine and when there are small amounts this is microalbuminuria, signalling a leaky glomerulus, that kidney structure where blood is filtered and impurities ejected as urine and the remainder retained and recirculated. Several though not all (672) studies have shown that South Asians, even those without DM_2, are more prone to proteinuria and microalbuminuria than comparative populations including White Europeans(673, 674). This is unsurprising as these problems are more common in those with DM_2, and South Asians have more of this. South Asians without DM_2, however, may also have more microalbuminuria(674). This raises a question—is it possible that early renal dysfunction might predispose South Asians to CVD? Or, is it more likely that the same processes that lead to CVD and DM_2 also lead to renal dysfunction? I veer towards the latter view. If that is correct, once we implement effective measures to prevent and control CVD and DM_2 we will also reduce much of the problem of renal failure.

The common mechanisms might include inflammation, endothelial dysfunction, or hyperglycaemia leading to damage to the microcirculation. Whatever is the cause, microalbuminuria, or other markers of renal dysfunction, especially in a South Asian person without DM_2, is a sign of a raised risk of CVD and DM_2. Actions that reduce the risk factors for CVD, DM_2, or microalbuminuria (e.g. reducing obesity and glycaemia) are likely to benefit all three outcomes. Overall, I judge the evidence to show renal dysfunction and failure is important in relation to CVD and DM_2 in South Asians but that it is not itself a dominant, primary cause of their particular susceptibility at the population level.

8.10 Thyroid dysfunction: an under-investigated postulate

Thyroid insufficiency as an important cause of CHD in South Asians is an example of an idea that has not been properly investigated. In 1985 Fowler responded to McKeigue et al.'s paper showing that the high risk of CHD in South Asians could not be explained(675), making the unexpected comment that 'this should cause no surprise'(676). He postulated that the high risk of CHD in Asian women could be explained by their high incidence of autoimmune thyroiditis. Further, he noted that impaired thyroid function may be a survival advantage in the 'Third World' but a disadvantage in an affluent society. He appealed to younger investigators to pursue this idea with a trial of thyroxine for the prevention of CHD in women.

To my knowledge this idea and trial has not been pursued. How do we evaluate this and similar postulates (a hypothesis would be better developed than this). I think we need to consider these ideas thoughtfully, but also sceptically, lest we deviate from more promising paths. The first question we might ask is whether subclinical hypothyroidism is established as important in the causation of disease as advanced hypothyroidism is(677). Epidemiological studies indicate a weak association between indicators of low thyroid activity and CHD(677), and this 'risk factor' has not made its mark in the ranks of factors of likely causal importance.

The second question is whether there is evidence for Fowler's claim that (South) Asian women have a very high incidence of autoimmune thyroiditis. There is no evidence to my knowledge that it is. The third question is whether studies of CVD in South Asians have shown an association with thyroid function, and again, the answer is, to my knowledge, no. The fourth question is whether this would also apply to South Asian men, for if not, it is not a rounded explanation as not only South Asian women are at high risk.

So, we conclude that a postulate forcefully proclaimed in a prominent journal has not garnered support more than 30 years later. This does not make it wrong, just an unlikely candidate explanation. The same likely applies to the many ad-hoc explanations we hear and read about.

8.11 **Milk and lactose intolerance**

Humans are the only mammals that drink milk in adulthood. The enzyme required to break down the sugar lactose in milk is lactase which is found on the surface of the small intestine. In its absence the lactose in milk is not broken down to its constituents of glucose and galactose and hence it is not absorbed in the small intestine and goes to the large intestine where it is broken down and metabolized by bacteria with adverse health consequences(119, 678). People who are short of this enzyme in adulthood are lactose intolerant. In fact, this is the normal adult biological state. These people tend to avoid milk altogether, to drink small amounts of it, or take milk products where the lactose has already been partially digested through fermentation (e.g. cheese, yoghurt) or has mostly been removed (e.g. butter or ghee as they are the fat component of milk and lactose is mostly in the non-fat component).

Genetic mutations in some human populations allow lactose to persist into adulthood and people possessing then can drink large quantities(119, 679). These are accumulated through genetic selection over many generations in populations where ample milk is available, i.e. in herder and dairy farming communities. The prevalence of the gene variant that allows lactose persistence has risen from about zero to nearly 100% in Northern European populations in about 7000 years. The extra survival and reproductive advantages from milk consumption were, clearly, exceptional possibly because the extra calcium and protein from milk prevented osteomalacia and pelvic narrowing in women. The white skin of Northern Europeans allowing more production of vitamin D for a given amount of sun exposure evolved at about the same time. The nutrition and calcium were, clearly, advantageous to survival and reproduction.

The consumption of dairy products has recently soared across the world because of their cheap production using industrial-scale dairy farming and special breeds of cows and other dairy animals. Milk and its products, especially by-products such as lactose powder, have become amongst the cheapest and most sought-after foods in affluent societies, and these products are rapidly adopted by South Asians, whether migrating abroad or from rural to urban areas(346, 463, 472, 680).

Between the 1960s and the 1980s, as the centrality of blood lipids in the development of CHD was established, the diet-heart hypothesis gained strength, with a strong focus on cholesterol, notwithstanding controversy(681). The simple idea was that eating a high saturated fat diet led to a rise in blood cholesterol and other lipids, and that promoted atherosclerosis. Dairy products are high in saturated fats and were incriminated on first principles by this reasoning. As we discussed in relation to diet (Section 7.7) the role of cholesterol has withstood scrutiny but the role of dairy products has proven to be complex. It now seems that the kind of fats in dairy are neutral and perhaps even beneficial in relation to CVD and DM_2 even though LDL-C is raised. This matter remains controversial(463, 464, 472).

South Asians are commonly lactose intolerant(682, 683). There are exceptions in places where dairy farming is established, especially Northern India. Most South Asians consume milk in small amounts or as fermented products such as yoghurt and paneer (a kind of soft cheese). Nonetheless, the consumption of both traditional milk products and European-type milk products is increasing fast across South Asia and in South Asians abroad(433, 493). Emigrant South Asians in affluent countries are immediately exposed to low-cost dairy products both while shopping and eating out. Furthermore, many non-dairy foods are processed to include, quite unexpectedly, dairy products such as lactose powder, milk powder, and whey powder(434, 678).

Given these two observations—dairy is a rich source of saturated fats and most South Asians are lactose intolerant—I have observed an anti-dairy body of opinion, including by distinguished cardiologists focused on the rise of chronic diseases. Some South Asian patients are being advised by some cardiologists to stop drinking milk and Indian dietary guidelines also steer us to reduced milk consumption either directly or indirectly.

Could it be that increasing exposure to dairy in a largely lactose-intolerant population might be a trigger for the epidemic of CVD and DM_2? I think this is unlikely but it cannot be discounted. The arguments against it include these: 1) even South Asians in the Punjab, who are from relatively lactose-tolerant dairy farming communities, are at very high risk of CVD and DM_2; 2) Dairy foods, especially in the fermented products popular with South Asians are, seemingly, neutral or even beneficial in relation to CVD; 3) Lactose intolerance mostly causes problems in the gastro-intestinal tract. There is some animal and clinical evidence that it can promote cardiac arrhythmias(678) but it has not been quantitatively linked to atherosclerosis or insulin metabolism.

There is a modern line of research, echoing that of the Victorian era when bowel function was a central concern of doctors, on disturbance of bowel flora as a cause of chronic diseases. It is too early to evaluate the significance of this for the epidemic of CVD and DM_2. Lactose intolerance, of course, causes bowel flora disturbances when lactose is consumed(678, 679).

Direct studies of the role of lactose intolerance in CVD and DM_2 in South Asians are limited though Jeffrey Segall articulated a clear hypothesis that a combination of lactose intolerance and insulin resistance promoted glycation of arterial wall proteins to which lipoproteins become attached, thus causing atherosclerosis(684). Segall paid especial attention to the patterns of CVD in South Asians and other similarly insulin resistant populations. Nonetheless, the evidence in general populations argues against this, even although studies on South Asians are not available.

I think that criticisms of milk consumption in relation to CVD and DM_2 in South Asians, whether in relation to lactose intolerance or not, are premature. That does not, however, mean it is innocent in the broader context of dairy-related foods, especially those processed with sugars, other fats, and other chemicals. Dairy products are likely to have an adverse effect through increased food intake and weight gain as they are often consumed as part of energy dense, processed foods, as most clearly demonstrated in emigrant South Asians(345, 680, 685). Weight gain is the result, and the consequences of that were reviewed earlier (Section 7.9).

8.12 Anatomical and physiological explanations

I have considered some aspects of anatomy and physiology, e.g. the lower height, lesser muscle mass, and tendency to central obesity of South Asians. In addition I have noted the possible effects of low birthweight on the structure and long-term function of organs, e.g. the smaller number of nephrons and possibly also fewer insulin-producing islets of Langerhans in the pancreas. Whether South Asians do, indeed, have anatomical differences in the pancreas, and pancreatic reserve, is not clear but clearly their pancreatic function is vigorous for they produce high levels of insulin. It seems improbable that such anatomic differences could explain the very high levels of DM_2. Organs such as the pancreas, like the kidney and liver, have considerable functional reserve. Whether these kinds of factors are causally important is not clear and we will return to that question in Chapter 9.

Similar observations have been made on the cardiovascular system itself. Studies on this topic have been sporadic. The topics we will consider here are the dimensions and functions of the heart, the size, and particularly diameter of the coronary arteries, the nature of the atheroma in the arteries, intima-media thickness, and arterial stiffness.

The heart is, generally, smaller in South Asians than in White Europeans. This is, however, a function of body size, and it is proportionate to that(686). This is entirely analogous to women having smaller hearts than men. This difference in heart size has no evident implications for South Asians' susceptibility to CVD. In studies in London South Asians had altered left ventricular function, high left ventricular filling pressure, and more concentric modelling(214). These observations may be important for diagnosis and clinical management but their significance for understanding disease causation is unclear.

Several studies have examined the structure of the coronary arteries in South Asians with special attention to the diameter of the lumen(687–690). Most of them find the diameter of the lumen to be comparatively small, but in line with the size of the heart and body. Hassaan et al. observed that South Asians in the US had narrower lumens and more diseased arterial segments(688). Lip pointed out that atheroma looks more severe in narrower arteries(689). Again, this is what we find when comparing men and women, and, again the differences do not seem to be important. It is noteworthy that women have much less CVD than men despite such anatomical differences.

One important measure of atheroma and future risk of adverse cardiovascular outcomes is intima-media thickness (IMT). This is usually measured in the carotid arteries. Given South Asians' high rates of CVD the prior expectation is that IMT would be comparatively high but it is not(691–693). From this surprising finding arises the question of whether the nature of atheromatous lesions in South Asians is different. Studies have suggested that atheroma is more diffuse in South Asians than Europeans, leading to the concept of a generalized, low-grade inflammation of the endothelium with diffuse low-grade atheroma(694, 695). Measures of the amount of atheroma have not, overall, found an excess in South Asians(696–699).

The arterial tree of South Asians is comparatively stiff, and this has been observed in both childhood and adulthood(398, 399, 561, 700–702). Box 8.1(p 196) summarizes a recent review of the evidence on this topic and Figure 8.1 is a simple conceptual diagram of how arterial stiffness might relate to CVD. The meaning of these observations is unclear but I return to it in Chapter 9.

Overall, the amount of research on anatomical and physiological differences in the vascular system is small. The limited findings do not point to these differences being especially important in explaining South Asians' tendency to CVD.

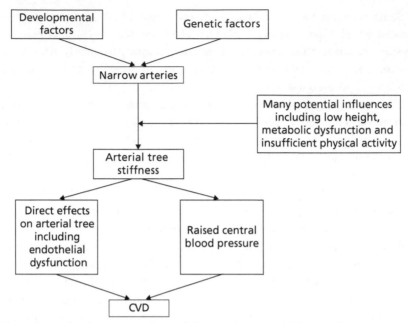

Figure 8.1 A simple, conceptual causal diagram for the possible role of narrower, stiffer arteries in South Asians.

The main exception to this generalization is arterial stiffness but that could be a coincidence or consequence rather than a cause, though interpretation would be easier if we knew the reasons and consequences. In one study the authors thought it was simply a reflection of differences in height(703).

In discussing BP I considered the possibility that in South Asians BP centrally might be higher even while that is not so for peripheral BP. Central BP is higher when there is arterial stiffness. There is modest evidence that this is the case and it may be especially relevant for the risk of stroke(398).

Differences between ethnic groups in anatomy and physiology of the kind above are sometimes relevant to the clinical care of individual patients, e.g. when going for surgery or clinical testing. They are unlikely to be an important explanation of South Asians' raised risk of CVD at the population level.

8.13 **Miscellaneous risk factors**

The attempt to explain South Asians' susceptibility to CVD and DM_2 has, as we have seen, generated many ideas. This section is relatively brief given the number of topics considered and its purpose is to be comprehensive.

8.13.1 **Other co-morbidities**

Diseases tend to go together with one causing or amplifying the effect of another. Our key example is in the role of DM_2 in causing and amplifying CVD and another is renal impairment doing the same. Might there be other co-morbidities, other than those we have considered, that will provide the explanation? For example, iron metabolism with a deficiency (anaemia) or an excess (haemachromatosis) are relevant both to CVD and DM_2. Anaemia is very common in South Asians, even in those living in wealthy countries abroad, especially women(704, 705). Another set of diseases related to CVD are the autoimmune disorders, e.g. thyroiditis (see Section 8.10), rheumatoid arthritis, and systemic lupus erythematosus. It seems improbable that these examples are serious candidates in our search for explanations but we should be open to other possibilities.

8.13.2 **Other genetic explanations: non-coding DNA and telomeres**

We considered genetic explanations in Chapters 2–4 but, notwithstanding interesting ideas and data, the genetic case was not compelling. Genetic knowledge is advancing fast and the conclusion might change, especially as the understanding of mechanisms for gene–environment mechanisms advances. We know very little about the non-coding parts of DNA (sometimes disparagingly called junk DNA) but we have learned that ethnic variations are greater there than in the genes. Another area of interest is the telomere, which can be thought of as the cap at the end of the chromosome. Telomere shortening is associated with premature ageing(706, 707). It is possible that South Asians' susceptibility to CVD and DM_2 is related to genetics but in ways, not necessarily the two here, that remain obscure.

8.13.3 **Other lifestyles and behaviours**

In studying CVD and DM_2 we usually focus on a few of the multiplicity of lifestyles and behaviours that characterize South Asian populations, especially those that distinguish them from others. Many lifestyles and behaviours remain to be investigated. One emergent area of study, for example, is sleep. Sleep is critical to health and poor and disrupted sleeping patterns are associated with cardiometabolic dysfunction(708). There is little evidence on this in South Asians. It seems unlikely that there are sufficient systematic differences in sleep between South Asians and other populations to explain the heightened susceptibility to CVD/DM_2. Cooking practices may be a promising area of work, especially given the high-heat cooking including loss of vitamin C, and the B_{12}/folate imbalance hypotheses(107, 639). I have considered high-heating cooking and vitamin B12 in some depth already.

8.13.4 Other biochemical disturbances

There are so many molecules—literally hundreds—associated with CVD and DM_2, and others emerging, that it is difficult to evaluate them in any population, never mind South Asians alone(76). Among those we have not considered earlier except in passing but that have been a focus of studies on South Asians are adiponectin(162), endotoxins(643, 652), and cellular adhesion molecules(650). More will be discovered, especially through the area known as metabolonomics, where all the products of genes are being mapped and linked to health states. It is likely that most of the biochemical changes are a consequence of the processes that lead to CVD and DM_2 rather than causes of them. For example, adiponectin is secreted by fat cells and it increases sensitivity to insulin. It is reduced by a high glycaemic diet. Adiponectin levels are comparatively low in South Asian populations and this has caused sporadic interest. The point is that this is one of numerous biochemical differences that are likely to be a consequence of factors such as fat composition and distribution and diet, which are themselves more likely to be important in disease causation.

8.13.5 Toxins in soil and food

We considered the possible role of advanced glycation end-products and trans fats (Section 7.5) that are created in the process of cooking, especially at high heats. These kinds of substances have been linked to CVD and diabetes. Arsenic is known to cause CVD but fortunately it is in small concentrations in most environments, although not so rare in some places including rural parts of Bangladesh. The possibility that there are specific toxins that are raising CVD and DM_2 risk in South Asians needs to be considered. Given the risk is seen in diaspora populations, some of whom such as Surinamese Indians emigrated several generations ago, such postulated toxins are likely to be in the cuisine as, obviously, other routes of exposure will be too variable across generations and geographies, e.g. air pollution even although it is undoubtedly important for CVD(322). Surinamese Indians, after many generations, still hold to traditional cooking methods and preferences(598, 709).

8.13.6 Breast-feeding

Breast milk is the optimal nutrition for babies, and has important and demonstrated health advantages, including enhancing immunity against infections. In South Asia whether in rural or urban areas, compared to the developed, industrialized countries breast-feeding rates are high. On first principles, we would expect cardiovascular benefits to both the breast-feeding mothers and to their infants. The benefits to the mothers, especially in helping to lose pregnancy-related weight, are not contentious.

The evidence in relation to cardiometabolic benefits to babies is unclear. Breast-feeding is associated with slightly lower BP in later life and, less consistently, with other cardiovascular risk factors(710). By contrast, breast-feeding, especially when it is prolonged, has been shown to be associated with stiffer arteries in infants, as shown in work on the distensiblity of the radial artery(711). This observation has been supported in experiments on baboons. One plausible explanation is that breast milk is high in cholesterol and other lipids, which is not surprising given their importance in nutrition and especially brain development, particularly in early life. These lipids form fatty streaks in the arteries. Fatty streaks would be expected to diminish once weaning starts, assuming that the lipid content of the post-weaning diet would be low. If, however, the post-weaning diet is rich in saturated lipids the expected removal of the fatty streaks might not occur. This is more likely to occur in urban settings where high fat diets are more likely to be consumed even by infants.

While the significance of these observations for the epidemic of CVD in South Asians is unclear, it is notable that adult South Asians do have more arterial stiffness than we would expect. Overall, while we might hope that more and longer breast-feeding along with many other benefits would protect South Asians from CVD, this might not be so and the opposite needs to be considered.

8.13.7 **Cortisol**

Cortisol is the corticosteroid hormone that is most commonly measured in human studies. Corticosteroids are produced by the adrenal glands and have numerous functions. Severe excess leads to Cushing's disease and severe deficiency to Addison's disease. Cushing's disease leads to abnormalities that are like those of metabolic syndrome, the condition originally named as Syndrome X by Reaven (see Chapter 1). Cortisol is also raised in response to stress and this is especially important in chronic stress. Corticosteroids have also been implicated in developmental programming. Ethnic variations in cortisol have been studied, including in South Asians. In South Asians cortisol levels tend to be similar or lower than in reference populations and in the Mysore birth cohort there was no association between adult cortisol and birthweights(712–714). Cortisol levels are lower in the presence of higher adipose tissue possibly because more cortisol is then bound to the glucocorticoid receptor. There is no clear evidence that corticosteroids are directly important in the susceptibility of South Asians to CVD and DM_2 via any of the mechanisms above.

8.13.8 **Alcohol**

Alcohol is one of the most contentious and heavily studied of the CVD risk factors but less so for DM_2. There are long-standing and popular claims that low to moderate consumption of alcohol, and especially red wine, has cardiovascular health benefits(62, 481, 715). There is some animal research and theoretical data to back this up. Similarly, alcohol does have hypoglycaemic effects and there is experimental evidence that an alcoholic drink with a meal reduces postprandial glucose levels(480). Alcohol, however, has many adverse health effects when consumed immoderately including for CVD, that it does not find a place in risk reduction advice.

Large sections of South Asian society (Muslims, Sikhs, Hindus, and Jains) have prohibitions and taboos on alcohol, especially for women. Overall, the proportion of alcohol abstainers is high in South Asian societies. There are, of course, exceptions, with much variation, e.g. despite the prohibition of alcohol in their religion Sikh men, at least abroad, have a reputation for their alcohol consumption and there is evidence to support this(10, 716). The matter is highly complex but it probably has little bearing on South Asians' susceptibility to CVD and DM_2. It does not explain differences and sometimes similarities between South Asian men and women from different countries or religions, and between South Asians and White Europeans. The little evidence there is on whether the purported benefits of alcohol for CVD apply to ethnic minority groups, including South Asians, is not, unlike most populations, clearly supportive of this (479, 717).

In my view, the most important explanation for the protective effects of alcohol is that people who are able to control their alcohol consumption to one or two modest drinks/day also have other favourable life circumstances and lifestyles that are the more important factors. In other words, the association is confounded(715). It is possible, however, that those who do not drink alcohol substitute other more harmful beverages, e.g. sugary drinks.

8.13.9 **Consanguinity, caste, and other forms of inbreeding**

In Chapter 1 briefly traced the history of *Homo sapiens* and the migration from East Africa to South Asia. In evolutionary terms modern humans are a young species and as a result of this and the fact that the emigrations were of small bands of people, we are all highly inbred with much admixture(37, 718). In South Asia, by no means uniquely, there are some ingrained customs that have promoted further inbreeding. Among the most important of these are marriage within caste, and within this, among biraderi (clans based on occupation and thus related to caste); and consanguineous marriage, most commonly between cousins and uncles and nieces(719, 720). Consanguinity of this kind has been, and still is, common across the world.

The advantages and disadvantages of such social and cultural practices leading to inbreeding are much debated and studied(720, 721). The question here is whether South Asians' susceptibility to CVD and DM_2 might be attributable to inbreeding. The study of the association between inbreeding and chronic diseases and their biological risk factors is a recent occurrence (the effects on genetic disorders is well documented). Ground-breaking studies of inbred island populations have shown some modest associations with CVD risk factors such as BP and cholesterol(718, 722, 723). In a case–control study in Pakistan, Ismail et al. found a very strong association between consanguinity and MI, which seems implausible(724). The role of inbreeding is in my view, at present, unclear. Our best pointer is that even in South Asian groups where inbreeding is much less acceptable, e.g. in Sikhs, CVD and DM_2 are very common.

Though Sikhism forbids the use of caste, in practice this prohibition is often not followed, and most marriages have been within biraderi(719, 720). These practices have been common through the ages yet the epidemic of CVD and DM_2 have emerged in the last few generations and are still rare in the rural areas where inbreeding is greatest. Pending further research, which may influence matters, I do not prioritize this explanation.

8.14 **Conclusions**

The interest and scale of the challenge of explaining the epidemics in South Asians of CVD and DM_2, and of rising adiposity, is reflected in the range of formal hypotheses (Chapters 2–5), the examination of contextual factors (Chapter 6), the re-appraisal of established causes (Chapter 7), and the continued exploration in many directions as reflected in this chapter.

The inference we can make with confidence is that there is not a stable and settled view on the question of why CVD and DM_2 epidemics occur and especially on why they seem to affect urbanized South Asians disproportionately given their patterns of known causal factors. As I stated in Chapter 1, either South Asians have more of the known causes, or they are more affected by them, or there are causes that we have not linked to the problem we are investigating. This has echoes of Donald Rumsfeld's famous line about (I paraphrase) (a) known knowns, (b) known unknowns, and (c) unknown unknowns. Clearly, in relation to CVD and DM_2 in South Asians there is much on (a), a moderate amount on (b) and probably a great deal of (c).

The main message from this chapter is that there is ongoing creativity in the development of ideas and both scholarly and research activity. Mostly, ideas are initially developed, pursued, and promoted with enthusiasm but when interest wanes as the promise is unfulfilled, we are left without a verdict on their importance. The scientific literature becomes cluttered as a result of this. Overall, it is unlikely that any of the factors considered in this chapter are sufficient, on their own, to explain South Asians' susceptibility to CVD and DM_2 It is still, however, important to consider them for at least three reasons: 1) this consideration might promote research to provide stronger evidence either to support or reject the idea; 2) it might help to generate new lines of thinking e.g. of other potential toxins or infections; 3) some of these ideas might be important as part of a complex causal process.

In Chapter 9 I will attempt a synthesis of the hypotheses and the empirical evidence together with the views of leading scholars and researchers who have been working on this subject.

Box 8.1 Vascular dynamics: arterial stiffness and arterial wave reflection

Faconti L et al. Do arterial stiffness and wave reflection underlie cardiovascular risk in ethnic minorities? JRSM Cardiovascular Disease 2016;5:1–9 (399).

My introductory remarks

Most of the general explanations for South Asians' heightened susceptibility to CVD and DM_2 tend to converge on metabolism and metabolic dysfunction, especially insulin resistance and adipose tissue function. Ideas have, however, been generated on the role of cardiovascular anatomy and function and have been presented in an empirical rather than theoretical way. Mostly, these have not found a place among the top-ranking explanations. One of the most important of these ideas is arterial stiffness.

The paper

Faconti et al.'s review question is, in effect, postulating a hypothesis, even though their work focuses on empirical evidence. They note that the excess risk of CVD in ethnic minority populations (the focus being on South Asians and Black Africans and Caribbeans) has not been explained. They

Box 8.1 Vascular dynamics (continued)

recommend examining targets organs, especially arteries, and not just risk factors.

When the peripheral arteries are stiff the pulse wave created when the ventricles of the heart pump the blood into the circulation (systole) travels faster than when the arteries are flexible. The pulse wave is reflected back from the peripheral arteries faster too, so there is a greater than normal rise in central BP, i.e. in the large arteries like the aorta. Coronary arteries supplying the heart are mostly filled during the resting phase of the heart, i.e. diastole, unlike the rest of the circulation when arteries are filled during systole. With arterial stiffness diastolic BP may decrease, reducing blood flow through the coronary arteries. There may also be damage to the small arteries and arterioles from such stiffness.

Several ways of measuring arterial stiffness are available including pulse wave velocity. Data by ethnic group on such measures are rare. As age and BP are the two most important factors for arterial stiffness, evidence that ethnic minorities have greater arterial stiffness needs to adjust for these factors. Furthermore, it is also important to know whether arterial stiffness is a consequence of other CVD risk factors, or augments their effects, or acts as an independent cause.

Ten studies, seven including South Asians, were reviewed by the authors. The conclusion was that the role of arterial stiffness in CVD risk in South Asians was unclear, at least as reflected in pulse wave analysis measures.

The case was re-examined with the augmentation index, a more complex measure that is independent of arterial stiffness, which, essentially, measures the additional BP added by the backward pulse wave that follows the forward one. The evidence that this might be important comes mainly from Singapore where Indians had lower BP than in the Chinese but had a higher augmentation index. Overall, however, the evidence was limited.

My concluding remarks

Although this is not a fully articulated hypothesis, it is clear that the authors are seeking a general factor, particularly one that acts in early life. Their review concludes that for South Asians the evidence is limited and inconclusive. There are several similar ideas based on circulatory system structure and function. Differences can be observed but whether they are causes, consequences, or coincidental tends to remain unclear. These kind of ideas are important because they examine the cardiovascular system directly and not via the lens of the metabolic system, even although that may be involved.

Chapter 9

A causal synthesis and models

9.1 Chapter 9 objectives are to:

1. Recapitulate on the main themes arising in earlier chapters, and create a life-course based synthesis that connects the ideas and hypotheses into a coherent whole, while setting aside the improbable or unnecessary explanations.
2. Consider how the genetic, developmental, socio-economic, lifestyle, and other factors discussed earlier may affect biochemistry, physiology, and ultimately cause the damage that leads to disease.
3. Outline potential pathways to pathology that can be described in conceptual causal diagrams.
4. Summarize discussions with scholars and researchers worldwide.

9.2 Chapter Summary

For diseases to occur the damage done by the causes must exceed the body's repair mechanisms, or lead to incomplete or faulty repair. This damage is initiated by disturbances in physiology or biochemistry, e.g. high blood glucose or LDL-cholesterol. Such changes may alter the anatomy, e.g. stiffening and narrowing of the arteries and creating endothelial dysfunction. These kinds of changes may lead to minor (endothelial dysfunction) or major pathology (atherosclerosis) and ultimately disease, e.g. atherosclerosis leading to thrombosis in the coronary artery causing a heart attack. The process is lengthy, usually stretching across several decades, so it is useful to utilize the life-course framework. There are likely to be trigger points at different parts of the life-course that are influential in enhancing disease susceptibility, This chapter synthesizes explanations that are relevant to each of diabetes, CHD, and stroke and to all three collectively, setting out potential pathways in causal diagrams. The explanations are based on the premise that genetic, socio-economic, and psychosocial backgrounds are enabling/predisposing factors and not primary. The causes are considered to be specific changes that impact through arterial dysfunction and metabolic dysfunction. The starting point is that the known causes of CVD and DM_2 also apply to South Asians. The key question then is what additional factors account for their raised susceptibility. This synthesis emphasizes glycation of tissues, possibly leading to arterial stiffness and microcirculatory damage. In addition to endothelial pathways to atherosclerosis an external (adventitial) one is proposed, i.e. microcirculatory damage to the vasa vasorum, the network of arterioles that supplies nutrients to the larger arteries themselves. This, then, leads to atherosclerosis and CVD. DM_2 plays into this pathway, not through insulin resistance, but through glycosylation and dyslipidaemia. The cause of the high prevalence of DM_2 in South Asians is difficult to explain. The explanation may lie in protective factors in Europeans as much as in detrimental ones in South Asians. The high glucose level is considered as an allostatic mechanism controlled by the brain. Beta cell failure still needs to be explained. In addition to the concept of ectopic fat in the liver and pancreas being the cause of this, two additional ideas are proposed, i.e. firstly, microcirculatory damage and secondly, glycation, mostly likely by dietary factors including neoformed contaminants, e.g. AGEs. This synthesis de-emphasizes the thrifty genotype and thrifty phenotype families of hypotheses. It moves from an emphasis on insulin and insulin resistance to the effects of glucose and other chemicals on tissues through glycation and microcirculatory damage. The discussions with scholars provided a consensus that the causes of South Asians' susceptibility to CVD and DM_2 were complex and unresolved. Generally their views chimed with earlier discussions, and did not clash with the synthesis here.

9.3 Introduction: a recapitulation of the main points in Chapters 1–8, and introduction to the nature of this synthesis and the inclusion of international scholars' perspectives

Extensive biomedical and epidemiological research, as summarized in Chapter 1, 7 and 8, especially, has demonstrated how and why CVD and DM_2 occur in all populations. This research has pursued four main lines of enquiry: describing the pathology, examining related biochemical and physiological changes, the pursuit of risk factors through demonstrating their statistical association with diseases, and the development and testing of causal hypotheses and theories, often in animal experiments and sometimes in clinical trials in humans.

Humans across the world, when living modern lifestyles, are extremely prone to CVD and DM_2 and these are among their commonest and most severe diseases(725, 726). All humans therefore, must be genetically susceptible to these diseases. Obviously, if human were genetically resistant to these diseases they would be rare or non-existent, e.g. the brain disease scrapie is common in sheep but not in humans. This human genetic susceptibility to CVD and DM_2 is uncovered in the circumstances of modern life styles. (Other mammals, especially in captivity as pets and zoo animals, also develop these diseases.)

Most of the research on CVD and DM_2 has been done on White European origin populations, mostly in the US and North West Europe, partly because the epidemics of these diseases struck these populations early (from the 1920s on) and partly because these places lead biomedical and epidemiological research. The study of international and ethnic (or racial) variations was incorporated into CVD and DM_2 research programmes in the 1950s, a strategy that proved especially valuable as the epidemic spread across the world, including to low- and middle-income countries. The causal knowledge developed in White European origin populations has been shown to apply reasonably well across the world(85). This knowledge is, however, complex, with many unanswered questions, and puzzling features. In seeking to understand why South Asians have so much CVD and DM_2 we need to start with the established general knowledge. When we come to unanswered questions we then look for additional understanding. This additional understanding, in turn, could help to solve the remaining puzzling questions in the general understanding.

In this book I have set out, albeit briefly, the clinical pathology, the scale of the problem of the CVD and DM_2 epidemics in South Asians, and the favoured explanations (Chapter 1). I then moved to some fundamental hypotheses addressing the question of why humans, including South Asians, are so prone to these diseases (Chapter 2–5). Most explanations have focused on obesity, insulin, insulin resistance, and dysglycaemia. In Chapter 6 I sketched out the broad population context, including the socio-economic and psychosocial changes as societies urbanize, which is the context within which the epidemics are occurring in South Asians. Then, in Chapter 7, I examined the established risk factors (presumed or demonstrated causes), which explain a great deal, but not everything and not why South Asians have more CVD and DM_2 than White European populations who have as much, if not even more, exposure to these factors. In Chapter 8 I explored a wide range of additional observations and ideas, some articulated to help explain the high risk of CVD and DM_2 in South Asians. In this chapter, I synthesize the evidence and seek to bridge the gap between the knowledge of pathology, causal hypotheses, and specific postulated or established risk factors.

A synthesis is of value if it produces a simpler and more insightful account than that which considers the separate components. To do this requires making judgements on what is likely to be important. One of the required tasks is to set aside unlikely explanations. The remaining explanations need to be coherently linked. Table 9.1 lists such explanations. The result of the synthesis is a scientific story, where there are main and minor characters, and a chronological plot. This scientific detective story is less about 'who done it?' and more 'how might it have happened?' The resulting textual story is re-told in relatively simple conceptual causal diagrams as in my four-stage model explaining South Asians' susceptibility to DM_2(96). The causal basis of DM_2 is complex but not when compared to CVD. I start with separate models for atherosclerotic CHD and stroke (CVD), and DM_2. (I see haemorrhagic stroke in South Asians as a separate entity with a different causal basis, with the exception of hypertension, that is outside the main enquiry in this book.)

The life-course approach offers an appealing and pragmatic frame for considering chronic disease where the development is over several decades and possibly straddles generations. This perspective is especially relevant given the prominence of the DOHAD hypothesis in explanations of susceptibility to CVD and DM_2 especially in South Asians.

As I reached this stage I spoke to 22 leading scholars and researchers and asked for their views on the causes of the susceptibility of South Asians to either or both of CVD and DM_2. The discussions were done mostly by Skype and lasted 30–60 minutes. My views were not divulged so their accounts were independent of mine. The appendix has a brief account of each discussion agreed with the scholars/researchers. I have produced a digest of these discussions within this chapter and considered how they alter my main conclusions (Section 9.7).

Table 9.1 An overview of the main ideas explaining the epidemic of CVD and DM_2 in South Asians considered in this synthesis and my assessment of the level of support for them

Ideas supported by literature and scholars	Ideas with promise and needing research	Ideas that are often presented but needing de-emphasis
◆ Fitness/physical activity low ◆ Muscle mass low ◆ Relative adiposity and central deposition of fat ◆ Ectopic fat, especially hepatic ◆ Excess energy consumption, with generalized adiposity ◆ Dietary imbalance with insufficient food/vegetables and protein and high levels of starchy, simple carbohydrates ◆ TFAs high *(renewed emphasis)* ◆ Glucose high ◆ Glycosylation, possibly by glucose in combination with other like glycosylating agents *(new emphasis)*	◆ High heat cooking and other factors leading to neoformed contaminants such as AGEs, with many effects including glycosylation *(new emphasis)* ◆ Damage to the microcirculation of the artery (vasa vasorum) *(new emphasis)* ◆ Arterial stiffness/raised central BP *(new emphasis)* ◆ Rapid increase in risk factors promoting allostasis, not homeostasis *(new emphasis)*	◆ The migratory process itself ◆ Socio-economic factors as specific explanations ◆ Genetic variation as a specific explanation ◆ Developmental factors/thrifty phenotype ◆ Thrifty genotype ◆ Mitochondrial efficiency ◆ Insulin/insulin resistance ◆ Inflammation ◆ Thrombotic tendency ◆ Infections

9.4 **A simple conceptual causal framework**

In Figure 9.1 I have outlined the main, broad causal forces that we have considered in Chapters 1–8. These forces are general, and not specific to South Asians, but they underpin more specific explanations developed in Figures 9.2, 9.3, and 9.4. In examining these figures as much emphasis should be given to what is missing as to what is present. As we move from the general to the specific this becomes more explicit. In Figure 9.1, it is clear that I have given the central role to the environment in its broadest sense and placed genetic and

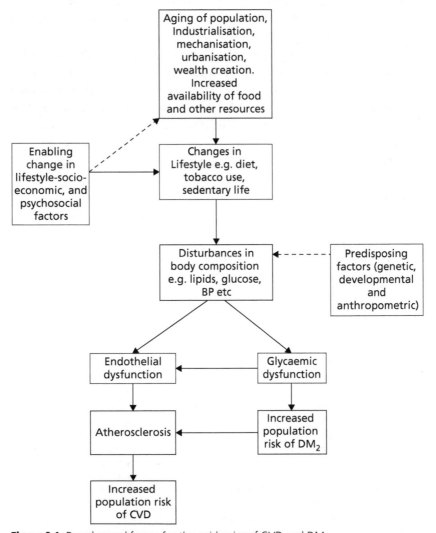

Figure 9.1 Broad causal forces for the epidemics of CVD and DM_2.

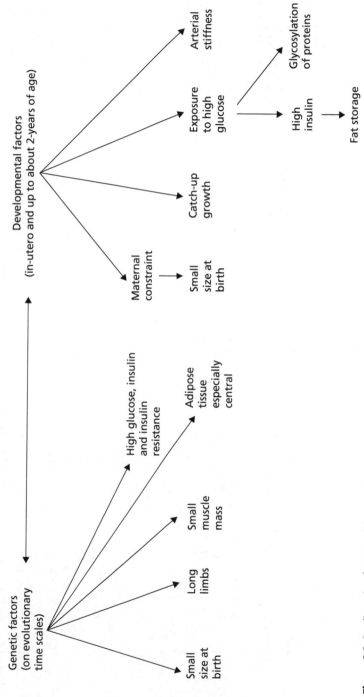

Figure 9.2 Predisposing factors with special relevance to South Asians.

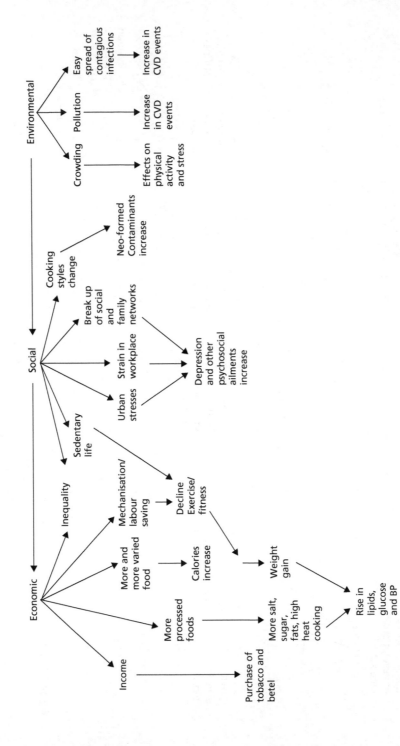

Figure 9.3 Enabling socio-economic and social factors with special relevance to the South Asian context.

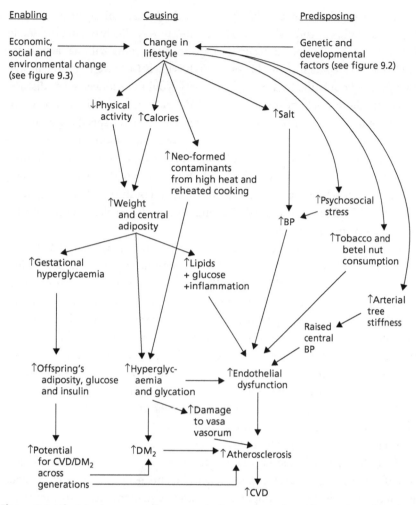

Figure 9.4 Lifestyle changes as the causes in the context of enabling and predisposing factors.

developmental factors as promoters that allow the specific causes to have their effects. The arrow from these promoters to the body disturbances is a broken one to signify that the effects are indirect.

Genetic and developmental factors affect anatomy, physiology, and biochemistry. The key point, however, is that these have little direct effect at the population level on disease outcome. Equally, there are socio-economic and social changes that, in themselves, are not causal for disease outcomes at population level. These forces come into play through lifestyle change, and the process of wealth creation, industrialization, mechanization and urbanization is important in accelerating the change of lifestyle but such change can occur even in villages. The changes in lifestyle seen in modernization are likely but not inevitable. If they were not allowed to occur, perhaps through some national action, the CVD and DM_2 epidemics would not occur. It is likely that, even without lifestyle change, the population in the wealthy society would live longer so, as diseases of ageing, there would be an increase in CVD and DM_2 overall because of the demographic transition, but the rise would not be seen in a specific age-group.

Changes in lifestyle lead to changes in body composition, physiology, and biochemistry (especially important being an increase in some lipids). In turn, these cause minor pathology such as endothelial dysfunction which eventually leads to atherosclerosis and CVD, and dysfunction in the regulation of glucose leads to DM_2. DM_2 leads to further changes in lipids, accelerating endothelial dysfunction, and atherosclerosis.

In South Asia, and especially in emigrant South Asians, there has been a particularly rapid move to affluence, urbanization, mechanization, and lifestyle change(23, 24, 46, 321, 324, 727). Razum and colleagues' ideas on the rapid emergence of the epidemiological transition in emigrants are relevant here(375). Their concept proposes that in the presence of rapid change, the chronic diseases with relatively short times between exposure to the cause and the signs of disease (incubation period), e.g. DM_2, occur first, while those with long incubation periods (e.g. cancers) lag behind. The general concept seems apt for South Asians, within South Asia or distant countries.

The question now, given the framework in Figure 9.1, is what is particular about South Asians that makes them so prone to CVD and DM_2 when the circumstances promote rapid lifestyle changes?

Figure 9.2 develops the promoting/predisposing factors section of Figure 9.1. The division in Figure 9.2 of influences that are genetic and developmental is arbitrary but it helps in simplifying a complex matter. These are interacting influences, as clarified in the top line, with arrows between genetic and developmental factors. The genetic profile of South Asians has developed on evolutionary time-scales as discussed in Chapter 2–4. The influence of developmental factors is transgenerational but probably with diminishing effects over two to three generations (unless the stimulus is maintained). The genetic and development factors influence each other (directly in the case of genes influencing development and via epigenetic mechanisms in the case of development influencing genes). The figure places emphasis on anthropometry—body size, shape, muscle-mass, and adipose tissue distribution. High glucose, insulin, and insulin resistance are also emphasized. A factor I have, unusually, emphasized and placed under developmental factors is arterial stiffness (it may be partly related to characteristics such as height that are genetic). It may be partly related to small body size. In addition to the usual effects of glucose I have emphasized glycosylation of proteins.

Low metabolism, a thrifty metabolism, an active immune system, neurobehavioural explanations, and specific genes acting directly on DM_2 or CVD pathways are not in Figure 9.2 explicitly. These are not, however, to be forgotten because they offer possible explanations for the characteristics shown in Figure 9.2.

The important point is that none of these predisposing factors, whether in Figure 9.2 or not, singly or collectively, is causing the CVD and DM_2 epidemics in urbanized South Asians. We know this because atherosclerotic CVD and DM_2 are not common in South Asian populations with these same predisposing factors who are still living in traditional, rural ways(729, 730). Interestingly, while DM_2 in such populations can be shown to be virtually non-existent by OGTT, the signs of potential CVD are present even when clinical CVD is low. Autopsy studies across the world, including in South Asian countries, show that atherosclerosis can be present, even common, in populations where the clinical outcomes are not common(373, 731–733). This fits with the earliest observations from the 19th century that a combination of atherosclerosis and other factors leading to thrombosis or instability of atherosclerotic plaque is needed to cause clinical outcomes such as MI or ischaemic stroke(331).

Figure 9.3 develops the pattern of relations of enabling social and economic factors. As with genetic and developmental influences interacting, so it is with economic, social, and environmental factors. Not only do they interact with each other (indeed the boundaries between them are arbitrary) but they also interact with genetic and developmental factors. A rise in income, for example, gives access to more, more varied, and highly desirable and tasty processed foods. It also permits people to purchase expensive foods including oils, flesh, eggs and milk and to cook food at prolonged, high heat and even repeatedly. Food can be kept for very long periods of time either refrigerated or frozen, but during this time AGEs and other neo-formed contaminants will gradually increase naturally. The regular and larger-scale purchase of substances such as alcohol, tobacco, and betel nut is made possible by increasing wealth. The disturbance of social and family networks and new ways of working may lead to strain and depression that may increase risk of CVD and DM_2. In urban environments, economic inequality increases and this social context is associated with adverse cardiovascular outcomes. The urban environment is highly mechanized and a sedentary lifestyle is possible and even promoted by high population density, mechanized transport, and lack of green and other open spaces. Air pollution, and urban infections, including influenza, accelerate CVD events probably by increasing risk of thrombosis at the site of pre-existing atherosclerosis (322, 643).

In Figure 9.4 the changes in lifestyle causing CVD and DM_2 are given in the midst of the enabling and predisposing factors. The pace of change may be important in its own right although the evidence suggests that the actual extent and amount of exposure, not the rapidity of change, is the important determining factor, but this will be considered further in Section 9.5.

Figure 9.4 mostly sets out the well-established pathways, i.e. changes in lifestyle risk factors leading to endothelial dysfunction and then atherosclerosis, and separately to hyperglycaemia. The established pathways are via increased use of tobacco, diet, weight gain, physical inactivity, psychosocial stress, and inflammatory processes triggering CVD events and rise in BP.

There are, however, five potential causal factors in Figure 9.4 that do not get emphasis in standard accounts that I think do deserve emphasis in relation to South Asians, i.e. gestational hyperglycaemia affecting both the mother in later life and the fetus through its life-course, betel nut consumption, neo-formed contaminants, stiffness of the arterial tree, and lastly a novelty especially in relation to CVD in South Asians, microcirculatory damage to the vasa vasorum(69, 71–75). I hypothesize this as an alternative route to atherosclerosis, i.e. disruption of the blood supply to the artery (i.e. the vasa vasorum) and not merely or only with endothelial dysfunction.

In Section 9.5, I will consider whether these conceptual causal paths are enough to explain South Asians' susceptibility to CVD and DM_2 and if not, I will consider which of the other ideas examined in this book need to be incorporated. Then, I consider what ingredients might still be missing and how we are going to find them.

In Chapter 1, I introduced the concept of the scattered pieces of a jigsaw puzzle that needed to be connected (Figure 1.1). I now tackle this challenge. Although CVD is more complex than DM_2, surprisingly, I find it easier to place the pieces of the CVD puzzle into a coherent picture, albeit with more pieces and potentially more pieces missing, than for DM_2. For this reason, I consider CVD first, then DM_2, and finally the common ground between them.

9.5 CVD: fitting the pieces of the puzzle

My task is like completing a jigsaw puzzle where the pieces from many puzzles have been mixed up, with many being unnecessary, and some necessary ones removed. In Figure 1.1, I illustrated this concept with nine categories of factors from which the causal picture is to be constructed. Perhaps the first task is to try to remove the pieces that do not seem to be part of the jigsaw we are solving. Then we have to find the platform—a table–to place and fit the pieces that remain.

Figure 9.5 shows the result of my solution for CVD and Figure 9.6 is for DM_2. The platform is the genetic, anatomical, physiological, and biochemical basis of human life that South Asians almost wholly share with other populations. All human diseases have a foundational genetic basis which underpins the platform. This does not preclude some specific genetic pieces in the jigsaw itself as well as on the platform but I have not found the need for this because no important specific differences have been found to justify this. On this platform I overlay a cloth—the socio-economic and social circumstances in which the population is living. The main pieces of the jigsaw can now be put in place, i.e. the major cardiovascular risk factors. Figure 9.7 shows the traditional risk factors—tobacco, hypertension, raised LDL-C, inactivity, obesity, depression, etc—as the shaded but unlabelled pieces. This will leave a few, albeit important, gaps, i.e. on the particular susceptibility of South Asians to CVD. What are these pieces? I propose these as follows:

♦ Glycation of tissues, particularly the vasculature, from hyperglycaemia from birth and IFG, IGT, and DM_2 later in life, compounded by the ingestion of compounds including, but not only, AGEs, in the cuisine(107, 734–737)

♦ Glycation leads to microvascular damage, possibly including the vasa vasorum (a new concept in the context of South Asians' health), allowing two pathways to atherosclerosis, the other being endothelial dysfunction, as illustrated in

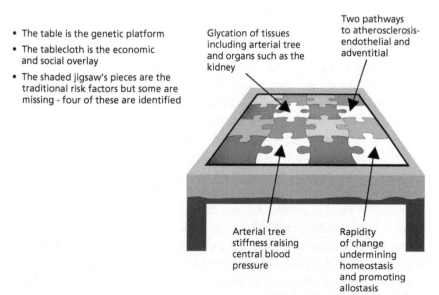

- The table is the genetic platform
- The tablecloth is the economic and social overlay
- The shaded jigsaw's pieces are the traditional risk factors but some are missing - four of these are identified

Glycation of tissues including arterial tree and organs such as the kidney

Two pathways to atherosclerosis-endothelial and adventitial

Arterial tree stiffness raising central blood pressure

Rapidity of change undermining homeostasis and promoting allostasis

Figure 9.5 The jigsaw puzzle analogy pinpointing the factors increasing susceptibility of South Asians to CVD.

- The table is the genetic platform
- The tablecloth is the economic and social overlay
- The jigsaw puzzle has some pieces missing - eight are proposed

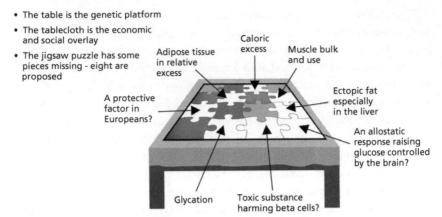

Figure 9.6 The jigsaw puzzle analogy for DM_2.

Figure 1.2 (68, 69, 71, 73, 75) Glycated products may also damage other organs, e.g. the kidneys, contributing indirectly to CVD(738, 739)

- Stiffness of the arterial tree partly caused by glycation, leads to raised central BP augmenting the risks(399)
- Rapidity of change in risk factors meaning that homeostasis is not achieved, leading to allostatic changes resetting the normal values, e.g. for weight, BP, cholesterol, etc(571, 740). The reduction in physical activity may be one of the most important of such risk factor changes, with a trial in South Asians showing the benefits of exercise are lost within days of stopping(589).

In this new synthesis, the long-standing emphasis on DM_2 and metabolic dysfunction as underlying a high risk of CVD in South Asians is retained but the emphasis is shifted from insulin and insulin resistance to the role of glucose in glycation of tissues. The role of glycated products in the cuisine is a relative newcomer to the clinical story, although studied carefully in laboratory and animal sciences. Arterial stiffness is in this synthesis is seen not merely as a consequence or marker of other factors, e.g. short stature, but especially through its effect on central BP, an important cause. I emphasize that these proposals do not undermine, in any way, the role of established risk factors. They offer a path to understanding South Asians' high susceptibility to CVD. The rapidity of change in lifestyles with unusually rapid re-setting of physiological norms in glucose, BP, LDL-C, adipose tissue with attendant inflammation, and other factors invokes and adds to the adaptation—dysadaptation concept by spelling out the pathways and invoking the mechanism of allostasis.

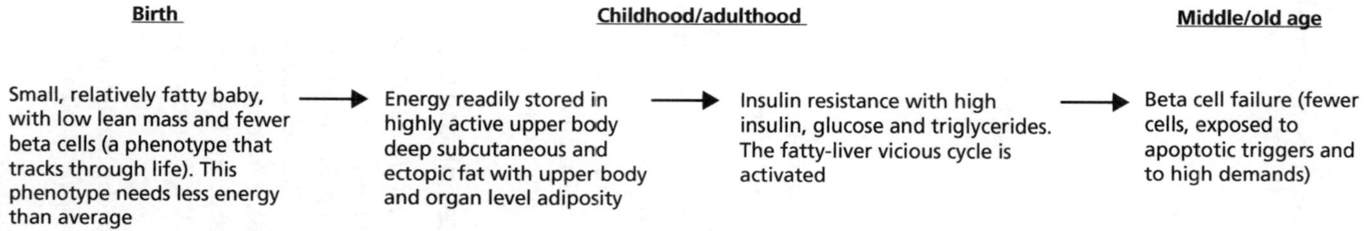

Birth

Small, relatively fatty baby, with low lean mass and fewer beta cells (a phenotype that tracks through life). This phenotype needs less energy than average

→

Childhood/adulthood

Energy readily stored in highly active upper body deep subcutaneous and ectopic fat with upper body and organ level adiposity

→

Insulin resistance with high insulin, glucose and triglycerides. The fatty-liver vicious cycle is activated

→

Middle/old age

Beta cell failure (fewer cells, exposed to apoptotic triggers and to high demands)

Figure 9.7 A four-stage model explaining the excess of diabetes in South Asians compared to Europeans.

Reproduced from Bhopal, RS. A four-stage model explaining the higher risk of Type 2 diabetes mellitus in South Asians compared with European populations. *Diabetic Medicine.* 30(1):35–42. Copyright © Raj Bhopal. Open Access.

In this account I have de-emphasized many previously heavily emphasized factors including the following:

- The stresses of migratory process in itself (as opposed to through altering lifestyles)
- Consanguinity
- Specific genetic polymorphisms
- Air pollution
- Alcohol
- Milk and lactose intolerance
- Specific dietary factors including vitamins, whether in excess or in deficit
- A generic pro-inflammatory state
- A high burden of infection
- A generic prothombotic state
- Insulin resistance
- Anatomical differences whether anthropometry or related to the cardiovascular system, e.g. narrow coronary arteries
- Numerous specific biochemical factors as being consequences of atherosclerosis or by-standers, excepting those parts of the accepted or likely causal pathways of LDL-C and triglycerides.

This synthesis is offered for critical scrutiny. In Section 9.7 I will summarize the views of a group of international scholars and see whether these support or alter this synthesis, which was prepared prior to such discussions.

9.6 DM$_2$: fitting the pieces of the puzzle

My paper providing a simple model (Figure 9.7) on the causes of the high risk of DM$_2$ in South Asians compared to White Europeans observed the paradox that more than 23 major risk factors had been identified but the conclusions of major reviews, including that of Ramachandran et al., were that the causes were still to be identified(78, 96). I noted some contradictions in the evidence, e.g. that the BMI of Bangladeshis is lower than in other South Asians and Europeans but their risk of DM$_2$ is higher. In essence the causal pathway proposed was:

- A comparatively low birthweight, relatively adipose South Asian baby with a low lean mass and possibly relatively fewer pancreatic beta cells is born
- This body type persists through the lifespan

- An excess of calories in urban environments leads to rapid, preferential deposition of fat in central and ectopic fat stores, rather than in superficial subcutaneous fat stores
- There is an exacerbation of the birth phenotype of high blood insulin, glucose, and triglycerides with fat deposition in the liver, creating a fatty-liver vicious cycle
- Pancreatic beta cell failure occurs from a combination of possibly fewer cells at birth and early life, high rates of cell death, and high demands, with DM_2 as the outcome.

This explanation drew entirely on the published literature and rested heavily on the DOHAD hypothesis but incorporated elements of others including the adipose tissue compartment and insulin resistance hypotheses. The role of fat in the liver in impairing glucose control was emphasized as was the finding that for some metabolic outcomes including glucose, insulin and insulin resistance, and triglycerides, South Asians need a BMI of about 22–24 to have the same levels as Europeans with a BMI of about 30. My paper emphasized that there is no inherent biological disadvantage in the South Asian phenotype of low birth weight, low muscle mass, and the central distribution of adipose tissue(96). It is the effect of the modern environment and lifestyle that is the problem.

This causal synthesis has, on reflection, two major strengths—simplicity and coherence. It is still in line with the evidence. It is, in my current view, incomplete and needing critical review and further development.

In Chapter 5 I found, to my surprise, unconvincing evidence for the DOHAD hypothesis. Putting on weight in later childhood and adulthood is clearly more important than intrauterine conditions as reflected in birthweight and similar markers. The importance of physical activity, muscular strength, and fitness has become clearer in recent years and seems of especial importance in South Asians. Evidence has emerged that, just as with BMI and waist circumference, the recommendations on physical activity based on Europeans may not apply. South Asians may need up to double the amount of physical activity recommended for Europeans. At a BMI of about 22 kg/m^2 and moderate to vigorous activity of 7 hours per week, including muscle toning and muscle building exercise, DM_2 would not be especially common in South Asians, as has historically been the case in rural, agricultural environments in South Asia.

Epidemiological and genetic evidence indicates that beta cell dysfunction, rather than insulin resistance, is the key problem for South Asians(123, 140, 157, 741–744). The question of why the beta cells fail is unresolved. The usual explanation is beta cell exhaustion. But, why would this occur? Mostly, tissues and cells respond to the need by growing, replicating, or becoming more efficient rather than either dying (apoptosis) or becoming exhausted. This kind of positive response happens with, for example, muscle cells. Indeed, people with DM_2 have high insulin before and many decades after diagnosis indicating a well-functioning beta cell mass. South Asians clearly have a responsive, active beta cell mass throughout most of their lives.

DM_2 'runs in families' and clearly so in South Asians but that does not imply there are special genetic mechanisms at work—genetic research shows mostly similar associations (with modest differences) between gene variants and DM_2(123, 140). As with the model for CVD, the genes provide the platform for DM_2 too on which we overlay the social and economic circumstances of the population. The question now is: given this platform what causes DM_2 to occur in South Asians so very commonly?

Figure 9.6 develops the jigsaw puzzle analogy for DM_2. Although CVD is more complex than DM_2, the large (about four-fold) difference in the prevalence of disease between South Asians and Europeans is more difficult to explain. The relative adiposity and low muscle mass are relevant but, in my view, not sufficient to explain this discrepancy. The figure proposes four, core concepts for making progress:

◆ Rather than looking for reason why South Asians have so much DM_2, we should look to why Europeans have less

◆ The brain may be setting or re-setting blood glucose at a higher level in South Asians, to optimize brain function for new kinds of behaviour as advocated by Watve (136) or to overcome difficulties in supplying nutrients to the brain, possibly because of microvascular impairment

◆ The higher blood and tissue glucose and other substances, possibly including AGEs and other neoformed contaminants in food, may be leading to microcirculatory damage

◆ This damage may, I hypothesize, include the microcirculation of the Islets of Langerhans in the pancreas, imparing blood flow and hence causing beta cell dysfunction that leads to DM_2.

Gerstein has proposed that the complications of diabetes are a result of microvascular problems leading to tissue ischaemia. However, he has not suggested that this might also be the reason for the occurrence of DM_2(70). Amongst others, Sattar and colleagues have pointed to the potential harmful role of ectopic fat in the pancreas(157, 562). This is a possibility though unproven. In a case–control study, Misra et al. found pancreatic volume was increased and it was correlated with body fat, but there was no direct measure of pancreatic adiposity (745) A recent review of ectopic fat including in the pancreas showed no evidence for an important role for pancreatic fat(533). It is hard, however, to see why ectopic fat should be harmful in the pancreas (unlike in the liver where it causes insulin resistance).

I don't think insulin resistance is the cause of beta cell exhaustion or failure and propose that we should be looking for substances that are compounding the effects of adiposity and damaging beta cells directly or via their micro-vasculature.

9.7 A summary of causal explanations offered by 22 scholars/researchers

Twenty two of 29 invited scholars/researchers from India, UK, Canada, US, and New Zealand participated in discussions (see appendix table 11.1 for names and web addresses for further information about them). The agreed summaries of discussions are also in the appendix. The discussants were invited to talk about DM_2 or CVD or both. The number of researchers/scholars working on this topic in a sustained way is quite small and they influence each other's views, so these cannot be considered to be independent. Indeed, much of this book is based on reading their work, so it is not surprising that even before these discussions I had covered, I believe, every explanation offered in the discussions.

There were three kinds of explanations offered: general hypothesis, general mechanisms, and specific mechanisms. These are summarized in Table 9.2 with the names of the people (given in alphabetical order) referring to them.

The overwhelming message from these scholars and researchers was that South Asians' susceptibility to CVD and DM_2 is a complex matter that cannot yet be explained, although we have much helpful knowledge about it. Only one specific explanation was proposed as a primary, explanatory factor for CHD in South Asians, i.e. lipoprotein(a) by Dr Enas Enas who has studied this factor carefully. Several other scholars who have also examined this factor in empirical studies did not endorse this view.

Explanations based on evolutionary effects over multiple generations and epigenetic, developmental effects over a few generations were mentioned commonly but, by contrast, the thrifty genotype and most other hypotheses considered in Chapters 1–4 were not.

In Table 9.2 I have listed some general observations that were not developed as hypotheses but offered mechanisms. The most frequently mentioned mechanism was life-course exposure to risk factors, perhaps around and from conception, e.g. high level of fetal exposure to glucose because of gestational diabetes mellitus.

Table 9.2 General causal concepts/explanations emphasized by scholars/researchers in the discussions

Causal concept/explanation	Scholars/researchers offering the explanation
Low pancreatic beta cell number/impaired development	Dorairaj Prabhakaran, Chittaranjan Yajnik, Salim Yusuf
Pelvic and other constraints to birth size	Jonathan Wells
DOHAD/thrifty phenotype/low birth weight and related markers/capacity load model	Sonia Anand, Caroline Fall, Jason Gill, Latha Palaniappan, Dorairaj Prabhakaran, Milind Watve, Jonathan Wells, Chittaranjan Yajnik, Salim Yusuf
Thrifty genotype	Alka Kanaya
Genetic polymorphisms specifically, including those relating to Lp (a))	Sonia Anand, Enas Enas (Lp (a)), Alka Kanaya (especially for DM_2), Kamlesh Khunti (for DM_2), Latha Palaniappan Paul McKeigue
Evolutionary changes from agricultural practices and famine ◆ Survival advantages ◆ Maintaining fertility	Venkat Narayan, Milind Watve, Alka Kanaya, Chittaranjan Yajnik
Variable disease selection hypotheses	Jonathan Wells
Neurobehavioural hypotheses, e.g. soldier-to-diplomat	Milind Watve
Adipose tissue compartment overflow	Alka Kanaya
Adaptation—dysadaptation over evolutionary timescales	Venkat Narayan, Jonathan Wells
Demographic and epidemiological transitions	Dorairaj Prabhakaran
Stressors around migration including racism (psychosocial factors)	Sonia Anand, Richard Cooper, Rajeev Gupta, Alka Kanaya, Karien Stronks
Social and environmental change and social group norms (e.g. inactivity and eating)	Karien Stronks
Insulin resistance (but not causal in itself)	Paul McKeigue
Pancreatic ectopic fat	Anoop Misra
Central adiposity, weight gain, obesity, ectopic fat	Sonia Anand, Caroline Fall, Jason Gill, Rajeev Gupta, Alka Kanaya, Sanjay Kinra, Anoop Misra, Dorairaj Prabhakaran
Diet a) with high glycaemic index and low protein b) harmful oils c) low fruit/vegetable content	Sonia Anand, Nita Forouhi, Rajeev Gupta, Paul McKeigue, Anoop Misra, Latha Palaniappan, Dorairaj Prabhakaran, Salim Yusuf
Cooking style with high temperature and TFAs and other adulterants	Rajeev Gupta, Dorairaj Prabhakaran

Table 9.2 Continued

Causal concept/explanation	Scholars/researchers offering the explanation
Diet—ingredient in food, possibly oils and other fats	Paul McKeigue
Micronutrient deficiency/imbalance	Venkat Narayan
Vit D deficiency/binding	Robert Scragg
Low alcohol use	Robert Scragg, Salim Yusuf
Metabolic perturbation that underlines both high CVD and metabolic syndrome	Paul McKeigue
Traditional risk factors	Sanjay Kinra
Risk factor thresholds vary	Dorairaj Prabhakaran
Life-time exposures to risk factors, e.g. to maternal gestational diabetes mellitus and hence hyperglycaemia	Sonia Anand, Caroline Fall, Nita Forouhi, Jason Gill, Sanjay Kinra, Venkat Narayan, Jonathan Wells, Salim Yusuf
Exposure to high levels of glucose	Sonia Anand, Richard Cooper, Rajeev Gupta, Kamlesh Khunti, Salim Yusuf
Low physical activity/sedentary lifestyle	Nita Forouhi, Jason Gill, Rajeev Gupta, Alka Kanaya, Kamlesh Khunti, Sanjay Kinra, Karien Stronks, Jonathan Wells, Salim Yusuf
Physical fitness	Jason Gill
Arterial stiffness	Sanjay Kinra, Robert Scragg
Central BP raised	Robert Scragg
Microvascular damage/dysfunction	Richard Cooper, Jason Gill
Lipid disturbances a) lipoprotein A to B ratio b) Some aspects of LDL-C	Sonia Anand, Paul McKeigue, Latha Palaniappan, Karien Stronks, Jonathan Wells, Chittaranjan Yajnik, Salim Yusuf
Muscle mass and function	Nita Forouhi, Jason Gill, Anoop Misra, Latha Palaniappan, Dorairaj Prabhakaran, Milind Watve, Chittaranjan Yajnik, Salim Yusuf
Infection burden	Dorairaj Prabhakaran
Inflammatory response	Kamlesh Khunti, Dorairaj Prabhakaran, Milind Watve
Pollutants ◆ Organic ◆ Air	Alka Kanaya Sanjay Kinra, Dorairaj Prabhakaran
Health care for prevention	Karien Stronks
Europeans may be the outliers for DM_2	Milind Watve, Salim Yusuf

Genetic factors, mostly gene–environment interactions rather than specific genetic polymorphisms, were also commonly discussed, usually with the caveat that this kind of work is at an early stage. The geographically widespread and persistent intergenerational susceptibility to CVD and DM_2 favoured a genetic basis according to Paul McKeigue even although it has been hard to pin down. Most scholars, however, thought the evidence in favour of a predominately genetic basis for South Asians' susceptibility was weak.

Jason Gill, alone, emphasized that disease outcomes can induce epigenetic changes and we cannot assume epigenetic changes cause diseases. The specific genetic link via Lp(a) was emphasized by Enas Enas.

Stress of one kind or another, including racism was, considered by a few people. Other general explanations were mentioned by only one or two people. Sanjay Kinra proposed that we need to study the traditional risk factors more carefully. Karien Stronks was alone in drawing attention to a relative lack of effective preventative health services.

Of specific risk factors and mechanisms in Table 9.2 the most common were:

◆ Patterns of adiposity and ectopic fat

◆ Lipid disturbances

◆ Long exposure to high levels of glucose

◆ Poor quality diets

◆ Muscle mass and function, physical fitness/activity and sedentary behaviours.

Among the other specific ideas noted were vitamin D deficiency, arterial stiffness with its consequence of raised central blood pressure, pancreatic ectopic fat, and pancreatic beta cell number and development.

Amongst these scholars there were some points of focus and much agreement, e.g. DOHAD, diet, physique, and physical activity. A lack of emphasis on some factors was surprising, given how they are emphasised in the scientific literature, e.g. lack of emphasis on genetics or insulin resistance.

The range of views, together with the candid admissions that the issues were complex, indicate that there is no generally agreed coherent explanatory framework (a theory) or set of risk factors for the questions under consideration.

Some of the newer ideas I have introduced in this book, e.g. microcirculatory damage and arterial stiffness were only occasionally mentioned by discussants and the vasa vasorum was not mentioned. I generally listened, and did not propose my views. However, on the occasions when I did raise them, e.g. microvascular damage of the vasa vasorum and raised central BP, scholars were interested and indicated they deserved further consideration.

9.8 **Conclusions**

This synthesis draws on theoretical work on hypotheses (Chapters 2–5), empirical work examining the distribution of risk factors and risk factor-disease-outcome relationships (Chapters 7–8), and broad analyses of the socio-economic and psychosocial backdrop to the epidemics of CVD and DM_2 (Chapter 6). The synthesis is supported by simple causal diagrams and a metaphor of solving a jigsaw puzzle. In Chapter 1 I introduced this metaphor with a scattering of the pieces of the puzzle and here I have offered a solution, albeit one still missing pieces.

Two important principles have underpinned this synthesis. First, given that all human populations are similar, and the demonstration that causes tend to be near-universally applicable, I have adopted the principle that if a factor X causes CVD (or DM_2) in one human population (say Europeans) it will cause it in another (e.g. South Asians). I think it is likely that even if the relations cannot be shown at one point of time, e.g. BMI and CVD, they will emerge, as sometimes co-factors are required. Given this principle, this synthesis can concentrate on what is different in South Asians especially in comparison with White Europeans.

The second principle is that I have attributed enabler or protector status to genetic, socio-economic, and psychosocial factors, rather than thinking of them as primary causes. The one exception is depression for which the evidence is strong. This is a contestable decision, but it allows me to concentrate on specific factors, nearly all related to lifestyle. This decision implies that there are no important specific genetic or socio-economic factors that are particular to South Asians. I think the research in these areas to date justifies this position as reasonable.

In my jigsaw puzzle metaphor, I have illustrated genetic factors as the platform. This platform is overlaid by the tablecloth of socio-economic and psychosocial factors. The pieces of the puzzle are presumed mostly to be the same as for European populations, but in some ways they are different. The causal diagrams (Figures 9.1–9.4 and 9.6) provide two kinds of information, i.e. what is absent (and hence demoted from the central narrative) and how the elements that are present link up.

The causes arise from lifestyle change, itself driven by industrialization, mechanization, and urbanization. The high susceptibility to CVD in South Asians is attributed to three specific factors and one general one. The three specific factors—glycation of tissues, endothelial (internal) and adventitial (external, microvascular) pathways to atherosclerosis, and arterial stiffness—may have a unifying underlying cause, i.e. a high exposure to substances that cause glycosylation. These include glucose and other sugars and neoformed contaminants in food including AGEs.

The general factor is the rapidity of lifestyle change leading to allostasis with resetting of physiological levels for glucose, blood pressure, etc, rather than the expected homeostasis. These factors sit alongside the traditional, accepted risk factors, e.g. smoking cigarettes/bidis, transfats, high LDL-C, etc. In the last 30–40 years the potential role of DM_2 and its precursors of IFG and IGT in the South Asian CVD epidemic has been emphasized. The previous emphasis, however, has been on insulin resistance (and more rarely on glucose itself(737)) rather than glucose as a glycating agent, glycosylation by other chemicals, and microcirculatory effects, as here.

The question of why South Asians have so much DM_2 and its precursors, including relatively high levels of glucose, needs to be resolved. It may be that the explanation lies in protective factors in Europeans as much, if not more, than risk factors in South Asians(137, 746). There are two important questions. First, why do South Asians have high fasting glucose levels? Second, why in later life do they get pancreatic beta cell failure leading to DM_2? The only good explanation I have found is that the high glucose may be an adaptive change to ensure delivery of high levels of glucose to the brain for optimal functioning. This is Watve's concept(102, 136). I don't, however, find the specific behavioural explanations for why this has occurred over evolutionary timescales convincing. It seems to me that it might be linked to size at birth. Beta cell failure is hard to explain. The concept that the beta cells become exhausted is not convincing. Why should that happen? One explanation is that the pancreas is infiltrated with ectopic fat. Even if that turns out to be so, why should such fat be harmful? I propose an alternative, i.e. that the damage to the pancreas is through the effects of glycosylation and microcirculatory damage. Alternatively, there may be other toxic chemicals, possibly neo-formed contaminants in food, e.g. AGEs.

This synthesis has implications for public health policy and practice, clinical care including preventive advice and care, and research. In the final chapter I examine and summarize global and South Asian approaches to the prevention and control of CVD and DM_2. I then distil existing specific guidance that has focused on the South Asian population. Finally, I modify this approach and guidance in the light of the evidence in Chapters 1–8, and this synthesis. I then set out some priorities for future scholarship and research, which by implication, if not explicitly, also inform us on what might be deprioritized.

Chapter 10

Implications for health policy, public health, health care, and research

10.1 Chapter 10 objectives are to:

1. Consider the implications of the synthesis in Chapter 9 for public health policy, public health practice, clinical practice, and research.
2. To integrate the guidance in the literature on the prevention and control of CVD and DM_2 with particular reference to South Asians.
3. Make recommendations to prevent the further rise of the epidemics of diabetes, CHD and stroke, especially in rural areas of South Asia and in future generations.
4. Reflect on the research agenda arising.

10.2 Chapter summary

Many policy documents exist on how to control the epidemics of chronic diseases globally, and there is a growing body of guidance that focuses on South Asian diaspora populations and South Asian countries. This guidance can be summarized as: apply particularly vigorously the internationally agreed CVD and DM_2 prevention and treatment strategies, with actions at a lower than usual threshold of risk factors. The problem is that achieving such strategies is extremely difficult even in high resource environments such as the UK, and for the population there and doing so for South Asians specifically would be even tougher. Most of the guidance is centred on individual level behaviour change. The challenge is to produce focused, low cost, effective actions, underpinned by clear, simple, and accurate explanations of the causes of the phenomenon. Setting aside popular but probably non-causal explanations is important.

The key messages for both professionals and the public are that the high risk of CVD and DM_2 in urbanizing South Asians is real but not inevitable. It is not innate or genetic. Similarly, the risks are unlikely to be acquired in utero, birth, or infancy, and programmed in a fixed way. Rather, exposure to risk factors in childhood, adolescence, and most particularly in adulthood is the key. In addition to studying the established causes and especially the thresholds at which they have their effects—tobacco, high BP, obesity, physical inactivity, diabetes mellitus, LDL-cholesterol, and psychological disorders such as depression—we need to research additional factors. Insulin resistance and high natural insulin, topics that have been the centre of attention, are likely to be markers and not direct causes.

More focus is needed on the content of the diet, muscle bulk, and the amount and nature of physical activity. The preparation of food and the production of neo-formed contaminants need close examination, especially in association with glycosylation of tissues by hyperglycaemia. Atherosclerosis in South Asians may be accompanied by arterial stiffness with raised central BP. Combination of both endothelial dysfunction and microvascular damage to the vasa vasorum needs consideration as causes of atherosclerosis.

A public health strategy targeted at mostly individuals and families is unlikely to work either well or fast enough. The priority should be national legislation and policy that alters environments to reduce exposure to risk factors and increase exposure to protective factors. Preventative health care needs to be targeted to reduce tobacco use, overweight/obesity, hypertension, exposure to transfats, exposure to glycating agents, and LDL-levels. Actions are required to increase physical activity, muscle strength, fitness, and diets with complex carbohydrates and uncooked or lightly cooked foods, especially vegetables and fruits. Causal explanations offer a means for controlling the epidemics of CVD and DM_2 in South Asians globally.

10.3 Introduction: approaches to intervention, the state of the art, and the need for a new causal synthesis

The history of medicine and public health shows that when the cause(s) of a diseases or health problem are understood, effective interventions usually follow, albeit sometimes slowly. Recent examples of this principle with both medical and public health consequences include the discoveries that 1) gastric ulcer (and gastric cancer too) is not, as long-believed, a complex matter resulting from stressors but an infection with particular strains of the bacterium *Helicobacter pylori*, and 2) that cancer of the cervix is mostly the result of an infection by the human papilloma virus. These recent discoveries add to historical ones around previously mysterious nutritional diseases such as scurvy (vitamin C deficiency) and pellagra (niacin, vitamin B_3 deficiency), and cancers caused by smoking cigarettes. The prevention, control, or cure of such problems becomes logical, rational, efficient, and effective as a result of causal knowledge. Causal knowledge is, rightly, the jewel in the crown of all scientific disciplines(27, 747).

Unfortunately, for CVD and DM_2, whether generally or in South Asians, specific causal knowledge of the kind in the above examples is not yet available but it will be. As considered in Chapter 1, causal thinking on these conditions is based on a complex model of interrelating risk factors. The complexity is partially captured by the web of causation as shown in Figure 10.1(27) This web of causation is for CHD but similar ones could be constructed for stroke and DM_2. The figure emphasizes that there are many relevant factors that are interconnected, only some causally. Even more importantly, it emphasizes the connections between risk factor-to-disease, disease-to-risk factor (reverse causality), and risk factor-to-risk factor. To take an example, smoking cigarettes may both cause CHD directly and by impairing physical activity through damaging the lungs and causing breathlessness and inhibiting exercise. CHD also has effects on some of its risk factors, e.g. by causing shortness of breath or chest discomfort that inhibits physical activity, that may then promote obesity and then high BP, which in turn affects both CVD and DM_2. The development of DM_2 will worsen CHD, and vice versa, with a downward spiral in health.

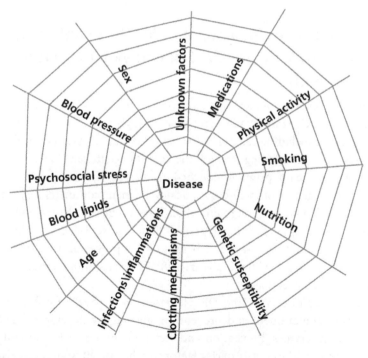

Figure 10.1 Web of causation and coronary heart disease.
Reproduced with permission from Bhopal, RS. (2016) *Concepts of Epidemiology*. Oxford, UK: OUP. Copyright © 2016 OUP.

Currently, we operate on the multifactorial model for CVD and DM_2. In future new causal knowledge will bring greater clarity and in turn better interventions, exactly as has happened with other complex diseases where the specific causes were pinpointed. Nevertheless, the current multifactorial model works very well for pragmatic healthcare and public health interventions at both an individual and population level for CVD and DM_2.

Models are simplifications of reality and that is their strength. Their role is to promote reflection, condense understanding, and point to possible actions. In Chapter 9 we examined a causal synthesis which is just one possible causal model. In this chapter we consider how this synthesis might help in public policy, public health, health care and research. This synthesis rests on 70 or more years of intense research and scholarship internationally. Scholars, researchers, policy makers and practitioners have also worked hard in developing strategies and practical actions to control and prevent CVD and DM_2. The challenge is to refine and improve the existing guidance in the light of the new synthesis. Before I do this, I need to sketch out, broadly, the current approach and directions in these arenas.

10.4 Public health policy, public health, health care, and research: principles underlying the current approach

Health policy internationally, whether through the UN, WHO or other influential players such as the World Bank, places a high priority on the control of chronic disease including CVD and DM_2, as these are seen as major health and economic threats, including through the costs of health care(111). The solutions, however, are not primarily couched in terms of fundamental issues such as changing the nature of socio-economic development, commercial enterprise or the phenomenon of rapid urbanization. There is no international policy, for example, promoting ruralization to prevent these disease(51). Even if there was such a policy, it would not work as urbanization has proven unstoppable across the world in the last few hundred years(748). It is a fact of modern life, which shows no sign of reversing.

Health policy for CVDs and DM_2 is based on established public health strategies of containment and prevention, and on the development of effective health services. Prevention and containment for CVD and DM_2 are based squarely on the control of risk factors, i.e. healthy lifestyles, and also on health care, e.g. for smoking cessation, and drug treatment to prevent, halt, or slow disease progression. These strategies have been developed, advanced, and tested in wealthy industrialized countries where the CVD and DM_2 epidemics are long-established but the same ideas are being implemented, albeit with refinement and local adaptation, in South Asian countries(23, 47, 62, 744, 749, 750).

The experience in wealthy, industrialized countries in Europe and the US is that the incidence of CVD can be reduced through risk factor control, and the risk of death and severe disability can be diminished by early treatment(751–753). These strategies were expected, in modelling studies, to reduce cardiovascular mortality by about 80%. Remarkably, this has been achieved. Since the 1960s/1970s when cardiovascular mortality was at its maximum in North America and Northern Europe, we have seen remarkable declines in mortality rates though somewhat less so in incidence rates. The success of these strategies has led to over-optimistic claims that CHD will be rare in the UK by 2050. Presently, as longevity following the onset of CHD has increased so has the number of people with chronic complications such as angina and heart failure. About half of the decline in CVD mortality is attributed to lifestyle change and half to better health care(753, 754). These strategies are expensive but, with the main exception of death within hours or days following a first MI or stroke, are effective and cost-effective for CVDs(754).

For DM_2 success has been limited at a national scale as the disease is increasing everywhere, and this is particularly striking in South Asia, but it's preventability is demonstrable in trials, mostly on people at high risk, e.g. with IGT or IFG(50, 324, 744). The effectiveness of such interventions when scaled up on a large scale and put into routine care is less than in trial settings(755–757). Some limited evidence focuses on South Asian populations both in South Asia and in the South Asian diaspora(758–764). The effects of interventions in South Asians, clearly, are less than in White populations in Europe or North America(765, 766). The reasons seem to relate to the greater difficulties in achieving set goals, especially but not solely, in weight loss and increasing physical activity(763, 764). In contrast to CVD risk factors such as cigarette smoking and hypertension, which are declining in many countries, obesity and physical inactivity have risen sharply over the last 40 years. This has impeded efforts to control the epidemic of DM_2 and probably slowed the decline in CVD. Notwithstanding the limited empirical research evidence on their effectiveness in routine, non-trial settings, clear recommendations for the control of DM_2, as for CVD, are available as considered below.

10.5 **Current approaches and recommendations on the prevention and control of CVD and DM$_2$ in South Asians**

We will examine the recommendations with emphasis on those from the UK, the US, and India, and especially on the latter given it has published detailed guidance tailoring advice for South Asians.

There is a long history, going back at least 40 years in the UK, in the provision of guidelines for the primary prevention and management of CVD and DM$_2$ and to prevent recurrence and complications(477). As emphasized in Chapter 1 and subsequently the main problem in South Asians is a raised incidence of these diseases rather than worse outcomes(767, 768). For this reason, the focus here is on primary prevention, which reduces disease incidence rather than on secondary prevention or health care that improve outcomes after the disease occurs.

The outcome following the occurrence of CVD, surprisingly, given the high rates of DM$_2$ and contrary to a few early, local studies, seems to be similar or even better in South Asians than European or other comparison groups, at least in settings where good quality, equitable health care is available(4, 767, 769–773).

While the management of DM$_2$ is a great challenge in South Asians and HbA1c levels, in particular, seldom shift downwards(774), some outcomes are better (e.g. peripheral vascular disease, and possibly the detrimental effect on life expectancy), some similar (CHD and stroke), and some worse (retinopathy and renal disease)(516, 775–781).

The principles underlying the management of CVD and DM$_2$ are much the same across ethnic groups. Guidelines focusing on the clinical care of South Asians, however, usually emphasize the need to tackle these diseases especially vigorously in South Asians.

The traditional approach to the prevention of CVD is to identify and tackle individual risk factors. If BP is high, at a systolic value of 150 mmHg, the individual would be managed to reduce BP below the acceptable threshold, which is currently 140 mmHg. The management would be based on lifestyle advice such as to lose weight, increase physical activity, and reduce salt intake. If this was ineffective antihypertensive drugs would be prescribed. This traditional approach is still the dominant one across the world, notwithstanding guidelines advising otherwise as considered later in this section. To be successful this approach requires that people without symptoms or signs of CVD are identified before the onset of complications. This requires screening apparently healthy populations, either as they attend health or other services such as pharmacies, or in specially designed community screening programmes, and more usually a mixture of these.

The guidelines based on this kind of approach are inherently complex. I have summarized and integrated several sets of guidelines designed for South Asian populations in Table 10.1. These guidelines can be succinctly summarized as follows: South Asians should follow the principles of the prevention approaches developed mostly in European origin populations but their targets are more stringent. The guidelines from India, in particular, but also from other South Asian countries tend to be more stringent than those in the UK or USA(116, 117, 217, 418, 529, 749, 750, 782, 783). There is nothing unique to South Asians in these guidelines though there is greater emphasis on HDL-C, Lp(a) and triglycerides than in guidelines developed for general populations in the UK or the USA(784–786).

It is likely that the guidelines I have summarized in Table 10.1 are correct in principle. There are, however, several problems. First, it has been difficult to achieve behaviour change of the kind promoted in Table 10.1 anywhere and particularly in South Asian populations, although sometimes small-scale gains are reported(517, 760, 763, 764, 774, 787–790). The single risk factor change that has had an enormous impact in Northern Europe and North America is reduction in smoking of cigarettes, partly because the cardiovascular system is exquisitely sensitive to exposure to tobacco smoke(437, 753). The decline in smoking has been a response to a long, difficult, and costly programme of legislation, policy, education, and individual level services delivering counselling and medications. Education alone, whether at the population level or at the individual, has been shown to be of modest value.

Secondly, we do not have the evidence on either how to achieve the changes envisaged in these guidelines in large population, community settings, or on their costs and consequences. With all interventions there are side-effects and we do not know how benefits and disbenefits will line up. Even on an apparently desirable goal such as keeping the BMI in South Asians between 18.5 and 23, which will certainly bring the DM$_2$ epidemic to heel, may have other adverse consequences, e.g. on all-cause mortality, infections, and possibly even CVD. Third, one wonders whether some other, possibly more focused, approach might work better and at lower cost. We will return to that in Section 10.5.

The newer approach to the prevention of CVD is based on the management of predicted overall risk, rather than the individual risk factors(785, 791, 792). This same approach is under development for DM$_2$(793–795) but the account below focuses on CVD because we have much more experience of this. In this approach, we calculate the predicted risk using an algebraic equation that incorporates information about the individual, e.g. age, sex, and perhaps indicators of socio-economic status and risk factors, e.g. cigarette smoking, or

Table 10.1 Summarizing and integrating guidelines designed for the primary prevention of CVD and DM$_2$ in South Asians

Risk factor	Recommended action	Comment on recommendation	Source of guidelines
High BP	SBP <130 mmHg DBP < 80 (In DM$_2$, <120/70 mmHg)	This is slightly stricter than Misra et al. (2009) for diastolic BP (<85 mmHg)(421)	AAPI (Coronary Artery Disease Committee)(878)
Tobacco use	None in any form		Long-standing consensus worldwide
Diet	◆ Total fat 15–30 g; saturated fat <10 g ◆ <7% of energy from saturated fat ◆ <21% of energy from all fats	The type of fat is important and generic advice like this is under re-evaluation.	Indian Council of Medical Research 2009(879) Enas (from AHA Step II diet) (880)
	◆ No deep frying or re-heating of edible oils ◆ No foods with TFAs	This seems sensible but there are costs. It is sensible but zero trans fat is not possible	Kooner 1997(881)
	◆ Five plus servings of fruit and vegetable daily	This is sensible but costly for poor people	AAPI (CAD Committee)(878)
	◆ Avoid sugars, salt, and processed refined foods and drinks	This seems sensible but the effect on normal South Asian life is high.	
Overweight/Obesity	◆ Redefine cut-offs for South Asians so normal is BMI ≤23 kg/m^2 and waist ≤ 90 cm in men and ≤ 80 cm in women	These values are normal in traditional living rural South Asian populations but rare in urbanized and overseas South Asians, especially in women.	Misra et al. (2009)(782)

Physical inactivity	◆ 30 minutes daily moderate intensity activity ◆ 15 minutes work related activity daily ◆ Muscle strengthening exercises—15 minutes daily ◆ Vigorous activity to be added for additional benefit ◆ Children: 60–90 minutes (daily) of sport and physical activity	This level of activity is much greater than in European guidelines The idea of adding muscle strengthening is sensible.	Misra et al. (2009)(421) Misra et al. (2012)(217)
Hyperglycaemia	◆ HbA1c <6.5 ◆ Fasting glucose <5.5 mmol/l (<100 mg.dL)	These targets are challenging and yet sensible.	AAPI (CAD Committee)(878) Misra 2009(421, 782)
LDL-cholesterol and other lipids in the blood	Total cholesterol: ◆ <4.1 mmol/l (<160 mg/dL) ◆ LDL ≤ 3mmol/l ≤120 mg/dL) ◆ HDL >1.03 ≥40 mg/dL) ◆ Triglycerides <1.69 mmol/l (≤150 mg/dL)		Enas (418, 878) Misra 2009 (421, 782)

the level of LDL-C. The number of variables entered depends on which of the many available equations is used(791).

The equations are based on information gathered from cohort studies where the baseline measure, say, LDL-C, is related to disease outcome in a large population. If the study finds that a 1 mmol/l increase in LDL-C leads to a 25% increase in CVD, this is entered into the equation. This information is then extrapolated to the individual to create a single predicted risk, usually expressed as a percentage over 10 years, e.g. my risk is about 11% without family history included and 22% when it is included.

When such risk scores were introduced they were used to make decisions on who should be treated with drugs such as statins(796). A 30% 10-year risk was typically considered an appropriate cut-off for justifying such interventions. This cut-off dropped to 20%, especially as the costs of statins diminished and their efficacy and safety was established. Currently, there is advocacy for treatment at 10% or even lower predicted risk, i.e. at 1% or even less per year(797).

The art of CVD prediction is crude in any population(791). Most people who actually have a CVD event were not in the group predicted to have one (sensitivity or true positive proportion is low). The method depends on high quality, valid cohort studies and was pioneered by the Framingham study. There are at least a dozen widely used and endorsed equations from several cohort studies. None of these are based on specifically prospective South Asian cohort studies but a few have been tested in and adapted for South Asian populations, and new equations are being actively sought for multiethnic populations(792, 798–802).

I calculated my own risk using about ten of the main equations available on the internet. The variability of the result with 10-year risk from 7% to 22%, alone, raises questions about these methods(803). This kind of variability has been demonstrated both worldwide and in South Asian settings. Different calculators produce wildly varying predicted risks and, as we don't know which estimates are correct, their value in South Asian populations is unclear.

The logical basis of the prediction equation method is clear but we should remember the calculator provides a probability in a population, e.g. 12%. In contrast, the information is used at an individual level, where the event will either occur or not (0% or 100% probability). There is a logical gap and leap required that is not easy to bridge but it needs to be to gain informed consent from the patient. The calculation of numbers needed to treat (strictly, prevent) can be helpful to patients and clinicians alike, though these tend to be quite large and they don't necessarily make the decision easier(804).

Despite these qualifications there are merits of the prediction equation approach. This prediction method of engaging with the prevention and control of CVD has several advantages, including its potential to target limited resources to those in greatest need. These include a simpler assessment process and a simpler way of communicating with patients and communities. The prediction equations have been incorporated into easy-to-use internet and other platforms so members of the public can enter their own data and explore the predicted results of taking particular actions, e.g. stopping smoking.

The prediction methods are based on standard, established risk factors. Many studies have shown that adding other (so-called novel) risk factors, including genetic variants, does not materially improve the score(801, 805). None of the prediction models are based on South Asian cohort studies, and are less accurate in South Asian populations than in the European origin populations. The UKs Q-risk model (now in its third version) is based on a large dataset from general practice (primary care) records. In terms of addressing the needs on a range of ethnic groups in a multi-ethnic society (including UK South Asians) it is the best available(798, 806–809). This calculator's equations would need to be modified for use in South Asia settings but there is evidence that it works reasonably well there too(807).

The research on this topic concurs that most risk predictors are underestimating CVD risk in South Asians. Given the result of Forouhi et al.'s study, it is not surprising—important factors for South Asians are missing from the equation(1). Several solutions have been offered summarised in table 10.2 including these:

a) Double the calculated risk

b) Add 10-years to the actual age of a South Asian person before calculating

Table 10.2 Suggestions on the use of risk scores in South Asians

Authors (Year of publication)	Source of recommendation	Recommendation	Comment
Enas et al.(882)	1st Indo-US summit on CHD (2007)	◆ Double the calculated risk	It seems a slightly exaggerated response
Aarabi(883)		◆ Screening to start at 18 years of age ◆ Add 10 years to the age of the South Asian person	Reasonable but ambitious
JBS 1 and 2(884, 885)		◆ Multiply predicted risk by 1.4	This multiplication seems about right
Q-risk (JBS 3) (785, 806)		◆ Include ethnicity as a variable in risk calculation	In the long term, this seems the right approach and an alternative to creating prediction algorithms for each ethnic group

c) Multiply the calculated risk by 1.4

d) Include ethnicity as a variable within the prediction equation. This, of course, needs cohort data to assess the associated relative risks.

While there is much enthusiasm for this prediction approach, and it has been widely adopted, as with many medical technologies, there is no evidence that it is any more effective, or cost-effective, than the traditional approach of tackling individual risk factors. In common with other approaches, there is the issue of human behaviour. One of the most important decisions resulting from this approach is targeting statin prescriptions at those at high risk. Unfortunately, even in this high-risk group many, perhaps as much as 50%, discontinue their treatment. Indeed, discontinuing such treatment is very common even among those prescribed it following a diagnosis of CVD, where the benefits are greatest(797, 810).

In the next section, I examine the difficulties of moving recommendations from research, to policy to behaviour change in populations and individuals, as a prelude to an adjusted set of recommendations.

10.6 **Impediments to the implementation of recommendations**

The guidelines discussed in Section 10.3 and summarised in table 10.1 are excellent in theory. The problem is the practical one of implementation and achievement of the goals. While the behaviour of individuals and populations changes, and sometimes surprisingly fast, guiding change in a particular direction is immensely challenging. For example, eating chicken was a rare event in Europe in the late 1950s but is becoming an everyday one now. By contrast, a strong recommendation emphasized over recent decades for eating five portions of fruits and vegetables per day remains quite rare with hardly any change. The reason for this kind of discrepancy is the presence of countervailing forces, including human preferences, and insufficient individual, societal, and governmental support. In addition, there is often lack of knowledge, experience, person-power, and facilities to achieve the desired change.

These general points could be illustrated in relation to any of the major risk factors considered in Chapter 7 and the recommendations in Table 10.1. I will illustrate them in relation to diet and weight for the reason that this affects the entire population, and is an issue of special, symbolic, and sometimes religious significance in South Asian cultures. The impediments and challenges, however, are universal and not in any sense restricted to South Asians. For example, in the US and the UK, especially Scotland, upwards of 60% of the adult population is overweight or obese on WHO standards despite decades of research, public health policy, and services to combat the problem(62, 387). The potential good fortune for South Asians is they may be able to learn from the failures in this regard in North America and the UK.

The research evidence is limited but, nonetheless, it is already clear that South Asians across the world, whether children or adults, respond minimally or not at all to individually targeted advice to avoid weight gain or reduce weight(493, 760, 811). Indeed, and remarkably, a high proportion of people gain weight even while participating in weight loss interventions(764, 812).

As we have already considered, in South Asian cultures (and many others) being lean rather than slightly overweight is commonly perceived as a problem. The opportunity to eat tasty food, especially as part of family and community life is rightly seen, especially at celebrations, as a blessing(455, 457). The freedom from economically harsh times, and hunger, that are still commonly witnessed in the hundreds of millions of poor South Asian people, is also perceived as a blessing. The cuisines of South Asian countries are famed for their quality, economy, health-giving properties, and taste and are coveted, including by hundreds of millions of non-South Asians who come across them.

It is also a blessing to be freed up from manual work, as in South Asia especially it tends to be low paid and often in harsh heat outdoors. These insights are shared by people brought up in South Asian cultures. As a plump baby, child, and young adolescent I was seen as a model of good health. My late mother became concerned when I shed most of my fat in my post-adolescent growth spurt. These personal observations, insights, and anecdotes on diet, weight, and physical activity in South Asians have been demonstrated in many qualitative studies. It is interesting to find ethnic differences in perception about adiposity. South Asian women, in particular, are less likely to perceive themselves as overweight when they are, compared with White European women(164, 813). Their preferences are for plumper bodies. These preferences are, undoubtedly, changing across generations(814). In Norway, it was shown that South Asians are less likely to lose the weight they gain during pregnancy in the post-partum period, for unknown reasons, even although they are more likely to breast-feed(815). Are the reasons biological or cultural? We don't know, but I would judge the latter explanation is correct.

The challenge of the individual behaviour change approach is further compounded by the low levels of knowledge of human biology, anatomy, and on the causation of disease in a large proportion of the South Asian population

(370, 371, 458). A mixing of traditional concepts of health and disease, including ancient systems of medicine such as Ayurveda and Unani, with modern medicine is also an issue. For example, the matter of hot and cold foods (and other traditional concepts) is important in many South Asian cultures but it is not about the temperature of the foods but of the effects they have on the person, and in a complex way, not just on heating or cooling the body physically(598, 816, 817). Nutrition advice needs to be nuanced and informed in these circumstances. Clinicians also need to be aware that even their most educated patients may be using traditional forms of healing alongside the prescribed medications(818, 819).

The above account is by no means defeatist. Rather, it calls for a new approach, where the onus for behaviour change is not solely on individuals but is accepted by society as a whole, with alteration of the environment being the primary tool, and targeted individual change merely the back-up, secondary approach(23, 323, 463, 820). It is worth noting that this is also the case worldwide and not just a matter for South Asia. A good example of the kind of action that has brought rapid success are changes in subsidies on fats and oils in Mauritius (subsiding soybean oil rather than palm oil) and in Poland (reducing trans and other hydrogenated fats) and promoting fruits/vegetables(821, 822). There is no place where individual-based lifestyle change approaches have succeeded, except with meagre returns for high investment. The one arguable exception to this rule is smoking cessation but even that has been achieved in the context of societal changes including banning of cigarette advertising, restricting sales in many ways, and severe restrictions on smoking in public spaces and indoor environments. Before examining how the research synthesis allows us to modify existing recommendations I consider some of the lessons from the research on CVD and DM_2 in South Asians in the last 40 or so years.

10.6.1 Lessons from the past for future research on CVD and DM_2 in South Asians

Although the problems have been sporadically brought to attention, South Asian countries have been slow in responding to signals that there was an imminent epidemic of CVD and DM_2. Arnold's history of diabetes in South Asia shows that even around the year 1900 physicians were writing that wealthy Indians were highly prone to diabetes mellitus(84). It is not clear why research, public health policy, and medical care did not converge to understand and tackle DM_2 earlier. There was, certainly, distraction by the now rejected concept that this was a tropical form of diabetes mellitus. There was, understandably, difficulty in prioritizing this health problem given the many others of infections, maternal and child health mortality, and nutritional deficiency, a controversy that continues(823). It is noteworthy that the matter was brought to international attention by the publication of the survey of diabetes mellitus in Southall, London by Mather and Keen in 1985(35). The extraordinary high prevalence of diabetes mellitus in the predominantly Punjabi population in Southall was echoed by the not quite so high but still problematic levels of the disease in the Darya Ganj area of old Delhi, India reported in 1986(36).

For CVD, the reaction was even slower. The possibility that CVD, and especially CHD, might be a problem for South Asians was not in the public's or professionals' consciousness. In the 1950s evidence emerged from Singapore and Uganda that Indians were highly prone to CHD compared with other ethnic groups they lived alongside(374, 416). This evidence was soon augmented by epidemiological studies in South Africa, , the UK, the Caribbean, and Fiji(57, 824–826). Subsequently, UK researchers, led by Marmot and McKeigue, initiated a wave of both ideas and research that has provided impetus for work across the world, including major international studies such as INTERHEART and PURE(14, 85, 221, 323).

Having conducted empirical research in New Delhi, India in 1962, Padmavati published a major review including the prescient remark that India provides a fertile ground for a CVD epidemiologist (827, 828). Padmavati concluded that CHD prevalence was still low but was more common in the upper classes, noting that 32% of their dietary calories were from fat. In 1962 Wig et al. reported that in 151 people dying from suicide and other causes unrelated to CVD in Northern India, there was significant atheroma in 70–90%(829): A few community surveys and a large number of hospital-based case series(830–834) were done.

The Jaipur Heart Project established by Gupta et al. published key cross-sectional, data from about 2003 onwards, with subsequent extension of similar studies across India(327, 835–837). Potentially globally important research by R B Singh and colleagues, sadly, was placed under a shadow by questions of research integrity which is why I have not cited these publications. (https://www.bmj.com/content/suppl/2005/07/28/331.7511.281.DC1; accessed eighth of May 2018) Intriguing work on 1.15 million Indian railway workers by Malhotra gave implausible results including much more IHD in South India but more risk factors in North India(833). The results were accepted at face value and used to develop hypotheses that seem to me to be implausible(834, 838).

One early, small cohort study was published in 1993 by Chadha et al(839). Unfortunately, no large-scale Framingham-like cohort study was established, and case–control studies were local and mostly small. As South Asian countries are major contributors, the global INTERHEART studies have recently filled the knowledge gap in case–control data and the PURE studies are doing so for cohort data(85, 323).

Outside South Asia, too, cohort studies on South Asian populations have been late in starting though the conversion of the Brent and Southall cross-sectional studies into the cohort SABRE study has made an important advance(1, 98, 99). The West of London LOLIPOP cohort study, which has been reporting on subgroups and also genetic variations in relation to diseases, has huge potential for filling many gaps in our knowledge as the number of outcome events grows with time(123, 840). Evaluated and published randomized interventions for either DM_2 and CVD outside South Asia have been sparse, and late arrivals(760, 764, 774, 787, 841). Even non-randomized evaluations of interventions reporting intermediate or final outcomes are rare in the literature(789, 842, 843). Presumably, most such interventions are not evaluated or their results are not published.

I have discussed how interventions targeted at individuals to change their health-related behaviour tend to be costly, often completely ineffective, and sometimes modestly effective(460, 787, 811, 844-846). This is particularly true for CHD while there has been more promise with the prevention of DM_2 through screening to find people with IGT (or IFG) and offering fairly intensive support. Some of the work has been on South Asian populations in South Asian countries as well as overseas. These are early days but, in comparison with studies of general populations in Europe and North America, such interventions have been less effective in South Asians in these countries(764, 841). Studies in India have shown some promise. The best known example is the Indian Diabetes Prevention Trial in Chennai where a 28% reduction in progression from IGT was seen in the intervention compared to the control group(763). This effect is about half that observed with similar interventions in the US and in Finland (765, 766).

The PODOSA trial set in Scotland showed a 1.6 kg weight loss compared to controls (actually 1.1 kg as the control group put on 0.5 kg) in a 3-year home-based dietitian led intervention focusing on diet and physical activity(764). While disappointing, this result on weight loss was better than in the Indian Diabetes Prevention Programme where there was none(763). Subsequent similar trials have shown either no weight loss or amounts similar to PODOSA. A worldwide systematic review has been published on weight loss in South Asian adults and children(760). Mostly, interventions had no or little effect, a conclusion endorsed by a second review.

The relatively promising results seen in Chennai, India are not necessarily replicable across South Asia, or even India, as there are several particular circumstances there including long-established research units and diabetes services led by charismatic and dedicated professionals(762, 763).

There may also be a publication bias in this field of enquiry with ineffective intervention studies not being published.

I conclude from this overview of about 60 years of research that empirical work has been small-scale, slow in starting, and catalysed by researchers working on the South Asian diaspora. The research has also been underpinned by the approaches, hypotheses, and findings of classical work conducted in North America and Northern Europe, such as the Framingham study(330).

In relation to the development of theories and hypotheses to explain the epidemics of DM_2 and CVD the literature, whether from South Asia based or overseas scholars interested in South Asians, is dominated by hypotheses developed for non-South Asian populations, i.e. the thrifty gene, the thrifty phenotype, and even more so insulin resistance, even in 2018 when these hypotheses have been demonstrated to be over-emphasized(17, 30, 76, 95). Predictably, a paper on the subject of CVD and DM_2 on South Asians will refer to a reference to one or all of the above three hypotheses but not as ones to be rigorously tested but assumed to be important. The voices of critics who have pointed to the lack of evidence or logical foundation of the argument have generally not been heard. Kennedy Cruickshank, for example, has over the last 20–30 years repeatedly published his observation that insulin resistance is not a cause of CVD, including in South Asians(847). Even though the research of one of the leading proponents of this hypothesis, Paul McKeigue, failed to find support for the hypothesis(1), it continues to be influential and cited(30).

In recent years we have seen hypotheses papers focused on South Asians, e.g. the adipose tissue compartment hypothesis, mitochondrial efficiency, behavioural switch (soldier-to-diplomat), and high-heat cooking(101, 102, 107, 147). New foci of risk factor research have also arisen, e.g. B_{12}/folate balance in utero and early life(287, 630). We have also observed tailoring of general hypotheses for South Asian populations in particular, e.g. the capacity load model of Jonathan Wells inspired by the thrifty phenotype(205). This is a sign of vigour and development in the field, though none of these ideas has yet matured.

Overall, we can see there have been impediments to concerted policy and public health action including a lack of priority given other demands; insufficient resource, infrastructure, expertize, and motivation to undertake the necessary large-scale, long-term cohort studies in South Asian countries; and, a reliance on concepts, methods, and hypotheses developed on studies of European origin populations in North America and Europe. While there are some who are not yet persuaded, mainly because of the ongoing problems with infection, malnutrition, and child health problems, there is a move to increase the quantity and quality of research, public health, and clinical practice in relation to non-communicable diseases in low and middle income countries including those of South Asia(23, 749, 750).

We need creativity, independence of thought and action, checks on integrity, and critical appraisal of evidence and hypotheses. The uncritical acceptance of appealing ideas is an impediment. Ideas that are not in line with evidence need to be set aside to make room for better ones. The greatest of such simplistic ideas, in my view, is that South Asians' propensity to DM_2 and CVD is 'genetic'. Aside from what that means, it is not plausible that diseases that wax and wane over a few decades are genetic in the sense we usually understand the term, i.e. primarily caused by specific gene variants. Equally, it is not plausible that a condition which is rare is one area and common in another, perhaps 10-miles away, both with the same ancestry, is genetic. This is not to deny that every condition has a genetic susceptibility but that is a different matter. Accepting that the epidemic of CVD and DM_2 in South Asians is not genetic permits us to progress, and not be deflected by the allure of genetic explanations(112).

10.7 Implications of the research synthesis for the recommendations

10.7.1 Changeability of risk factors and intermediate outcomes

Although CVD and DM_2 are chronic diseases and can be induced and reversed over long time scales, the risk factors are highly malleable to change, especially given environmental change. This is obvious for risk factors like physical activity and cigarette smoking, where the CVD benefits occur quickly, and true though less obvious for dietary factors such as salt and olive oil intake. It is not obvious for complex metabolic traits like hyperglycaemia or lipid profiles but it is true there too. The classic demonstration of this was in Australian aborigines but it is relevant to all populations including South Asians. O'Dea et al. observed with careful measurement that in urbanized Australian Aborigines just a few weeks of living in the rural, traditional lifestyle led to massive improvements in their cardiometabolic profile(314). Over 8 kg of weight loss occurred in 7 weeks and glucose levels went from an average of 11.6 mmol/l (above the cut-off for DM) to 6.6 mmol/l. This kind of change can dramatically cut the risk of CVD and eliminate DM_2. Of course few people can transform their lives so much.

The same kind of result has been achieved in both DM_2 prevention and DM_2 treatment by diet studies(848). Generally, a 7–15kg weight loss would eliminate DM_2 in most people with that diagnosis. This kind of weight loss, however, is more difficult in South Asians than in the more overweight White Europeans where these effects have been shown. I now consider whether similar dramatic changes might apply to South Asians. I am reflecting on the recommendations in two parts—the established risk factors in Section 10.7.2 and the newer ideas I have introduced in Section 10.7.3.

10.7.2 Established risk factors and thresholds

The main question here is whether the thresholds for action are lower for South Asian than other comparison populations, usually of European origin. In relation to DM_2 and in adults this is largely agreed for thresholds for overweight and obesity(86). There is early evidence that thresholds differ for physical fitness, muscle mass, and physical activity(585). If confirmed there will be severe challenges to overcome to develop, and implement at population level, effective interventions to increase aerobic and anaerobic physical activity in South Asians. The small experience of trying to do this has been disappointing. Fortunately, walking is highly acceptable to South Asian men and women, especially as a group activity(587, 849). At 3 miles per hour, walking uses about three times the energy of resting and is moderate physical activity. Walking may be a major part of the solution, especially in groups adding social benefits to those of exercise(849). Arguably, this is the top public health research priority, i.e. gauging the minimum necessary fitness and activity programme for South Asian children and adults and developing and evaluating cost-effective interventions.

There may be similar variances in thresholds for other risk factors, e.g. for BP in Bangladeshis particularly, and serum LDL-C and plasma glucose and its capacity for glycation in all South Asians. Clarity on this is likely to emerge as cohort studies in South Asians report on disease outcomes in relation to risk factor thresholds.

Of the other CVD factors in Table 1.4, diet will be a top research priority perhaps with an examination of the balance of ingredients, e.g. carbohydrates, proteins, fats, fibre, and micronutrients possibly related to fruits and vegetables and severe vitamin D deficiency. There is considerable controversy in this area which is being augmented by the results of the PURE study(408, 469, 850). The nature of food preparation is considered separately in Section 10.7.3.

Of the causal factors in Table 1.5 for DM_2, considerable work is already underway on genetics, the distribution of adipose tissue and adverse fetal and early life development. This work needs more focus on the pancreas. Most of the gene variants associated with DM_2 relate to beta cell function. The question of why beta cell failure occurs is critical and specific answers are needed, and not general answers such as cell fatigue. The question of whether South Asians' pancreas is adversely affected by ectopic fat is important and if so why and how. Physical activity and muscle function, as discussed in relation to CVD above, are equally important to DM_2.

The possible effects of tobacco metabolites as toxins damaging the pancreas (among other organs) needs to be researched with appropriate emphasis on the way tobacco is used in South Asia including as bidis and chewed tobacco whether as part of paan or not. The adverse effect of paan-type concoctions even when tobacco is not included, also merits closer study(379, 851).

10.7.3 The newer ideas needing further exploration: neo-formed contaminants, arterial stiffness, the vasa vasorum microcirculation, and homeostasis/allostasis

In solving a puzzle or mystery, especially in medical research, the generation of ideas is important. If promising, these can be developed as hypotheses. The problem arises when these are prematurely, widely promulgated and elevated to the status of facts. Genetic differences, low birthweight, insulin resistance, and central obesity are, in my view, examples of such ideas that, in the absence of solid understanding, have been promoted beyond the evidence for them. I would not want the same to happen for the new ideas I have introduced.

Like many others, I have placed strong emphasis on South Asians' diets. Quite a number of small-scale trials on specific ingredients, e.g. cinnamon, cashew nuts, fibre, protein supplements, and rice have been done in South Asian populations(466, 468, 852–854). It is hard to gauge where this work will lead but it needs replication and further development.

With colleagues I have studied the cooking process, starting with frying but broadening to high-heat cooking(107). The topic has already been discussed earlier. It is, I propose, a top priority to study the neo-formed contaminants in South Asian foods(377, 433). Some of them, like AGEs, are likely to interact with high levels of glucose in the glycosylation of proteins and tissues like collagen. Others such as TFAs catalyse atherosclerosis. There are likely to be a multiplicity of effects, possibly on LDL-C and other lipids considered causal for CVD. A brief research agenda for this topic has already been published(107).

I have taken an interest in arterial stiffness partly because of my longstanding curiosity on how Bangladeshis who have an average low BP have high rates of stroke(396). As someone with no standard CV risk factors at all I was intrigued by the fact my arteries were comparatively stiff in 1999 and again when re-tested in about 2012 by my research colleagues. There is no good explanation for why there is such stiffness in South Asians, although there are a number of suggestions including anthropometric differences, variations in cardiovascular risk factors, vitamin D deficiency, and others(293, 399, 700, 701, 855). There is evidence of an association between arterial stiffness and impairment of blood flow in the major arteries to the brain(398).

Glycosylation of tissues as considered above offers a pathway to arterial stiffness—AGEs are known to stiffen issues(107). AGEs also harm the kidneys and South Asians have a great deal of renal dysfunction, which promotes CVDs creating a vicious cycle(734, 738, 739). The reasons for, and consequences of, arterial stiffness in South Asians deserve greater attention.

In my medical school in the 1970s pathologists showed me in post-mortems that atheroma plaques are patchy and much or most of the coronary artery is healthy. There was no explanation for why, though concepts of stress points and blood flow turbulence were among explanations considered. It could be, to some extent, random, perhaps a result of some kind of trauma at a particular place. Out-of-the-blue, I found a new explanation by a surgeon—the idea being that atherosclerotic plaques occur where the arterial blood supply (via the vasa variorum) is poor(68), i.e. it is a defect in the microcirculation. I found that this concept had been proposed before(75). There is a very small literature on this microcirculation in relation to atherosclerosis(69–75).

There is a very important implication of this possibility, i.e. that damage to the artery does not solely occur from the endothelium inwards but from the outer lining of the artery, the adventitia, inwards. Several studies have found, surprisingly, that there is no evidence of any excess problem with the intima and media, the inner linings of the artery, in South Asians (including children) compared with other populations(398, 691–693, 856, 857). We now need to examine in South Asians the outer lining, the adventitia, which is by far the most complex layer of the arterial wall(71, 73, 858).

South Asians are prone to microcirculatory disorders, a tendency that is usually attributed to hyperglycaemia, e.g. retinopathy. Hyperglycaemic retinopathy is associated with plasma glucose levels of 11.1 mmol/l and above, and this is the rationale for the WHO definition of DM_2 demonstrated using an OGTT(859). Yet, we know people with IGT (glucose 7.8–11.1 mmol/l), and less clearly so, people with IFG, have higher risks of CVD than people with normoglycaemia(526, 860). Indeed, hyperglycaemia is associated with cardiovascular outcomes with no clear threshold(523, 524, 736). It is plausible, if not highly likely, that some microcirculatory beds are adversely affected by lower levels of glucose than 11.1 mmol/l. In the follow-up to the Southall study, hyperglycaemia has been linked with high rates of stroke in South Asians(780). The effects of glucose might be compounded by a greater tendency to glycosylation in South Asians because of other glycosylating agents, AGEs from high heat cooking only being one source(107, 488, 489, 861, 862).

If there is a process causing microcirculatory damage in South Asians, it might affect the pancreas and especially the circulation to the islets of Langerhans and hence impairment of the beta-cells. The process could also affect the kidneys(738).

There is a mystery of why South Asians with DM_2 have less peripheral vascular disease than White Europeans with DM_2(697, 778). One possible explanation is differences in the microcirculation supplying the arteries of the lower limb. I have consulted surgical colleagues and others interested in the microcirculation but I can find no evidence on this particular issue, although there is evidence that the microcirculation differs in different vascular beds(73). It may be that South Asians have a vasa vasorum in the peripheral arteries that is more resistant to microcirculatory damage than that in White European origin populations.

The final area I have chosen is more general, i.e. changes that overcome homeostatic mechanisms and induce the allostatic response. Intuitively, we would expect our metabolism to be set according to local circumstances through a process of adaptation. Indeed, this is the core idea behind the DOHAD hypothesis. If something changes later in life our metabolism might be unprepared (dysadaptation). As we have discussed many bodily functions are under strong homeostatic control. Many, clearly, are not. LDL-C is not as it is about 1 mmol/l at birth and typically 3–5 mmol/l by adulthood and often much higher, and fluctuates quite a lot according to lifestyle, particularly diet. If it rises particularly fast is that an extra risk? Alternatively, might having high cholesterol in early life protect you in later life? We really don't know but experimental evidence indicates this phenomenon is seen in pigeons(227).

When a measure resets to a different value, that is allostasis. Allostasis occurs with many measures, e.g. BP and weight though clearly there is a tipping point when pathology results. It is common for BP to reset itself in adults from an average systolic value of about 120 mmHg to 130 and even 140. A gain of weight, say of 2 kg after a holiday, can sometimes become long term or permanent.

South Asians have changed fast, whether on migration abroad or from rural to urban areas, or by rapid urbanization. Is the rapidity of change important in itself? This is plausible but in several population studies it is not clear that it is, and for weight there is evidence that it is the lifetime burden of overweight that matters more rather than a switch in status(563, 863). This is akin to smoking—being a smoker from the age of 9 years does not protect you compared to starting smoking at 29 years of age—the opposite is true. The evidence is limited, especially in South Asians, but the concept is powerful and needs more research than hitherto on a broad range of risk factors.

10.8 Effectiveness and sustainability of interventions in practice: the transferability of knowledge to South Asians

Interventions that actually manage to reduce CVD and DM_2 risk factors give results similar to those expected on theoretical knowledge of disease causation, whether in people merely with risk factors or people with adverse health outcomes already(586, 588, 760, 787, 845, 864). The problem is that in practice, and even in clinical trial settings, the interventions usually lead to, on average, small or unsustainable, short-term changes. Sometimes, there is no change at all(340). That is not to deny that some individuals change greatly but, surprisingly, others change in adverse ways even during the active intervention phase. Why would people, for example, put on substantial amounts of weight after having consented to healthy eating interventions to bring about weight loss(764)? We need to understand this mysterious phenomenon. One explanation offered to me is that the healthy eating programme brings food to the subconscious and conscious mind and this, at least sometimes, has the opposite of the desired effect.

The benefits of lifestyle interventions tend to fade away, sometimes within days of the intervention stopping, as shown in relation to physical activity and insulin resistance in South Asian population in London(589). This has now been documented and observed in numerous locations and populations worldwide. To reiterate and re-emphasize, this is not a reflection of our causal knowledge of CVD and DM_2 but of our knowledge of how to achieve lasting behaviour change in human populations, and a great deal of work is underway to improve this including on cross-cultural adaptation so interventions work better in ethnic minority and socio-economically deprived populations(865–870).

Very little behaviour change intervention research has been published specifically on South Asian populations so there is uncertainty on whether the above observations apply to them but it is a reasonable assumption. The little published research indicates that it may actually be harder to achieve behaviour change in South Asian populations than in comparable European origin populations(760, 763, 764).

In achieving sustainable change Whelan et al. identified 11 core principles(871, 872) that I have summarized as:

♦ Adopt multiple strategies in multiple settings
♦ Plan for long-term sustainability
♦ Base interventions on evidence

- Ensure there is capacity to deliver
- Engage those needing to be involved, including the communities
- Evaluate the work
- Embed the findings into policy
- Adapt and evolve the interventions in the light of evaluation
- Diversify the sources of funding
- Secure leadership
- Recruit champions to the cause.

Whelan's principles seem a sound starting point for scholars, researchers, interventionists, and practitioners to follow and adapt in the context of South Asians and their susceptibility to CVD and DM_2.

10.9 Conclusions

The call to arms against the spread of the chronic diseases has been made repeatedly in, and in recent years even more stridently than ever to, the lower and middle income countries where the epidemics of CVD and DM_2 are growing fast and where most cases of these disease already occur. South Asia is, in the judgement of major international agencies, at the epicentre of this global epidemic (notwithstanding some doubts about this created by the lack of high quality, valid, population data)(23, 47, 62, 111, 725).

Actions to describe, prevent, control, and tackle the epidemics is underway in South Asians, albeit with a slow start and perhaps even reluctantly given the many other demands on limited public resources, which rightly are targeted at the poorest in society, and at the most amenable conditions, e.g. infections (823, 873). In recent years CVD and DM_2 in South Asia have been mainly problems of the more affluent groups and more affluent locations(24, 327, 727, 874–877). As with many aspects of these epidemics, we can be confident that they will follow the pattern seen in Europe and North America and soon hit the poorest people hardest and they will have the triple burden of poverty, infections, other diseases of poverty, and the chronic disease that follow even the most modest adverse changes in lifestyle arising from socio-economic and environmental change.

South Asia has, however, great advantages compared with, for example, the US, the UK, and Finland in the 1940s and through to the 1960s when the epidemic of CVD struck in these places. The advantages include these:

- A wealth of reliable knowledge on causation
- Much published experience on legislative, policy, public health, and health care interventions that do and do not work, including some work on South Asian populations

- Backing from international and national institutions, including the UN and WHO
- Traditional values, behaviours, and lifestyles that are antidotes to these diseases
- Effective medications (e.g. statins, BP medications), and
- Huge populations that have still not changed their traditional lifestyles so are still at low risk.

The epidemics of chronic diseases can be restrained but not stopped. These epidemics have been described by Ban Ki-Moon, recently the secretary general of the UN, as a public health emergency in slow motion. To tackle the epidemics we need the same urgent response we apply to any emergency. The first requirement for any effective response is a careful examination of the causes—the topic and goal of this book.

Appendix

Discussions with scholars and researchers

The scholars consulted are listed in Appendix Table 11.1.

Appendix Table 11.1 List of people participating in discussions

	Title and Name	Country of workplace	URL for their workplace and CV
1.	Prof Sonia Anand	Canada	https://fhs.mcmaster.ca/medicine/cardiology/faculty_member_anand.htm
2.	Prof Richard Cooper	US	https://www.sheffield.ac.uk/scharr/sections/ph/staff/profiles/richard
3.	Dr Enas Enas	US	https://doctors.advocatehealth.com/p/enas-a-enas-downers-grove-cardiology
4.	Prof Caroline Fall	UK	https://www.southampton.ac.uk/medicine/about/staff/cf.page
5.	Prof Nita Forouhi	UK	http://www.mrc-epid.cam.ac.uk/people/nita-forouhi/
6.	Prof Jason Gill	UK	https://www.gla.ac.uk/researchinstitutes/icams/staff/jasongill/
7.	Prof Rajeev Gupta	India	http://people.du.ac.in/~rgupta/about.html
8.	Prof Alka Kanaya	US	http://whcrc.ucsf.edu/people/alka-kanaya-md
9.	Prof Kamlesh Khunti	UK	https://www2.le.ac.uk/offices/press/research . . . profile . . . 1/professor-kamlesh-khunti
10.	Prof Sanjay Kinra	India/UK	https://www.lshtm.ac.uk/aboutus/people/kinra.sanjay
11.	Prof Paul McKeigue	UK	https://www.ed.ac.uk/profile/paul-mckeigue
12.	Prof Anoop Misra	India	http://www.anoopmisra.com/
13.	Prof Venkat Narayan	US	https://www.sph.emory.edu/faculty/profile/#!KNARAYA
14.	Prof Latha Palaniappan	US	https://profiles.stanford.edu/latha-palaniappan
15.	Prof Dorairaj Prabhakaran	India	https://www.phfi.org/faculty-a-researchers/654

	Title and Name	Country of workplace	URL for their workplace and CV
16.	Prof Robert Scragg	New Zealand	https://unidirectory.auckland.ac.nz/profile/r-scragg
17.	Prof Karien Stronks	The Netherlands	www.uva.nl/en/profile/externe-medewerkers/amc/.../stronks-karien/stronks-karien.htm
18.	Prof Milind Watve	India	http://www.iiserpune.ac.in/people/facultydetails/61
19.	Prof Jonathan Wells	UK	http://www.ucl.ac.uk/ich/research/population-policy-practice/People/wells-jonathan
20.	Prof Chittaranjan Yajnik	India	https://www.danishdiabetesacademy.dk/pr/storytelling/first-5-years/ranjan-yajnik
22.	Prof Salim Yusuf	Canada	http://www.phri.ca/people/dr-salim-yusuf/

Sonia Anand (SA) 13/11/17

Introduction

SA agreed with the observation of a susceptibility of South Asians to both DM_2 and CHD. She explained this as a consequence of especially long exposure to cardiometabolic risk factors, perhaps even starting in utero and transmitted intergenerationally.

Explanations

SK thought the high risk of CHD (e.g. MI as one major outcome) had been well explained in the case–control Inter-Heart Study (Joshi et al.) by a combination of DM_2, apolipoprotein B to A ratios, and central adiposity as reflected in waist/hip ratios. By contrast, as I pointed out, the risk ratio rose rather than attenuated on adjustment for such risk factors in the SABRE (Southall and Brent Revisited) Cohort Study.

SA then reflected on cardiometabolic outcomes including DM_2, with a focus on exposure to glucose in utero given the propensity of South Asian mothers to gestational diabetes mellitus (GDM), and their infants' relatively low birth-weight and relative adiposity even at birth (the thin-fat phenotype). South Asians also have more fat in ectopic depots including the viscera, liver, pericardium, and possibly the pancreas. This state, with high glucose and insulin resistance, could lead to beta-cell failure, the end step for DM_2.

SA considered the nature of beta cell failure. Why should such cells fail? At present the answer is unknown but she identified genetic factors, lipotoxicity from ectopic fat, and a diet with high glycaemic index and low protein as potential pathways. Such diets might have effects through the life-course and promote central adiposity and low HDL, and may predispose to GDM.

SA then reflected on what the underlying forces for the observed phenotype might be. She identified genetic factors as an avenue that needs deeper exploration notwithstanding the lack of clear progress so far. Similarly, the gene–environment interaction could manifest through epigenetic changes and go across the generations. The programming of adult disease through early life experiences (DOHAD hypothesis) was identified as potentially important.

SA then discussed the most popular of the ideas offered by the public, i.e. stresses of migration. This kind of stress is very difficult to measure. In her PhD work she examined some biomarkers of stress finding that cortisol levels were not raised in South Asian populations though norepinephrine (adrenaline) levels were raised. On reflection SA thought racism and discrimination could be important stressors for migrant populations, but were little studied.

Conclusion

SA has participated in several multi-ethnic studies of various designs in the Canadian and international settings. The main message from this discussion was that while clear cut explanations are not available there is good understanding of pathways to CHD and DM_2, entailing early and unusually prolonged exposure to causal factors.

Postscript

SA offered to examine her data sets for unpublished data, including on cortisol and the risk of CHD in Chinese in the Canadian setting.

Richard Cooper (RC) 19/09/17

Introductory comments

RC has worked on ethnic variations in cardiovascular diseases and related problems especially blood pressure (BP), and also diabetes mellitus (DM). His specialist area within this topic has been hypertension and BP in African-American and African origin populations, both in African countries and abroad. This discussion aimed to seek lessons to be generalized to other ethnic groups, especially South Asians.

RC's perspectives

RC emphasized that measurement of the phenotype and the risk factors is difficult and we should be circumspect about the validity of the data, one example being the unlikely report of Mozambique having the highest level of BP in the world.

RC agreed that BP in rural Africa is usually low and rises somewhat, in line with expectation given increases in risk factors, in urban Africa. It is the out-of-Africa populations that have particularly high BP but even here it is a mixed picture. In Jamaica, Cuba and other Caribbean locations the BP of African origin population is on a par with White American populations.

BP is not uniform across the US and varies by place, time, and population. The African American populations have about 4 mmHg higher BP than White Americans. This is in line with findings on African origin populations in Canada and Europe. Contrary to expectation, the same was true of African origin people (not Black African-Americans) living in the US and studied in NHANES. This said, the levels of BP in these populations were still lower than the levels recorded historically in Finland and Russia.

Explanations

RC said there was no clear explanations for the phenomenon above, despite so much study. Indeed, we may never find an answer or may find it in an unexpected place (in analogy as for peptic ulcer).

RC considered genetics, epigenetics, psychosocial factors (especially racism), and nutrition. Genetic explanations have been examined in detail. At this point this arena is not promising.

Epigenetic and telomere-related explanations require a knowledge of environmental factors interacting with the genome, leading to difference in the epigenome.

In picking areas with the most promise RC emphasized nutrition (fruits, vegetables, salt, frying) and psychosocial factors, though both posed formidable challenges in accurate measurement.

RC concurred that microvascular damage, possibly from hyperglycaemia, could be related to atherosclerosis.

Observations on South Asians

Some of the points above are directly pertinent to South Asians, e.g. difficulties in measurement and of explanation. On specific matters RC didn't think the low HDL-C and high triglyceride levels in South Asians were explanatory of their high risk of CVD. Hyperglycaemia over long periods, preceding the onset of DM_2, was seen as a more promising line.

Enas Enas (EE) (30/10/17)

Introduction

As a cardiologist EE saw aggressive, atherosclerotic heart disease in young people (under 40 years) without traditional risk factors. While DM_2 might be important in causation it was not the key factor int this age group.

Explanations

EE does not favour explanations based on traditional risk factors. He has observed that South Asians tend to have high levels of the more recently studied, so-called emerging risk factors. In South Asia they are also exposed to high levels of indoor and outdoor air pollution.

Of all the risk factors EE picks LP (a) as the key to understanding CHD in South Asians. In his practice over the past 25 years, he found Lp(a) explaining about 90% of otherwise unexplainable, malignant CHD in young Indians. Lp(a) is under strong genetic control so if EE's view is correct we have a genetic explanation for South Asians' susceptibility to CHD. He referred to recent, unpublished analysis of INTERHEART where about 7000 cases of MI and similar numbers of controls were compared in seven populations. The association of hp(a) with MI was present in all except the African origin group and the odds ratio was highest in South Asians.

EE reflected on why his long-standing emphasis on Lp(a) has not been accepted by researchers and scholars more widely. One explanation is that there are 42 isoforms of the molecule, and the small isoforms are associated with CHD and the large ones are not, so measuring total Lp(a) is not enough. Measurement of LP(a) isoforms is not necessary in clinical practice but one should use an assay method that is not affected by isoforms' size. Since LP(a) levels are stable after age 2, one measurement is sufficient for risk stratification. Lp(a) testing need not be repeated, especially since currently there is no approved LP(a) lowering therapies.

Although established risk factors do not explain the higher CVD risk in South Asians, they are extremely important; indeed, the management of elevated LP(a) is simply more aggressive control of the established risk factors, particularly lipids. LDL-C levels can be lowered safely to very low levels (<25–30 mg/dl, i.e. less than 1 mmol per litre).

Prediction algorithms

EE referred to several UK studies showing that the observed CVD risk is about 50% higher in South Asian men and about 100% higher in South Asian women, even when established risk factors are entered into a prediction model. EE believes that algorithms incorporating LP(a) need to be studied. In the meantime, EE recommends including a calibration factor, e.g. adding 10 years of age or multiplying the estimated risk by an appropriate factor, e.g. times 1.5–2 depending on the algorithm.

Conclusion

Lp(a) has been studied in general and South Asian populations alike. It is a candidate that could explain a genetic susceptibility in South Asians, with lifestyle and environmental factors providing the trigger. EE emphasized it is time to study this risk factor again with modern methods.

Caroline Fall (CF) 23/10/17

Introductory remarks

CF judged that the evidence in favour of the developmental origins of health and disease (DOHAD) was stronger for DM_2 than for cardiovascular diseases. The central concept is that some deficiency in utero, probably nutritional but not solely so, leads to impaired development of key tissues of which she prioritized the pancreas, kidney, muscle, and liver. Birthweight is merely one marker of such a deficiency. The impairment may be initiated by several factors, e.g. over- and under-nutrition, steroids in pregnancy, and toxins such as indoor smoke and endocrine agents. The evidence is clear cut in animals, where the changes can be induced with modest interventions. The changes were transferred intergenerationally in animals, probably through epigenetic mechanisms.

Animal studies have shown specific defects in these tissues, resulting from manipulation of fetal nutrition, ranging from reduced numbers of pancreatic islet cells and impaired vascularization of the islets to reductions in the expression of insulin signalling proteins.

The DOHAD hypothesis in relation to South Asians

If their small birthweight is a signal of some deficiency that affects the fetus, then the hypothesis could apply to most South Asians. Given the effects are seen across several generations, it is possibly not surprising that birthweight of South Asians born in favourable socio-economic circumstances are not rising (as in the offspring of South Asian origin mothers born in the UK). There may be some non-nutritional fetal constraints that remain unknown.

The data from birth cohorts in South Asia fit the DOHAD hypothesis. It is clear, however, that a combination of low birth weight and later rise in adiposity (even small amounts) is the highest risk state. The inference from this is that South Asians should gain weight in the first 1–2 years of life but after that should not cross weight for height centiles. In addition to weight gain, other risk factors, e.g. tobacco, may also have greater adverse effects so, in effect, a low birth weight is an indicator of a phenotype especially sensitive to risk factors.

At present it is not known whether interventions can alter the course of events. Indeed, it is unclear what interventions are required. CF was cautious because interventions in pregnancy that lead to weight gain might even increase DM_2 in adulthood. So, trials are needed. (In passing, CF noted that a higher birth weight is associated with a higher incidence of cancers and that, as a generalization, South Asians have both low birthweights and low rates of cancer.)

Ongoing and recent trials

CF was aware of three trials in South Asia, in which the aim was to improve maternal nutrition and health, with a long-term view of reducing non-communicable disease risk. One has been reported. Potdar et al. supplemented the diets of women prior to conception. Birthweight was raised in women of normal or high BMI (>18.5), and the prevalence of gestational diabetes was halved.

The second trial is of B_{12} supplementation in adolescent boys and girls and is led by CS Yajnik. The outcome will be the effects on their offspring. The results are awaited.

The third trial is a multifaceted intervention in rural Mysore. The fieldwork is currently being planned.

These and other trials are needed to help judge the role of the DOHAD hypothesis in South Asians.

Conclusions

CF's judgement is that the DOHAD hypothesis is important in relation to DM_2 in South Asians but the state-of-art is not sufficiently developed to quantify its role accurately, to conclude cause and effect, or to implement public health interventions. In this case, more research is needed.

Nita Forouhi (NF) 08/01/18

Introductory remarks

Nita Forouhi (NF) observed that even though current research is not finding specific genetic differences in South Asians to explain their high risk of CHD and DM_2, these outcomes result from an interaction between genetic and non-genetic factors. There is still much genetic research to do before we can evaluate its importance. NF noted that genetic effects might be through specific phenotypes, e.g. body composition or lipids and these need further study. She also noted the potential importance of fetal and child developmental factors and also the environment including air and soil pollutants. Finally, NF emphasized that potential causes could have varying effects across places and ethnic groups, taking the example of fish consumption and DM_2. This was protective in North America, neutral in Europe, and adverse in East Asia. The different associations might relate to different kinds of fish, toxins, cooking methods, etc. NF then focused on diet and physical activity as especially important in explaining South Asian susceptibility to CHD and DM_2.

Specific explanations

NF thought that the interrelated issues of low muscle mass, muscular strength, fitness, and physical activity were underemphasized in research and were important. These factors have not been measured accurately in research in South Asians so their importance is not assessable on past research. In addition to epidemiological understanding, we need social science research to understand the reluctance and difficulties of exercising in South Asian populations.

NF believes that the foods and drinks taken are the key to understanding disease outcomes, more so than the constituents. Research on the prospective relationship between food and CHD/ DM_2 is not available in South Asians. Generally, macronutrients from different sources have different effects, e.g. fatty acids from plants, dairy products, and different kinds of meat differ in their chemical composition and effects. It is not helpful to speak of fats or even saturated fats as one entity. A high fat diet is probably fine if it has much mono or polyunsaturated fat.

South Asian diets have high carbohydrate that is generally refined and oils that are potentially harmful, e.g. processed oils such as Vanaspati, with substantial TFA content. Fruit and vegetable content of South Asian diet tends to be low. Some saturated oils used in South Asia, e.g. coconut oil may not be harmful even though on first principles they may be expected to be. There is new evidence emerging on this. The concerns about high omega-6 levels in South Asians remain controversial. NF pointed to evidence that linoleic acid, a major contributor to omega-6 levels was inversely associated with CHD outcomes.

The combination of low physical activity and poor diet may promote GDM that has effects on adult disease that go across the generations in South Asians.

Conclusions

NF concluded that the causes of CHD and DM_2 are complex and the reasons for the susceptibility of South Asians to these diseases is still unclear. Within the broader context of an array of genetic and environmental influences, NF selected two clusters of risk factors as the ones for emphasis, i.e. a physical activity, muscle mass, fitness, and an imbalance in the consumption of foods.

Jason Gill (JG) 11/12/17

Introduction

After agreeing there was a susceptibility in South Asians, JG proceeded straight to explanations but he did point out that the pattern we see in South Asians i.e.

early onset DM_2 is not unique to them, e.g. it is also seen in African people in Malawi. The inference is that the explanation(s) are likely to be generalizable.

Explanations

JG observed that as the prevalence of SNPs associated with DM_2, and the strength of the association with outcomes, are both similar in South Asians and European-origin populations a genetic basis to South Asians' susceptibility is, perhaps surprisingly, not being supported by research. Most of the genetic variants seem to be related to beta-cell function.

The attention is turning to epigenetic changes, quite likely fitting with the ideas of the developmental origins of adult disease (DOHAD). Some evidence has emerged of differences in epigenetic markers in South Asians and Europeans in middle age but JG queried whether these were a precursor or consequence of hyperglycaemia.

There is indirect evidence in favour of the importance of the DOHAD hypothesis, e.g. the thin-fat Indian baby phenotype, which is more about a relative paucity of lean tissue as there is no excess of fat (just 'fat sparing'). Muscle bulk, strength, physical fitness, and physical activity are important in relation to glucose metabolism. JG referred to Eastwood et al.'s data where adjustment for lean tissue, statistically, greatly narrowed differences between South Asians and White Europeans. In another related study, Ghouri et al. found that adjustment for differences in VO_2 max (a measure of fitness) also statistically accounted for much of the difference in insulin resistance. Muscle in South Asians, therefore, burns less fat but why? The oxidative enzymes seem similar. JG suggested it could be an issue of capillaries not dilating sufficiently or not transporting nutrients to muscle efficiently. If so, this would point to a microvascular dysfunction. I then shared thoughts on possible dysfunction in the microvasculature supplying the coronary arteries.

JG emphasized a point brought to his attention by Venkat Narayan that low muscle mass may merely be a marker for a cause and not the cause itself, e.g. a factor X that led to low muscle and poor development of beta cells.

JG shared unpublished data from the GlasVEGAS study where young South Asians and White European men were given food and encouraged to gain weight. The weight gain was about 1.4 BMI units in both groups. The early indications are that there was no difference in tendency to visceral fat deposition in the two groups. Strikingly, however, White Europeans' weight gain was 30% lean mass whereas South Asians' weight gain was nearly all adipose tissue. Adverse metabolic effects were seen in South Asians but not in Europeans. Fat deposition in the pancreas may be impairing beta cell function, eventually leading to beta cell exhaustion.

Conclusion

JG concluded that the causal story has not been finished. We have many ideas that interrelate in complex ways. This discussion placed special emphasis on epigenetic changes in early life, muscle and its use, and acquisition of adipose tissue. A simple genetic explanation was considered unlikely.

Rajeev Gupta (RG) 06/11/17

Introduction

Rajeev Gupta (RG) has seen a great deal of premature, symptomatic CHD in people under 40 years and even under 30 years. While this is apparent in the city RG noted that similar problems, though less common are present but might not be diagnosed in rural areas. He and his colleagues have been developing explanations centred around migration from rural to urban areas.

Explanations

The commonly stated view that South Asians are genetically prone to CHD has not been, as yet, substantiated by research. RG pointed out that Indians have a lower rate of the genetic disorder familial hypercholesterolaemia than Europeans. Nonetheless, there are possibly gene–environment interactions that are ill-understood, possibly relating to metabolism.

Of environmental explanations, RG emphasized three, i.e. physical inactivity, diet/adiposity, and stress. A reduction in physical activity is a common and rapid consequence of increased wealth in the urban environment. The sedentary lifestyle is popular in India and, together with a change in diet, this leads to cardiometabolic problems.

The diet in urbanized India is high in refined carbohydrates and leads to dyslipidaemia, especially high triglyceride levels. Moreover, the cooking of food is at high temperature and reduces the health benefits of vegetables. RG also emphasized the high amount of TFAs in Indian food, especially street food. RG also flagged up that there may also be other adulterants in food (including in fruits). He picked out the example of the School Food Programme as an example of a poor quality diet that is largely carbohydrate.

This kind of diet together with sedentariness leads to abdominal adiposity (the toxic fat concept) and cardiometabolic abnormalities. RG identified the role of DM_2 and its precursors in the pathogenesis of CHD in Indians.

RG then identified the stress of migration, with reduced family support and social networks as an explanation. He emphasized the stress of striving to achieve (John Henryism) as an example of a stressor, and the stress of living in cramped, built-up city environments.

Conclusions

In concluding RG mentioned that prevention efforts are limited, health care is patchy, and patients' compliance with medical advice and drug prescriptions is poor, and these factors mean tackling the problem is difficult. RG's explanations, based on decades of observations and research, show the complexity of the issues. RG's emphasis on dietary components (e.g. TFAs) and possible contaminants (not specified) was noteworthy. He and his colleagues have been studying carefully the rapidity of the social/epidemiological transition in India with particular reference to cardiovascular risk factors. The trends are worrying, e.g. National Family Health Survey data from 1998 to the present show a doubling of obesity prevalence.

Alka Kanaya (AK) (16/10/17)

Introductory remarks

AK utilizes the socio-ecological model ranging from individual risk factors through to public policy. She assesses that the evidence shows a modestly raised genetic risk for DM_2, particularly in relation to gene variants relating to beta cell function. Although the equivalent genetic evidence for CVD is weaker she thinks we will uncover it. On this background susceptibility, South Asians' behaviours and social circumstances lead to high risk of DM_2 and atherosclerotic heart disease, though in the populations AK is studying, not of stroke.

AK is studying South Asians of mostly Indian origin who have comparatively high socio-economic status. Nonetheless, they have the typical high risk described in South Asians in other urbanized settings.

Explanations

AK placed emphasis on insufficient physical activity, poor diet, and psychosocial stressors, including racial discrimination. The populations she studies are well educated and have high incomes so she does not ascribe the South Asian susceptibility to low socio-economic status. There are three major dietary patterns that are consumed by US South Asians: a mainly traditional South Asian one with much frying, 'Western' processed varieties, and a more prudent fresh fruit and vegetable pattern. Each of these patterns are similarly prevalent in the MASALA cohort study that she leads.

Reflections on general hypotheses and risk factors

AK thought elements of general hypotheses may be relevant and she picked out the thrifty gene and adipose tissue overflow hypotheses (noting that South

Asians had less pericardial fat than comparison populations in the MASALA/
MESA) Studies.

In relation to established risk factors she did not find in her MASALA/MESA
studies much support for a special role in prediction of atherosclerosis or incident CVD events for:

- Lipid sub-fractions including Lp(a)
- Inflammatory markers
- Adipokines.

She is prioritizing as promising:

- Organic pollutants (effect on beta cell function)
- Genomic and epigenetic risk
- Rapid accumulation of coronary calcium in the arteries.

Conclusion

AK clearly sees that explaining the susceptibility of South Asians to DM_2 and
CVD is work in progress. This said her emphasis is on a slightly raised genetic
risk which is greatly amplified by three major, environmental sources of risk,
i.e. insufficient physical activity, a diet that predisposes to these outcomes, and
psychosocial factors.

Kamlesh Khunti (KK) (21/09/17)

Introduction

KK started with a potential important general point: that clarity on the causes
of the approximately three-fold greater risk of DM_2 in South Asians has not
increased since we last discussed it 8 years ago. However, there have been several new explanations and risk factors in the literature. He was not optimistic
of rapid causal progress as we need to understand the causes of DM_2 in all/any
population, not just South Asians.

Areas for emphasis

In the discussion KK put the greatest emphasis on these areas:

1. A life-long raised glucose level causing micro- and macro-vascular damage,
   partly through endothelial dysfunction.
2. An augmentation of the above by an enhanced inflammatory response.
3. The observation that new drugs (GLP1 receptor and SGLT2 inhibitors) are
   effective in reducing cardiovascular risk, especially in South Asians, supports the above.

4. South Asians exhibit more sedentary behaviour and lower levels of moderate and vigorous physical activity, though they do more light physical activity. More studies using objective measures are needed.

5. Diet is probably very important but this needs more work using biomarkers.

6. Genetic studies show 8–10 SNPs that seem especially relevant in South Asians but as DM_2 is polygenic it is unlikely we will pinpoint the specific pathways.

Sanjay Kinra (SK) (26/10/17)

Introduction

SK emphasized that CVDs are multifactorial diseases. Various combinations of many factors may cause the biological changes leading to CVD. These combinations are likely to vary in different times and places.

Causal explanations

There may be a special susceptibility in South Asians to DM_2 but SK was less convinced about this for CVD. He had no convincing general explanations but of the plausible ones he would pick the effects of poor development in utero and early life for nutritional reasons.

This said SK placed emphasis on the established CVD risk factors. He thinks that these need to be measured more accurately than hitherto and in longitudinal studies over the life-course. SK was not confident about the results of studies showing that the excess risk in South Asians compared to other ethnic groups can't be explained in regression models. In addition to better designs and data, we need to include variables such as air pollution.

In the context of explanations centred around the major risk factors for CVD there are areas of special emphasis in South Asians and of these SK picked: early life nutrition being suboptimal, a propensity to central obesity and insulin resistance, and insufficient physical activity and fitness. These factors are more prominent in urbanizing environments.

SK reflected on general pathways including arterial stiffness. SK's studies have shown this is a potential problem and is a signal of premature vascular ageing. The explanation is not always clear but may be a result of body shape and size and different effects of BP on the vasculature.

Conclusions

SK thinks the primary explanation for the high risk of CVD in South Asians lies in the risk factors we know about. He thought there would be refinements through studies of specific matters, e.g. Lp(a) and transfatty acids, but these would add a small amount to our causal understanding.

Paul McKeigue (PM) (25/09/17)

Introductory comments

PM made two general observations that are relevant to this discussion. First, classically, in migrant health studies, the disease patterns converge over time and across generations. This is not the case for either CVD or DM_2 in South Asians. This suggests a strong influence of genetic factors and/or a persistent, long-lasting environmental exposure.

Second, CHD begain to decline rapidly about 1968 in the USA, Canada, and Australia. This fall is too large to have been explained by advances in medical care. The rise and fall was about 10 years later in Western Europe, and later still in Eastern Europe. In Japan and the Mediterranean countries the expected rise didn't occur. PM wondered about some ingredient in food that was distributed in different times in different groups of countries (trading blocs). In this context PM referred to trends in the use of margarine; some specific kinds of oil and fats including lard, reheating oil, deep frying and reusing oil repeatedly.

Explanations for South Asians' tendency to CVD and DM_2

Unlike many other populations, such as African Caribbeans with a susceptibility to DM_2, South Asians also have high rates of CVD. This leads to the search for a cause that is common to both outcomes.

In his and others' work in the 1980s, PM thought the common cause was the cluster of phenotypes now known as metabolic syndrome. Insulin resistance is closely linked to this. These were candidates as the common causes but follow-up of the Southall cohort has shown that biomarkers of metabolic syndrome (raised insulin, raised glucose, raised triglyceride and low HDL-C) do not explain the ethnic difference in CHD mortality. PM thinks that there may be a more subtle explanation for the coexistence of metabolic syndrome and high CHD risk in the same population. For instance, the metabolic syndrome may be an adaptive response to some unrecognized metabolic perturbation.

PM picked subtle features of lipid metabolism as his favoured underlying cause. South Asians have, characteristically, high triglycerides and low HDL-C, with little difference in LDL-C. Lipids are complex and PM thinks we need to study them in more detail with modern chemical methods and data analysis. For instance, modified LDL particles (containing oxidized lipid) are more atherogenic because they are taken up by the scavenger receptor.

PM discussed Lp(a) which is higher in African Caribbeans who have relatively low CHD, and small dense LDL-C particles which were not independently associated with CHD in the SABRE Study.

PM considered the role of glucose in micro- and macrovascular disease including my thoughts on damage to the vasa vasorum. The idea of microvascular damage to the vasa vasorum might make sense but the classic studies done in the 1980s showed that the risk of retinopathy does not increase unless the 2-hour post-glucose load plasma glucose is above 11 mmol/l. The risk of cardiovascular disease, however, was shown to increase at a lower threshold of Post-glucose load 2-hour glucose about 8 mmol/l.

Conclusions

PM thinks we should think of some factor that triggers a process that leads to atherosclerosis and DM_2, the latter possibly being a metabolic compensation/reaction in the process. He emphasized that the matter needs re-investigation with a focus on lipid metabolism and combining genetic and environmental perspectives in cohort studies.

Anoop Misra (AM) (17/10/17)

Introductory remarks

AM opened with a clinical observation based on his outpatient clinic: of some 45 patients with DM 10 were under 30 years old, and some were in their teens. He clarified that while the relative susceptibility of Indians (in India) to CHD and stroke still remained unclear the situation for an epidemic of DM_2 was stark.

Explanations

In 1991/2 the Indian economy was liberalized with multiple consequences, including the expansion of the highway network, with increased availability of goods including hardware (TV, mobile phones) and junk foods across the country. The distinction between rural and urban was blurred and a large migration of people from rural areas to urban areas also took place. The culture changed including an expansion in eating out.

In this context AM attributed the epidemic of DM_2 in South Asians to adiposity/obesity, with a propensity to abdominal adiposity and ectopic, especially hepatic, deposition of fat. This combination of events has disrupted metabolic pathways.

For DM_2 to occur a dysfunction of pancreatic beta cells is required (so-called beta cell fatigue). The cause of this is unknown but AM considers ectopic pancreatic fat to be the most likely explanation. Such fat may produce cytokines and other molecules that disrupt beta cell function. (Atrophic pancreatitis does occur in Indians but AM did not see that as a major explanation for the ongoing epidemic.)

He cited a study showing that at diagnosis people with DM_2 have larger than expected pancreatic volume, the extra probably being fat. The pancreas is very sensitive with even 2% loss of pancreatic fat improving its function.

AM judged that this is the dominant pathway to DM_2 in South Asians. He is not convinced there is in South Asians especially a genetic predisposition to DM_2 itself but it is probably important in adipose tissue distribution and the tendency to ectopic fat and in low muscle mass.

The preventive strategy emerging from this analysis emphasizes food habits and nutrition (including more protein), and physical activity incorporating both aerobic and resistance exercises.

Conclusions

AM agrees that the story is incomplete but it is unclear what the extra mysterious factor X is or how we uncover it. The explanations around adiposity, ectopic fat, muscle use and mass, and nutritional quality are the ones he emphasizes, pending further advances in knowledge.

Venkat Narayan (VN) 11/12/17

Introduction

K M Venkat Narayan (VN) took an eco-historical viewpoint that emphasized living conditions across hundreds and more likely thousands of years. He foresaw the role of agriculture, food availability, and the quality of food across generations as being fundamental to more specific explanations.

Explanation

VN observed that a settled agriculture lifestyle occurred early on the Indian subcontinent and as a result population size rose, as the hunter-forager type of lifestyle became less common. Skeletal examination suggests that height diminished over time, indicating that there may have been diminishing nutrition per person or a change, e.g. move to vegetarianism, or both. This kind of nutritional stress was exacerbated by periodic famine and this worsened during colonial rule.

Given these circumstances there may have been survival advantages in a phenotype where fat was preserved and blood glucose was high, or insulin secretion was reduced and where glucose was preferentially reserved for the brain. (RSB noted these ideas chime with Milind Watve's soldier-to-diplomat hypothesis). VN pointed out that Indian women with a BMI of as low as 15–17 remain fertile whereas White European women would probably not be so at such a BMI. Although, Pima Indians and Sub-continent Indians are both at roughly equal risk of DM_2, at given weight or glucose level, the Pimas are most insulin resistant while the Indians are more insulin deficient.

We reflected on whether these circumstances have led to genetic changes and if so which ones. VN postulated they could be epigenetic and cited work whereby following starvation in rats, metabolic changes in the offspring could be detected for more than 20 generations (Yajnik and other colleagues).

This historical adaptation of South Asian populations is exposed as disadvantageous from the perspective of CVD and DM_2 when there is a rapid economic and nutrition transition. Even modest changes—a small rise in BMI or decrease in physical activity—raises the risk. In South Asians DM_2 occurs frequently even at BMIs of less than $20kg/m^2$, e.g. in Chennai. VN noted a similarity in survivors of HIV infection who also get DM_2 at low BMIs.

Finally, given this broad explanation is sound, what biological mechanisms might be important? Obviously, if the epigenetic explanation is correct then that is one way of altering metabolism. There are alternatives in which micronutrients, e.g. a deficit of an amino acid such as lysine, could be a factor.

Conclusion

VN observed that this broad, environmentally driven explanation is generalizable to other populations, e.g. people in other parts of Asia, in sub-Saharan Africa, and African immigrants entering the US more recently. In essence the concept here is of adaptation and then dysadaptation but not in one lifetime, but over multiple generations.

VN also considered the clinical and public health implications, which, pending deeper understanding of specific causes, point to screening, and early detection of risk followed by vigorous management.

Latha Palaniappan (LP) (31/08/17)

Introductory comments

In the US there is no practical way of disaggregating South Asian subgroups, e.g. Indian, Pakistani, etc. In the US the predisposition of South Asians to DM_2 is clear cut but when using rates (or standardized mortality rates) CVD is either similar to or even lower than that in the reference non-Hispanic White population. LP and colleagues have shown that proportional mortality rates for CVD are high in South Asians indicating that CVD is comparatively common in this population relative to other causes of death, e.g. cancer deaths are low.

Explanations for South Asians' predisposition to DM$_2$

LP thinks the relatively low muscle mass in South Asians needs more emphasis, including studying the effect of muscle strengthening, especially in people with diabetes and yet normal weight. Muscle is a major user of glucose.

She also thinks there are dietary issues, possibly in the nature of carbohydrates, and the balance of them to fats and proteins. She has been involved in trials of 40% versus 60% carbohydrate diets. She also wonders whether the usual guidelines on caloric intake are too high for South Asians.

Explanations for predisposition to CVD

LP thinks the almost invariably low HDL-C and (sometimes) high Lp(a) need further investigation, notwithstanding current scepticism, especially on the causal role of HDL-C. She also thinks that the study of genetic contributions to ethnic differences in CVD and DM$_2$ needs to be pursued with larger samples of South Asians disaggregated into subpopulations. Future work should emphasize sequencing the whole genome, including understanding epigenetic modifications (i.e. methylation, deacetylation, telomeres) rather than the current genome-wide association study approach where the panels of SNPs have been selected mostly on their relevance in White European origin populations.

Finally, she referred to the fetal origins of adult disease hypothesis and we discussed the thin-fat Indian baby concept promoted by Chittaranjan Yajnik. She referred to US obstetricians' observations of South Asian babies being long and skinny but with prominent abdomens.

She thinks the epigenetic modifications may be the key to how the environment affects genetic expression, especially in the fetal origins of disease hypothesis.

Conclusions

This discussion underlined the view that there is no clear and compelling explanations for South Asians' tendency to DM$_2$ and CVD and more work needs to be done. Of the matters we discussed, muscle strength, volume and use was the one to focus most on.

Dr D Prabhakaran (DP) 29/01/18

Introductory remarks

DP emphasized the complex, multifactorial basis of the high incidence/prevalence of CVD and DM$_2$ in South Asians. He also pointed out the great heterogeneity of South Asians and that these diseases are at different points in their evolution in South Asia, indeed in different regions of India alone.

Causes seen on a large scale

In a bird's eye overview DP perceived three great, interacting forces. First, operations of the demographic and epidemiological transitions whereby better environments lead to an ageing population, and the control of infections and their replacement by other health problems including chronic diseases. Second, the influence of the social determinants of health of which he picked the infection burden and poor nutrition linked to lower birthweight with prolonged consequences including in adult disease. Third, the biological and lifestyle risk factors, which he thought had similar effects across populations but might operate at different thresholds, e.g. BMI.

DP thinks genetic factors play a small role in South Asians' susceptibility to CVD and DM_2.

Causes DP focused on

Having painted an outline DP pointed to some areas of particular interest. He thought the concepts of DOHAD, reflected in the low birthweight of South Asians, was important. He saw the consequences of this in terms of body composition (relative adiposity and low muscle mass) and possibly in cellular number and function, e.g. impaired pancreatic beta cell number and function. There is also a proinflammatory state in South Asians possibly related to dispose tissue and the exposure to infections. South Asians have seen an unusually rapid move to the epidemiological transition through socio-economic change, urbanization, and change of lifestyles. One of the results has been decline in the physical activity traditionally seen in agrarian life. The role of air pollution and other hazards from toxins, e.g. organic pollutants acting as endocrine disruptors, needs more emphasis in the modern context.

Lipids and adipose tissue were considered in some depth by DP. Adipose tissue in the liver—fatty deposition unrelated to alcohol—might be especially important in South Asians. The specific way dietary oils/lipids are consumed in India, for example, might be important. For example, specific combinations of free fatty acids and TFAs might be toxic through accelerating or triggering pathways to atherosclerosis or DM_2.

DP considered the composition and actions of the commonly used oils and solid fats used in India. Some are prone to conversion to TFAs. Overall, however, we cannot generalize about hazards of these lipids in Indian diets, including for either polyunsaturates or saturates.

Conclusions

DP used the analogy of a jigsaw puzzle. We already have many of the pieces that we need to put it together (RSB informed DP that Chapter 1 of this book introduces the scattered pieces of the jigsaw puzzle and this is put together in Chapter 9). In DP's vision the jigsaw puzzle is complicated but we have identified many of the pieces.

Robert Scragg (RS) 24/08/17

RS noted a few points of interest based on work in New Zealand that sometimes get little attention, e.g. a comparatively low alcohol use in South Asians and a higher pulse rate. We then focused on vitamin D deficiency and two of its potential adverse outcomes, i.e. dysglycaemia and arterial dysfunction as measured in pulse wave analysis.

Vitamin D and its role in dysglycaemia and cardiovascular disorders

Recently, randomized control trial evidence has augmented the knowledge from cohort studies. The idea from cohort studies that high levels of vitamin D (>50 nmol/l) might be beneficial is being undermined by randomized control trials. However, there is evidence that there may be benefits in people who are deficient in vitamin D, i.e. plasma vitamin D of <25 nmol/l. Since the proportion of South Asians with vitamin D deficiency is high, these observations might be particularly relevant to them.

More evidence will emerge in the next few years as the ongoing VITAL and D2D trials report, and in due course, are meta-analysed. It may be that plasma 25-OH D levels are not the important measure and that, for example, vitamin D binding protein is more relevant.

Robert discussed the Von Hurst trial(628) where insulin resistance in South Asian women was diminished by 4 k IU/day of vitamin D (this being the one trial in South Asians he was aware of).

The role of vitamin D in this area is still unclear though not as dramatic as implied by cohort studies. The benefits for dysglycaemia/CVD, if any, are likely to lie in people with low levels of vitamin D, a point relevant to South Asians.

Cardiovascular function

South Asians, including in New Zealand have, compared to Europeans, high arterial stiffness and raised central BP. A trial of vitamin D supplementation has shown improvements in arterial function (but not on BP or CVD outcomes) (613). Central arterial BP and pulse wave velocity predict CVD, adding precision to the Framingham equation. South Asians' arterial stiffness could arise from a combination of factors including low vitamin D and dysglycaemia, possibly acting via endothelial dysfunction.

Non-vitamin D effects of sunlight

While there is interest in the effects of sunlight on nitric oxide (and other pathways) a trial in Auckland showed no benefits in the relation to cardiovascular biomarkers of either UV A or UV B, though the latter doubled vitamin D levels(615).

Conclusions

The impairment of musculoskeletal and immune function in vitamin D deficiency is reason for ensuring that it is avoided. Given the high prevalence of deficiency in South Asians, and the possible benefits in glucose metabolism and arterial function, we need to keep an open mind on the role of vitamin D in predisposing South Asians to DM_2 and cardiovascular diseases.

Postscript

I drew Robert's attention to the high-heat cooking hypothesis(886); four hypotheses including high central arterial pressure and vitamin D deficiency(396) for Bangladeshis' propensity to stroke; and a trial of cod liver oil in London about 200 years ago(887).

Karien Stronks (KS) (16/10/17)

Introductory remarks

KS explained the issue as one where South Asians had a high but still unexplained susceptibility to CVD and DM_2, which translates into a higher incidence of disease when South Asian populations live in an environment that leads to unhealthy diets, physical inactivity, and stress. She argued that current studies primarily focus on the aetiology of these diseases and the role of individual risk factors such as diet. However, the mechanisms of disease causation might be different from mechanisms of preventing that disease (see also Kelly & Russo, Soc Health & Illness 2017). The perspective of the mechanisms of prevention of CVD and DM_2 shifts the focus from individual risk factors towards the social forces that shape these risk factors at a group level. This focus is imperative as a basis for designing effective measures to prevent this increased risk at population level from arising. She therefore pinpointed the central question as: what is it about the environment, together with social context, that raises disease incidence (as it is not an issue of case fatality)?

Explanations

KS emphasized the matter is complex and she noted some principles arising from complexity science, e.g. systems have their unpredictable dynamics, with feedback loops. She took the example of obesity. A factor leads to obesity in some individuals. These individuals have effects on others, i.e. there are collective effects. As obesity becomes common, it may become the norm and the new norm affects many people. In the South Asian context, she noted strong group pressures towards physical inactivity and, especially, eating for social purposes, not just for meeting nutritional needs. The mental brake that says I have had enough food is ineffective in the context of such social pressures and situations.

She favoured insufficient physical activity, overeating, and adiposity as the core factors but these had to be understood in their proper context: adverse socio-economic circumstances, living in a discriminatory society where there are social stressors, pressure for success within the community, and insufficient support within the health system for prevention which is more of a need for South Asians than in native, European-origin Dutch people.

Explanations she didn't support

KS didn't think there was a simple, single answer, e.g. eating too much of an ingredient such as rice. She was not drawn to any of the general hypotheses that focus on single explanations, e.g. genetics.

Value of risk factor association studies

KS considered knowledge about risk factors to be valuable for adjusting the timing, emphasis, and approach of preventive programmes, but only if placed within the context of the above-mentioned wider forces that shape these risks.

Conclusions

KS emphasized the need for context-specific solutions, taking the example of Bollywood dancing as a means of incorporating physical activity in the everyday lives of South Asians, based on knowledge on the mechanisms of disease prevention rather than of disease causation. In order to really understand and prevent the increased risk of CVD and DM2 in South Asians, we should look beyond the individual, and focus on the processes at the level of groups, society, environment, etc that shape individual risks.

Milind Watve (MW) (31/07/17)

MW emphasized that South Asians' propensity to DM_2 is shared with many populations and that people of Northern European origins may be the outliers. He pointed to three, possibly integrated explanations as follows:

1. Differential deposition of fat mass, with less deposition in peripheries and more centrally, possibly driven by climatic factors.

2. An evolution to a complex social life, possibly because of less time spent in food foraging and hunting in warm climates (typically 3 hours) leaving more opportunity for socializing. This could have led to the lower muscle mass in South Asians and favoured a 'diplomat' rather than 'soldier' kind of life. This permits more fuel for the brain, required to maintain complex social networks.

3. In cold climates people need to take shelter in winter and will be sedentary for much of the time. They would have evolved mechanisms to remain healthy through this period. In the tropics there is no such harsh environment and opportunity to evolve for sedentarism. Admittedly, there is not a great deal of evidence for this idea but it is worth considering.

MW speculated that South Asians' tendency to atherosclerosis may be promoted by circulating macrophages that are not being utilized in the peripheries for their usual roles, e.g. by the diminished number of insect bites and minor injuries. So, there is a pro-inflammatory state that is diverted for other, potentially harmful, purposes.

The hypotheses that MW would de-emphasize include the thrifty genotype and insulin resistance per se. This said he agrees that the complex of metabolic changes that accompanies insulin resistance is important. Diet has, in his view, been overemphasized too. Low birth weight (fetal origins/thrifty phenotype hypothesis) may be important because of low muscle mass, which needs more emphasis.

MW thinks the role of glucose has been overemphasized too. In discussing protein glycation by glucose and other agents he pointed out that slower protein turnover is important in this phenomenon, and that it is not simply a question of hyperglycaemia.

Comment by RSB

This discussion pointed to the complexity of the issues. There is, presently, no simple, clear explanation. This discussion put a strong emphasis on evolutionary adaptation.

Further discussion by email (7/8/17)

RSB asked about the widespread concept of beta-cell exhaustion and why cells would get exhausted. The response was: 'I don't believe that beta cells get exhausted. One reason is that the beta cell number goes up in hyperinsulinemia. Per cell insulin production doesn't go up. So any given cell is not working more to get exhausted. People have measured insulin transcription rates in rats and found that in hyperinsulinemic state, transcription per cell is reduced, not increased.

The other reason is what you said rightly. The body strengthens a tissue that is in use.'

Jonathan Wells (JW) 20/11/17

Introduction

Jonathan Wells' (JW) view is that the causes of chronic diseases such as CHD and DM_2 include important drivers that are societal. There are numerous influences leading to these diseases that have additive effects The causes cluster and cannot be teased apart easily–they can be thought of as parts of a complex jigsaw. Investigations can be at various levels. Jonathan's work has tried to bring an evolutionary perspective to physiological adaptations relevant to cardiometabolic disorders.

Explanations

The South Asian susceptibility to CHD and DM_2 starts in fetal life with the phenotype seen at birth. These influences may cascade across generations. The susceptibility has evolved but not necessarily genetically. Environmental and epigenetic mechanisms are likely to be important.

JW summarized the capacity load model that was inspired by Barker and Hales' thrifty phenotype hypothesis. Essentially, in this model capacity is developed in early life, e.g. numbers of nephrons, pancreatic beta-cell mass, cardiac structure, airway diameter, grip strength, etc. There are critical periods after which capacity cannot be extended easily and sometimes not at all. This capacity sets the limits to homeostasis, i.e. the ability to maintain physiological norms when under challenge. Birthweight is one important, composite marker of this capacity and is low in South Asians.

South Asians are thin at birth and as their body fat is, relatively, spared we see the thin-fat phenotype as emphasized by Chittaranjan Yajnik.

JW is a contributor to work submitted for publication suggesting the thin phenotype dates to ancient times, reflected in the skeletons found in the Gangetic plain. There is evidence that the height of Indians has diminished over the last 10,000 years, although data are sparse.

Together with their low metabolic capacity South Asians are being confronted with new stressors such as sedentary behaviours and increased caloric intake, especially from oils. (There are also challenges such as air pollution in and outside the home.)

These factors, both historical and contemporary, promote adiposity and especially central adiposity. From an evolutionary perspective, JW has argued that tougher environmental conditions favour fat deposition over linear growth, as abdominal adipose tissue funds immune function and peripheral adipose tissue funds reproduction in females. This helps explain the combination of short height and thin physique with preserved fatness in South Asians, exposed to unpredictable monsoon events.

Beyond this, JW has offered the variable disease selection hypothesis that proposes that gastrointestinal infections over evolutionary periods have further favoured deposition of fat centrally so the immune system has access to easily accessible stores of energy, thus potentially explaining the high waist-hip ratios of South Asians, who regularly encounter such pathogens in monsoon conditions. Catch up growth also tends to lead to truncal adiposity and is a related factor.

JW then discussed the role of the pelvis in birth weight. There are constraints on birth size and the short stature and thin aspect of South Asian women relate to smaller pelves and narrower birth canals, thus resulting in the birth of smaller babies. JW considered diet to contribute to low birthweights especially strict vegetarianism with a low level of protein, especially animal protein.

Metabolic capacity cannot be built up in late life. Further, humans may not have physiological mechanisms for handling excess of nutrients or reversing changes, e.g. weight gain. The modern circumstances of ample nutrition and long survival despite a sedentary life were rare in the past, so low capacity would seldom have been converted into overt health problems.

Conclusions

JW's capacity load model aligns with and develops the developmental origins of adult disease concept. The role of early life development, in JW's view, cannot be disentangled from related changes in later life, e.g. weight gain in adulthood. The essential point is that the early life development equips you to face later metabolic and other challenges. South Asians have not been equipped well for the metabolic challenges they are now facing, hence the toll of DM_2 and CHD. Large increases in metabolic load are now overwhelming the low metabolic capacity in many South Asians.

Chittaranjan Yajnik (RY) 22/11/17

Introduction

In general terms RY thinks the evidence for a genetic explanation for South Asians' susceptibility to DM_2 or CHD is unconvincing, especially given recent genome-wide association studies. While rare genetic variants may be uncovered and shown to be important they will not explain large-population level variations. This said RY believes epigenetic changes are important. These arise from complex gene-environment interactions that will take many decades to understand. RY favours a life course explanation founded on DOHAD.

Explanations

The life-course explanation needs to be set in the long-term, multigenerational history of the population. Archaeological evidence using skeletons shows that in the 19th to early 20th centuries the average height of Indians did not increase, whereas by contrast there was a 15 cm (6 inch) gain in height in European populations. This signals a stagnation in socio-economic development and especially in nutritional status. Over multiple generations there may have been pre-conceptional, peri-conceptional, intrauterine, and early life influences that left, through epigenetic change, a susceptibility to cardiometabolic disease. This susceptibility may be signalled by markers such as small birthweight, low muscle mass, relative adiposity, low nephron number, and impaired development of the beta cells of the pancreas. Famines, poor hygiene, weather, and the subordinated role of women were potential compounding factors.

This susceptibility would be exposed only when there were challenges to cardiometabolic homeostasis, especially via exposure in later life to high levels of nutrition and reduced physical activity.

Given this background we would predict that it would take several generations of socio-economic development, including good nutrition, for improvements to occur. RY has been studying this in the Pune Maternal Nutrition Study.

Data from the Pune Maternal Nutrition Study (PMNS)

This study is set in a typical, poor, rural, agrarian society. Since the PMNS started over 20 years ago the area's socio-economic fortunes have improved, for reasons including new water irrigation systems allowing crops such as sugar cane that provide new sources of income.

The data in PMNS now cross three-generations (F0, F1, and F2). The F0 mothers, on average, had a BMI of 18.1, were 1.52 m tall and were highly glucose tolerant on the OGTT done at 28 weeks of pregnancy. Their female offspring (F1) have grown 5 cm taller than their mothers and their BMI has risen. Their babies (F2) were born about 200g heavier than they themselves were at birth.

An OGTT at 28 weeks of pregnancy in F1 showed much worse glucose load handling than in F0. GDM was much commoner in F1 than in F0.

The interpretation of these unpublished results is difficult. However, they cause concern that socio-economic development may not lead to the anticipated benefits and may exacerbate cardiometabolic risk. This said, these are early results. Nonetheless, we concurred that they echoed what we see in

Indians overseas, e.g. the Surinamese Indians in the Netherlands, and Punjabis in Southall, London.

We need to think again about the issues beyond nutrition generally to micronutrients and nutritional balance.

Conclusion

RY's explanation is set in a historical, population setting with multigenerational effects that are more environmental than genetic. The answers are unclear at present but the life course perspective of the DOHAD hypothesis offers a potentially important perspective.

Salim Yusuf (SY) (17/10/17)

Introductory remarks

South Asian populations are akin to some others, e.g. Malays, so they are not outliers even amongst large population groups. In relation to DM_2 it may be that European origin populations are the outliers.

In SY's observations in Canada and internationally South Asians have relatively high DM_2 and MI but not, unlike in the UK, stroke. Explaining these variations is difficult.

Explanations

SY emphasized that despite careful searching genetic risk factors for MI have not been shown to cluster in South Asians. (Although not specified I think this point was generalized to DM_2 also).

Given this, our attention turns to non-genetic risks of which the most important seem to be: 1) relative physical inactivity, 2) a diet with high carbohydrate content and low in fresh fruits and vegetables, 3) no apparent cardio-protection from alcohol (a combination of consumption patterns and type of alcohol, i.e. liquor), 4) lifelong hyperglycaemia with early failure of beta-cells, 5) adverse adipose tissue distribution.

In line with the developmental origins of adult disease hypothesis there may have been influences on the pancreas that lead, in due course, to early dysfunction of beta cells. Such influences might include numbers of islets of langerhans or their formation. Intrauterine developmental factors might also lead to low muscle mass.

Other related observations

SY has re-examined the role of Lp(a) but the evidence suggests it has an incremental rather than highly influential role as a component of dyslipidaemia.

Other PURE data show South Asians have low risks of deep vein thrombosis and pulmonary embolus, and this argues against a tendency to thrombosis; rather, the opposite seems to be true.

Conclusions

SY reflected that despite studying the topic for about 25 years he has not come to a clear understanding of the ethnic variations we discussed today. Presently, we have to work with complex and sometimes paradoxical findings and explanations, with emphasis on lifestyle factors, of which physical activity and diet seem the most important.

References

The reference list is not a comprehensive bibliography on the subject of diabetes, CHD and stroke in South Asians which would be long, perhaps several thousands of articles. Rather, the reference list aims to include most papers and books that have offered explanations for South Asians' susceptibility to CVD/DM. These papers/books may not necessarily have, at the time, focused on South Asians but ones that have subsequently been utilized for such a focus. The references also prioritizes major reviews of the topic and guidelines that are designed for South Asians.

1. Forouhi NG, Sattar N, Tillin T, McKeigue PM, Chaturvedi N. Do known risk factors explain the higher coronary heart disease mortality in South Asian compared with European men? Prospective follow-up of the Southall and Brent studies, UK. Diabetologia. 2006;**49**:2580–8.

2. Paul SK, Owusu Adjah ES, Samanta M, Patel K, Bellary S, Hanif W, et al. Comparison of body mass index at diagnosis of diabetes in a multi-ethnic population: A case-control study with matched non-diabetic controls. Diabetes, Obesity & Metabolism. 2017;**19**(7):1014–23.

3. Lawder R, Harding O, Stockton D, Fischbacher C, Brewster DH, Chalmers J, et al. Is the Scottish population living dangerously? Prevalence of multiple risk factors: the Scottish Health Survey 2003. BMC Public Health. 2010;**10**:330.

4. Bansal N, Fischbacher CM, Bhopal RS, Brown H, Steiner MF, Capewell S, et al. Myocardial infarction incidence and survival by ethnic group: Scottish Health and Ethnicity Linkage retrospective cohort study. BMJ Open. 2013;**3**(9):e003415.

5. Bhopal RS, Bansal N, Fischbacher CM, Brown H, Capewell S. Ethnic variations in the incidence and mortality of stroke in the Scottish Health and Ethnicity Linkage Study of 4.65 million people. European Journal of Preventive Cardiology. 2012;**19**(6):1503–8.

6. Fischbacher CM, Bhopal R, Steiner M, Morris AD, Chalmers J. Is there equity of service delivery and intermediate outcomes in South Asians with type 2 diabetes? Analysis of DARTS database and summary of UK publications. Journal of Public Health. 2009;**31**(2):239–49.

7. Bhopal RS, Bansal N, Fischbacher C, Brown H, Capewell S. Ethnic variations in chest pain and angina in men and women: Scottish Ethnicity and Health Linkage Study of 4.65 million people. European Journal of Preventive Cardiology. 2012;**19**(6):1250–7.

8. Bhopal RS, Bansal N, Fischbacher CM, Brown H, Capewell S. Ethnic variations in heart failure: Scottish Health and Ethnicity Linkage Study (SHELS). Heart. 2012;**98**:468–73.

9. Bhopal R, Unwin N, White M, Yallop J, Walker L, Alberti KG, et al. Heterogeneity of coronary heart disease risk factors in Indian, Pakistani, Bangladeshi, and European origin populations: cross sectional study. BMJ. 1999;**319**:215–20.

10. Becker E, Boreham R, Chaudhury M, Craig R, Deverill C, Doyle M, et al. Health Survey for England 2004. The health of minority ethnic groups. London: The Information Centre; 2006.

11. **Greater Glasgow NHS Board.** Black and Minority Ethnic Health in Glasgow. Glasgow: Greater Glasgow NHS Board; 2006.

12. **Whybrow P, Ramsay J, MacNee K.** The Scottish Health Survey–Equality Groups. Edinburgh: The Scottish Government; 2012.

13. **Traci Leven Research.** 2016 Black and Minority Ethnic Health and Wellbeing Study in Glasgow. Glasgow: NHS Greater Glasgow and Clyde, 2017. Final Report.

14. **McKeigue PM, Miller GJ, Marmot MG.** Coronary heart disease in South Asians overseas: a review. Journal of Clinical Epidemiology. 1989;**42**(7):597–609.

15. **Bhopal R, Bansal N, Steiner M, Brewster DH.** Does the 'Scottish effect' apply to all ethnic groups? All cancer, lung, colorectal, breast and prostate cancer in the Scottish Health and Ethnicity Linkage Cohort Study. BMJ Open. 2012;**2**:e001957.

16. **Marmot MG, Adelstein AM, Bulusu L.** Immigrant mortality in England and Wales 1970–78. Causes of death by country of birth. London: HMSO; 1984.

17. **Reaven GM.** Role of insulin resistance in human disease. Diabetes. 1988;**37**(12):1595–607.

18. **Tillin T, Hughes AD, Mayet J, Whincup P, Sattar N, Forouhi NG,** et al. The relationship between metabolic risk factors and incident cardiovascular disease in Europeans, South Asians, and African Caribbeans: SABRE (Southall and Brent Revisited)—a prospective population-based study. Journal of the American College of Cardiology. 2013;**61**(17):1777–86.

19. **Zaman MJS, Shipley MJ, Stafford M, Brunner EJ, Timmis AD, Marmot MG,** et al. Incidence and prognosis of angina pectoris in South Asians and Whites: 18 years of follow-up over seven phases in the Whitehall-II prospective cohort study. Journal of Public Health. 2011;**33**(3):430–8.

20. **Nijjar A, Wang H, Dasgupta K, Rabi D, Quan H, Khan N.** Outcomes in a diabetic population of South Asians and whites following hospitalization for acute myocardial infarction: a retrospective cohort study. Cardiovascular Diabetology. 2010;**9**(1):4.

21. **Saposnik G, Redelmeier DA, Lu H, Fuller-Thomson E, Lonn E, Ray JG.** Myocardial infarction associated with recency of immigration to Ontario. QJM. 2010;**103**(4):253–8.

22. **Shrivastava U, Misra A, Mohan V, Unnikrishnan R, Bachani D.** Obesity, diabetes and cardiovascular diseases in india: public health challenges. Current Diabetes Reviews. 2017;**13**(1):65–80.

23. **Prabhakaran D, Jeemon P, Roy A.** Cardiovascular diseases in India: Current epidemiology and future directions. Circulation. 2016;**133**(16):1605–20.

24. **Dandona L, Dandona R, Kumar GA, Shukla DK, Paul VK, Balakrishnan K,** et al. Nations within a nation: variations in epidemiological transition across the states of India in the Global Burden of Disease Study. Lancet. 2017;**390**(10111):2437–60.

25. **Yusuf S, Reddy S, Ounpuu S, Anand S.** Global burden of cardiovascular diseases Part II: Variations in cardiovascular disease by specific ethnic groups and geographic regions and prevention strategies. Circulation. 2001;**104**:2855–64.

26. **Shearmur J, Shand J. Karl Popper:** The Logic of Scientific Discovery 2012. 262–86 p.

27. **Bhopal RS.** Concepts of Epidemiology: Integrating the Ideas, Theories, Principles and Methods of Epidemiology. Third edition. New York, NY: Oxford University Press; 2016.

28. **Ramaiya KL, Swai AB, McLarty DG, Bhopal RS, Alberti KG.** Prevalences of diabetes and cardiovascular disease risk factors in Hindu Indian subcommunities in Tanzania. BMJ. 1991;**303**(6797):271–6.

29. **Patel KCR, Bhopal, RS.** (Editors). The Epidemic of Coronary Heart Disease in South Asian Populations: Causes and Consequences. Birmingham: South Asian Health Foundation; 2004.

30. **Volgman AS, Palaniappan LS, Aggarwal NT, Gupta M, Khandelwal A, Krishnan AV,** et al. Atherosclerotic cardiovascular disease in South Asians in the United States: Epidemiology, Risk Factors, and Treatments: A Scientific Statement From the American Heart Association. Circulation. 2018;**138**:1–3.

31. **Gasevic D, Ross ES, Lear SA.** Ethnic differences in cardiovascular disease risk factors: a systematic review of North American evidence. Canadian Journal of Cardiology. 2015;**31**(9):1169–79.

32. **Kanaya AM, Kandula N, Herrington D, Budoff MJ, Hulley S, Vittinghoff E,** et al. Mediators of atherosclerosis in South Asians living in America (MASALA) study: objectives, methods, and cohort description. Clinical Cardiology. 2013;**36**(12):713–20.

33. **Gujral UP, Narayan KM, Pradeepa RG, Deepa M, Ali MK, Anjana RM,** et al. Comparing type 2 diabetes, prediabetes, and their associated risk factors in Asian Indians in India and in the US: The CARRS and MASALA studies. Diabetes Care. 2015;**38**(7):1312–18.

34. **Gupta R, Khedar RS, Gaur K, Xavier D.** Low quality cardiovascular care is important coronary risk factor in India. Indian Heart Journal. 2018; https://doi.org/10.1016/j.ihj.2018.05.002

35. **Mather HM, Keen H.** The Southall Diabetes Survey: prevalence of known diabetes in Asians and Europeans. BMJ. 1985;**291**:1081–4.

36. **Verma NP, Mehta SP, Madhu S, Mather HM, Keen H.** Prevalence of known diabetes in an urban Indian environment: the Darya Ganj diabetes survey. BMJ. 1986;**293**:423–4.

37. **Hellenthal G, Busby GB, Band G, Wilson JF, Capelli C, Falush D,** et al. A genetic atlas of human admixture history. Science. 2014;**343**(6172):747–51.

38. **Wall JD, Yang MA, Jay F, Kim SK, Durand EY, Stevison LS,** et al. Higher levels of Neanderthal ancestry in East Asians than in Europeans. Genetics. 2013;**194**(1):199–209.

39. **Dries DL.** Genetic ancestry, population admixture, and the genetic epidemiology of complex disease. Circulation: Cardiovascular Genetics. 2009;**2**(6):540–3.

40. **Ayub Q, Tyler-Smith C.** Genetic variation in South Asia: assessing the influences of geography, language and ethnicity for understanding history and disease risk. Briefings in Functional Genomics. 2009;**8**(5):395–404.

41. **Majumder PP, Basu A.** A genomic view of the peopling and population structure of India. Cold Spring Harbour Perspectives in Biology. 2014;**7**(4):1–10.

42. **Silva M, Oliveira M, Vieira D, Brandão A, Rito T, Pereira JB,** et al. A genetic chronology for the Indian Subcontinent points to heavily sex-biased dispersals. BMC Evolutionary Biology. 2017;**17**(1):88.

43. **Veeramah KR, Novembre J.** Demographic events and evolutionary forces shaping European genetic diversity. Cold Spring Harb Perspect Biol. 2014 Sep; **6**(9): a008516.

44. **McKeigue PM, Ferrie JE, Pierpoint T, Marmot MG.** Association of early-onset conronary heart disease in South Asian men with glucose intolerance and hyperinsulinemia. Circulation. 1993;**87**:152–61.

45. **Haider Z, Obdaidullah S, Ud Din F, Zubair M, Saleem M.** Prevalence of coronary heart disease in Pakistani patients suffering from maturity onset diabetes mellitus. Journal of Tropical Medicine & Hygiene. 1978;**81**(6):98–102.

46. **Shrivastava U, Misra A, Mohan V, Unnikrishnan R, Bachani D.** Obesity, diabetes and cardiovascular diseases in India: public health challenges. Current Diabetes Reviews. 2017;**13**(1):65–80.

47. **Yakoob MY, Micha R, Khatibzadeh S, Singh GM, Shi P, Ahsan H,** et al. Impact of dietary and metabolic risk factors on cardiovascular and diabetes mortality in South Asia: analysis from the 2010 Global Burden of Disease Study. American Journal of Public Health. 2016;**106**(12):2113–25.

48. **Jayawardena R, Ranasinghe P, Wijayabandara M, Hills AP, Misra A.** Nutrition transition and obesity among teenagers and young adults in South Asia. Current Diabetes Reviews. 2016;13(5):444–51.

49. **Saleheen D, Zaidi M, Rasheed A, Ahmad U, Hakeem A, Murtaza M,** et al. The Pakistan Risk of Myocardial Infarction Study: a resource for the study of genetic, lifestyle and other determinants of myocardial infarction in South Asia. European Journal of Epidemiology. 2009;**24**(6):329–38.

50. **Biswas T, Islam A, Rawal LB, Islam SM.** Increasing prevalence of diabetes in Bangladesh: a scoping review. Public Health. 2016;**138**:4–11.

51. **Fatema K, Zwar NA, Milton AH, Rahman B, Awal AS, Ali L.** Cardiovascular risk assessment among rural population: findings from a cohort study in a peripheral region of Bangladesh. Public Health. 2016;**137**:73–80.

52. **Hussain A, Vaaler S, Sayeed MA, Mahtab H, Ali SM, Khan AK.** Type 2 diabetes and impaired fasting blood glucose in rural Bangladesh: a population-based study. European Journal of Public Health. 2007;**17**:291–6.

53. **Yajnik CS, Joglekar CV, Lubree HG, Rege SS, Naik SS, Bhat DS,** et al. Adiposity, inflammation and hyperglycaemia in rural and urban Indian men: Coronary Risk of Insulin Sensitivity in Indian Subjects (CRISIS) Study. Diabetologia. 2008;**51**(1):39–46.

54. **Bhopal RS.** Migration, Ethnicity, Race and Health in Multicultural Societies. Second edition. Oxford: Oxford University Press; 2014.

55. **Bhopal R, Donaldson L.** White, European, Western, Caucasian, or what? Inappropriate labeling in research on race, ethnicity, and health. American Journal of Public Health. 1998;**88**(9):1303–7.

56. **Yeo KK, Tai BC, Heng D, Lee JM, Ma S, Hughes K,** et al. Ethnicity modifies the association between diabetes mellitus and ischaemic heart disease in Chinese, Malays and Asian Indians living in Singapore. Diabetologia. 2006;**49**(12):2866–73.

57. **Adelstein AM.** Some aspects of cardiovascular mortality in South Africa. British Journal of Preventive and Social Medicine. 1963;**17**:29–40.

58. **Wild SH, Fischbacher C, Brock A, Griffiths C, Bhopal R.** Mortality from all causes and circulatory disease by country of birth in England and Wales 2001–2003. Journal of Public Health (Oxford). 2007;**29**(2):191–8.

59. Tan KHX, Barr E, Koshkina V, Ma S, Kowlessur S, Magliano DJ, et al. Diabetes mellitus prevalence is increasing in South Asians but stable in Chinese living in Singapore and Mauritius. Journal of Diabetes. 2016;9(9):855–64.

60. Patel JV, Vyas A, Cruickshank JK, Prabhakaran D, Hughes E, Reddy KS, et al. Impact of migration on coronary heart disease risk factors: comparison of Gujaratis in Britain and their contemporaries in villages of origin in India. Atherosclerosis 2006;185(2):297–306.

61. Bhatnagar D, Anand IS, Durrington PN, Patel DJ, Wander GS, Mackness MI, et al. Coronary risk factors in people from the Indian subcontinent living in west London and their siblings in India. Lancet. 1995;345(8947):405–9.

62. Tzoulaki I, Elliott P, Kontis V, Ezzati M. Worldwide exposures to cardiovascular risk factors and associated health effects: current knowledge and data gaps. Circulation. 2016;133(23):2314–33.

63. Rajendran P, Rengarajan T, Thangavel J, Nishigaki Y, Sakthisekaran D, Sethi G, et al. The vascular endothelium and human diseases. International Journal of Biological Sciences. 2013;9(10):1057–69.

64. Chambers JC, McGregor A, Jean-Marie J, Kooner JS. Abnormalities of vascular endothelial function may contribute to increased coronary heart disease risk in UK Indian Asians. Heart. 1999;81:501–4.

65. Boon MR, Karamali NS, de Groot CJ, van SL, Kanhai HH, van der Bent C, et al. E-selectin is elevated in cord blood of South Asian neonates compared with Caucasian neonates. Journal of Pediatrics. 2012;160(5):844–8.

66. Jain P, Kooner JS, Raval U, Lahiri A. Prevalence of coronary artery calcium scores and silent myocardial ischaemia was similar in Indian Asians and European whites in a cross-sectional study of asymptomatic subjects from a UK population (LOLIPOP-IPC). Journal of Nuclear Cardiology. 2011;18(3):435.

67. Kanaya AM, Kandula NR, Ewing SK, Herrington D, Liu K, Blaha MJ, et al. Comparing coronary artery calcium among US South Asians with four racial/ethnic groups: The MASALA and MESA studies. Atherosclerosis. 2014;234(1):102–7.

68. Haverich A. A surgeon's view on the pathogenesis of atherosclerosis. Circulation. 2017;135(3):205–7.

69. Taruya A, Tanaka A, Nishiguchi T, Matsuo Y, Ozaki Y, Kashiwagi M, et al. Vasa vasorum restructuring in human atherosclerotic plaque vulnerability: a clinical optical coherence tomography study. Journal of the American College of Cardiology. 2015;65(23):2469–77.

70. Gerstein HC, Werstuck GH. Dysglycaemia, vasculopenia, and the chronic consequences of diabetes. Lancet Diabetes & Endocrinology. 2013;1(1):71–8.

71. Stenmark KR, Nozik-Grayck E, Gerasimovskaya E, Anwar A, Li M, Riddle S, et al. The adventitia: Essential role in pulmonary vascular remodeling. Comprehensive Physiology. 2011;1(1):141–61.

72. Ritman EL, Lerman A. The dynamic vasa vasorum. Cardiovascular Research. 2007;75(4):649–58.

73. Galili O, Herrmann J, Woodrum J, Sattler KJ, Lerman LO, Lerman A. Adventitial vasa vasorum heterogeneity among different vascular beds. Journal of Vascular Surgery 2004;40(3):529–35.

74. Martin JF, Booth RFG, Moncada S. Arterial wall hypoxia following thrombosis of the vasa vasorum is an initial lesion in atherosclerosis. European Journal of Clinical Investigation. 1991;21(3):355–9.

75. **Barger AC, Beeuwkes R, 3rd, Lainey LL, Silverman KJ.** Hypothesis: vasa vasorum and neovascularization of human coronary arteries. A possible role in the pathophysiology of atherosclerosis. The New England Journal of Medicine. 1984;**310**(3):175–7.

76. **Hopkins PN, Williams RR.** A survey of 246 suggested coronary risk factors. Atherosclerosis. 1981;**40**(1):1–52.

77. **Unnikrishnan R, Anjana RM, Mohan V.** Diabetes mellitus and its complications in India. Nature Reviews Endocrinology. 2016;**12**(6):357–70.

78. **Ramachandran A, Ma RC, Snehalatha C.** Diabetes in Asia. Lancet. 2010;**375**(9712):408–18.

79. **Taylor R.** Type 2 diabetes: etiology and reversibility. Diabetes Care. 2013;**36**(4):1047–55.

80. **Sinha S, Rathi M, Misra A, Kumar V, Kumar M, Jagannathan NR,** et al. Subclinical inflammation and soleus muscle intramyocellular lipids in healthy Asian Indian males. Clinical Endocrinology (Oxford). 2005;**63**(3):350–5.

81. **Forouhi N, Jenkinson G, Thomas EL, McKeigue P, Bhonsle U, Bell JD.** Insulin Sensitivity and Muscle Triglycerides: an in vivo Magnetic Resonance Study. The Smith Kline Beecham Research Symposium, 1999.

82. **Eastwood SV, Tillin T, Wright A, Mayet J, Godsland I, Forouhi NG,** et al. Thigh fat and muscle each contribute to excess cardiometabolic risk in South Asians, independent of visceral adipose tissue. Obesity (Silver Spring). 2014;**22**(9):2071–9.

83. **Anand SS, Tarnopolsky MA, Rashid S, Schulze KM, Desai D, Mente A,** et al. Adipocyte hypertrophy, fatty liver and metabolic risk factors in South Asians: the Molecular Study of Health and Risk in Ethnic Groups (mol-SHARE). PLoSOne. 2011;**6**(7):e22112.

84. **Arnold D.** Diabetes in the tropics: race, place and class in India, 1880–1965. Social History of Medicine. 2009;**22**(2):245–61.

85. **Yusuf S, Hawken S, Ounpuu S, Dans T, Avezum A, Lanas F,** et al. Effect of potentially modifiable risk factors associated with myocardial infarction in 52 countries (the INTERHEART study): case-control study. Lancet. 2004;**364**(9438):937–52.

86. **Misra A.** Ethnic-specific criteria for classification of body mass index: a perspective for Asian Indians and American Diabetes Association position statement. Diabetes Technology & Therapeutics. 2015;**17**(9):667–71.

87. **Bhopal R.** Epidemic of cardiovascular disease in South Asians. BMJ. 2002;**324**:625–6.

88. **Tan ST, Mills R, Loh M, Panoulas V, Afzal U, Scott J,** et al. Investigation of the validity of cardiovascular death certification amongst UK Indian Asians and Europeans. Heart. 2014;**100**(Suppl 3):A64-A.

89. **Pavkov ME, Hanson RL, Knowler WC, Bennett PH, Krakoff J, Nelson RG.** Changing patterns of type 2 diabetes incidence among Pima Indians. Diabetes Care. 2007;**30**(7):1758–63.

90. **Olabi B, Bhopal R.** Diagnosis of diabetes using the oral glucose tolerance test. BMJ. 2009;**339**:b4354.

91. **Lambert AM, Burden AC, Chambers J, Marshall T.** Cardiovascular screening for men at high risk in Heart of Birmingham Teaching Primary Care Trust: the 'Deadly Trio' programme. Journal of Public Health. 2012;**34**(1):73–82.

92. **Verma A, Birger R, Bhatt H, Murray J, Millett C, Saxena S,** et al. Ethnic disparities in diabetes management: a 10-year population-based repeated cross-sectional study in UK primary care. Journal of Public Health. 2010;**32**(2):250–8.

93. **Ben-Shlomo Y, Naqvi H, Baker I.** Ethnic differences in healthcare-seeking behaviour and management for acute chest pain: secondary analysis of the MINAP dataset 2002-2003. Heart. 2008;**94**(3):354–9.

94. **Neel JV.** Diabetes mellitus: a 'thrifty' genotype rendered detrimental by 'progress'? American Journal of Human Genetics. 1962;**14**:353–62.

95. **Hales CN, Barker DJP.** The thrifty phenotype hypothesis. British Medical Bulletin. 2001;**60**(1):5–20.

96. **Bhopal RS.** A four-stage model explaining the higher risk of type 2 diabetes mellitus in South Asians compared with European populations. Diabetic Medicine. 2013;**30**(1):35–42.

97. **Chambers JC, Obeid OA, Refsum H, Ueland P, Hackett D, Hooper J,** et al. Plasma homocysteine concentrations and risk of coronary heart disease in UK Indian Asian and European men. Lancet. 2000;**355**:523–7.

98. **Ranganathan M, Bhopal R.** Exclusion and Inclusion of nonwhite ethnic minority groups in 72 North American and European cardiovascular cohort studies. PLoS Med. 2006;**3**(3):e44.

99. **Tillin T, Forouhi NG, McKeigue PM, Chaturvedi N.** Southall and Brent REvisited: Cohort profile of SABRE, a UK population-based comparison of cardiovascular disease and diabetes in people of European, Indian Asian and African Caribbean origins. International Journal of Epidemiology. 2012;**41**(1):33–42.

100. **Yajnik CS, Chandak GR, Joglekar C, Katre P, Bhat DS, Singh SN,** et al. Maternal homocysteine in pregnancy and offspring birthweight: epidemiological associations and Mendelian randomization analysis. International Journal of Epidemiology. 2014;**43**(5):1487–97.

101. **Sniderman AD, Bhopal R, Prabhakaran D, Sarrafzadegan N, Tchernof A.** Why might South Asians be so susceptible to central obesity and its atherogenic consequences? The adipose tissue overflow hypothesis. International Journal of Epidemiology. 2007;**36**(1):220–5.

102. **Watve MG, Yajnik CS.** Evolutionary origins of insulin resistance: a behavioral switch hypothesis. BMC Evolutionary Biology. 2007;**7**:61.

103. **Engelgau MM, El-Saharty S, Kudesia P, Rajan V, Rosenhouse S, Okamoto K.** Capitalizing on the Demographic Transition: Tackling Noncommunicable Diseases in South Asia. Direction in Development; Human Development. Conference edition: The World Bank; 2011.

104. **Cappuccio FP.** Commentary: Epidemiological transition, migration, and cardiovascular disease. Internation Journal of Epidemiology. 2004;**33**:387–8.

105. **Forsdahl A.** Are poor living conditions in childhood and adolescence an important risk factor for arteriosclerotic heart disease? British Journal of Preventive and Social Medicine. 1977;**31**:91–5.

106. **Roswall N, Li Y, Sandin S, Strom P, Adami HO, Weiderpass E.** Changes in body mass index and waist circumference and concurrent mortality among Swedish women. Obesity (Silver Spring). 2016;**25**(1):215–22.

107. **Kakde S, Bhopal RS, Bhardwaj S, Misra A.** Urbanized South Asians' susceptibility to coronary heart disease: The high-heat food preparation hypothesis. Nutrition. 2017;**33**:216–24.

108. Rafnsson SB, Saravanan P, Bhopal RS, Yajnik CS. Is a low blood level of vitamin B12 a cardiovascular and diabetes risk factor? A systematic review of cohort studies. European Journal of Nutrition. 2011;50:97–106.

109. Wang L, Manson JE, Song Y, Sesso HD. Systematic review: Vitamin D and calcium supplementation in prevention of cardiovascular events. Annals of Internal Medicine. 2010;152(5):315–23.

110. Sukumar N, Rafnsson SB, Kandala NB, Bhopal R, Yajnik CS, Saravanan P. Prevalence of vitamin B-12 insufficiency during pregnancy and its effect on offspring birth weight: a systematic review and meta-analysis. The American Journal of Clinical Nutrition. 2016;103(5):1232–51.

111. World Health Organization. Global action plan for the prevention and control of noncommunicable diseases 2013–2020: World Health Organization; 2016.

112. Alper JS, Natowicz MR. The allure of genetic explanations. BMJ. 1992;305 (6855):666.

113. Gould SJ. The Mismeasure of Man. London: Pelican Books Ltd; 1984.

114. Barkan E. The Retreat of Scientific Racism. London: Cambridge University Press; 1992.

115. Defesche JC, Gidding SS, Harada-Shiba M, Hegele RA, Santos RD, Wierzbicki AS. Familial hypercholesterolaemia. Nature Reviews. Disease Primers. 2017;3:17093.

116. Iyengar SS, Puri R, Narasingan SN, Nair DR, Mehta V, Mohan JC, et al. Lipid Association of India (LAI) expert consensus statement on management of dyslipidaemia in Indians 2017: part 2. Clinical Lipidology. 2017;12(1):56–109.

117. Iyengar SS, Puri R, Narasingan SN, Wangnoo SK, Mohan V, Mohan JC, et al. Lipid Association of India Expert Consensus Statement on Management of Dyslipidemia in Indians 2016: Part 1. J Assoc Physicians India. 2016;64(3):7–52.

118. Jablonski NG. The evolution of human skin colouration and its relevance to health in the modern world. Journal of the Royal College of Physicians of Edinburgh. 2012;42(1):58–63.

119. Campbell AK, Waud JP, Matthews SB. The molecular basis of lactose intolerance. Science Progress. 2005;88:157–202.

120. Rosenberg NA, Pritchard JK, Weber JL, Cann HM, Kidd KK, Zhivotovsky LA, et al. Genetic structure of human populations. Science. 2002;298(5602):2381–5.

121. Anand SS, Xie C, Pare G, Montpetit A, Rangarajan S, McQueen MJ, et al. Genetic variants associated with myocardial infarction risk factors in over 8000 individuals from five ethnic groups: The INTERHEART Genetics Study. Circulation: Cardiovascular Genetics. 2009;2(1):16–25.

122. Chhabra S, DP. A, S V, Luthra K, rang R, SC n, et al. Study of apolipoprotein E polymorphism in normal healthy controls from northern India. Disease Markers. 2000(16):159–61.

123. Kooner JS, Saleheen D, Sim X, Sehmi J, Zhang W, Frossard P, et al. Genome-wide association study in individuals of South Asian ancestry identifies six new type 2 diabetes susceptibility loci. Nature Genetics. 2011;43(10):984–9.

124. Hopewell JC, Peden J, Saleheen D, Chambers J, Clarke R, Collins R, et al. Abstract 17979: a genome-wide association study of risk of coronary artery disease in european and south asian populations. Circulation. 2010;122(Suppl 21):A17979–A.

125. Chambers JC, Ireland H, Thompson E, Reilly P, Obeid OA, Refsum H, et al. Methylenetetrahydrofolate reductase 677 C→T mutation and coronary heart disease risk in UK Indian Asians. Arteriosclerosis, Thrombosis, and Vascular Biology. 2000;**20**(11):2448–52.

126. Cassell PG, Jackson AE, North BV, Evans JC, Syndercombe-Court, Phillips C, et al. Haplotype combinations of calpain 10 gene polymorphisms associate with increased risk of impaired glucose tolerance and type 2 diabetes in South Indians. Diabetes. 2002;**51**(5):1622–8.

127. Chambers JC, Elliott P, Zabaneh D, Zhang W, Li Y, Froguel P, et al. Common genetic variation near MC4R is associated with waist circumference and insulin resistance. Nature Genetics. 2008;**40**(6):716–18.

128. Scott WR, Zhang W, Loh M, Tan ST, Lehne B, Afzal U, et al. Investigation of genetic variation underlying central obesity amongst South Asians. PLoS ONE. 2016;**11**(5):e0155478.

129. Aidoo M, Terlouw DJ, Kolczak MS, McElroy PD, ter Kuile FO, Kariuki S, et al. Protective effects of the sickle cell gene against malaria morbidity and mortality. Lancet. 2002;**359**(9314):1311–12.

130. Neel JV. The Thrifty Genotype Revisited. New York: Academic Press; 1982.

131. Prasad DS, Kabir Z, Dash AK, Das BC. Childhood cardiovascular risk factors in South Asians: A cause of concern for adult cardiovascular disease epidemic. Annals of Pediatric Cardiology. 2011;**4**(2):166–71.

132. Neel JV. Update to 'The Study of Natural Selection in Primitive and Civilized Human Populations'. Human Biology. 1989;**61**(5/6):811–23.

133. Fee M. Racializing narratives: obesity, diabetes and the 'Aboriginal' thrifty genotype. Social Science & Medicine. 2006;**62**:2988–97.

134. McDermott R. Ethics, epidemiology and the thrifty gene: biological determinism as a health hazard. Social Science and Medicine. 1998;**47**(9):1189–95.

135. Speakman JR. The evolution of body fatness: trading off disease and predation risk. Journal of Experimental Biology. 2018;**221**(Pt Suppl 1).

136. Watve M. The Rise and Fall of Thrift. Doves, Diplomats, and Diabetes: a Darwinian Interpretation of Type 2 Diabetes and Related Disorders. New York: Springer Science+Business Media New York; 2013.

137. Sellayah D, Cagampang FR, Cox RD. On the evolutionary origins of obesity: a new hypothesis. Endocrinology. 2014;**155**(5):1573–88.

138. Wells JCK, Pomeroy E, Walimbe SR, Popkin BM, Yajnik CS. The elevated susceptibility to diabetes in India: an evolutionary perspective. Frontiers in Public Health. 2016;**4**:145.

139. Goodarzi MO. Genetics of obesity: what genetic association studies have taught us about the biology of obesity and its complications. Lancet Diabetes & Endocrinology. 2018;**6**(3):223–36.

140. Tabassum R, Chauhan G, Dwivedi OP, Mahajan A, Jaiswal A, Kaur I, et al. Genome-wide association study for type 2 diabetes in Indians identifies a new susceptibility locus at 2q21. Diabetes. 2013;**62**(3):977–86.

141. Kaufman JS, Dolman L, Rushani D, Cooper RS. The contribution of genomic research to explaining racial disparities in cardiovascular disease: a systematic review. American Journal of Epidemiology. 2015;**181**(7):464–72.

142. **Coronary Artery Disease (C4D) Genetics.** A genome-wide association study in Europeans and South Asians identifies five new loci for coronary artery disease. Nature Genetics. 2011;**43**(4):339–44.

143. **Minster RL, Hawley NL, Su CT, Sun G, Kershaw EE, Cheng H**, et al. A thrifty variant in CREBRF strongly influences body mass index in Samoans. Nature Genetics. 2016;**48**(9):1049–54.

144. **Loos RJ.** CREBRF variant increases obesity risk and protects against diabetes in Samoans. Nature Genetics. 2016;**48**(9):976–8.

145. **Speakman JR.** Thrifty genes for obesity, an attractive but flawed idea, and an alternative perspective: the 'drifty gene' hypothesis. International journal of Obesity. 2008;**32**(11):1611–17.

146. **Speakman JR.** A nonadaptive scenario explaining the genetic predisposition to obesity: the 'predation release' hypothesis. Cell Metabolism. 2007;**6**(1):5–12.

147. **Bhopal RS, Rafnsson SB.** Could mitochondrial efficiency explain the susceptibility to adiposity, metabolic syndrome, diabetes and cardiovascular diseases in South Asian populations? International Journal of Epidemiology. 2009;**38**(4):1072–81.

148. **Deane R, Ojo O, Zotor F, Amuna P.** The effects of ethnicity and environment on energy expenditure and body composition changes. Clinical Nutrition. 2002:128 [Abstract].

149. **Henry CJ, Rees DG.** New predictive equations for the estimation of basal metabolic rate in tropical peoples. European Journal of Clinical Nutrition. 1991;**45**(4):177–85.

150. **McMurray RG, Soares J, Caspersen CJ, McCurdy T.** Examining variations of resting metabolic rate of adults: a public health perspective. Medicine & Science in Sports & Exercise. 2014;**46**(7):1352–8.

151. **Nair KS, Bigelow ML, Asmann YW, Chow LS, Coenen-Schimke JM, Klaus KA**, et al. Asian Indians have enhanced skeletal muscle mitochondrial capacity to produce ATP in association with severe insulin resistance. Diabetes. 2008;**57**(5):1166–75.

152. **Cassell PG, Saker PJ, Huxtable SJ, Kousta E, Jackson AE, Hattersley AT**, et al. Evidence that single nucleotide polymorphism in the uncoupling protein 3 (UCP3) gene influences fat distribution in women of European and Asian origin. Diabetologia. 2000;**43**(12):1558–64.

153. **Martinez-Hervas S, Mansego ML, de Marco G, Martinez F, Alonso MP, Morcillo S**, et al. Polymorphisms of the UCP2 gene are associated with body fat distribution and risk of abdominal obesity in Spanish population. European Journal of Clinical Investigation. 2011;**42**(2):171–8.

154. **Pednekar MS, Hakama M, Hebert JR, Gupta PC.** Association of body mass index with all-cause and cause-specific mortality: findings from a prospective cohort study in Mumbai (Bombay), India. International Journal of Epidemiology. 2008;**37**(3):524–35.

155. **Sauvaget C, Ramadas K, Thomas G, Vinoda J, Thara S, Sankaranarayanan R.** Body mass index, weight change and mortality risk in a prospective study in India. International Journal of Epidemiology. 2008;**37**(5):990–1004.

156. **Pierce BL, Kalra T, Argos M, Parvez F, Chen Y, Islam T**, et al. A prospective study of body mass index and mortality in Bangladesh. International Journal of Epidemiology. 2010;**39**(4):1037–45.

157. **Sattar N, Gill JM.** Type 2 diabetes in migrant South Asians: mechanisms, mitigation, and management. Lancet Diabetes & Endocrinology. 2015;**3**(12):1004–16.

158. Chen Y, Copeland WK, Vedanthan R, Grant E, Lee JE, Gu D, et al. Association between body mass index and cardiovascular disease mortality in East Asians and South Asians: pooled analysis of prospective data from the Asia Cohort Consortium. BMJ. 2013;**347**:f5446.

159. Lee CM, Barzi F, Woodward M, Batty GD, Giles GG, Wong JW, et al. Adult height and the risks of cardiovascular disease and major causes of death in the Asia-Pacific region: 21,000 deaths in 510,000 men and women. International Journal of Epidemiology. 2009;**38**(4):1060–71.

160. Katzmarzyk PT, Leonard WR. Climatic influences on human body size and proportions: ecological adaptations and secular trends. American Journal of Physical Anthropology. 1998;**106**(4):483–503.

161. Yaghootkar H, Lotta LA, Tyrrell J, Smit RA, Jones SE, Donnelly L, et al. Genetic evidence for a link between favorable adiposity and lower risk of type 2 diabetes, hypertension, and heart disease. Diabetes. 2016;**65**(8):2448–60.

162. Mente A, Razak F, Blankenberg S, Vuksan V, Davis AD, Miller R, et al. Ethnic variation in adiponectin and leptin levels and their association with adiposity and insulin resistance. Diabetes Care. 2010;**33**(7):1629–34.

163. Bush HM, Williams RG, Lean ME, Anderson AS. Body image and weight consciousness among South Asian, Italian and general population women in Britain. Appetite. 2001;**37**(3):207–15.

164. Patel S, Bhopal R, Unwin N, White M, Alberti KG, Yallop J. Mismatch between perceived and actual overweight in diabetic and non-diabetic populations: a comparative study of South Asian and European women. Journal of Epidemiology and Community Health. 2001;**55**:332–3.

165. Harpsoe MC, Nielsen NM, Friis-Moller N, Andersson M, Wohlfahrt J, Linneberg A, et al. Body mass index and risk of infections among women in the Danish national birth cohort. American Journal of Epidemiology. 2016;**183**(11):1008–17.

166. Aune D, Sen A, Prasad M, Norat T, Janszky I, Tonstad S, et al. BMI and all cause mortality: systematic review and non-linear dose-response meta-analysis of 230 cohort studies with 3.74 million deaths among 30.3 million participants. BMJ. 2016;**353**:i2156.

167. Zaccardi F, Dhalwani NN, Papamargaritis D, Webb DR, Murphy GJ, Davies MJ, et al. Nonlinear association of BMI with all-cause and cardiovascular mortality in type 2 diabetes mellitus: a systematic review and meta-analysis of 414,587 participants in prospective studies. Diabetologia. 2017;**60**(2):240–8.

168. Global BMI Mortality Collaboration, Di Angelantonio E, Bhupathiraju ShN, Wormser D, Gao P, Kaptoge S, et al.. Body-mass index and all-cause mortality: individual-participant-data meta-analysis of 239 prospective studies in four continents. Lancet. 2016;**388**(10046):776–86.

169. Ni MC, Rodgers A, Pan WH, Gu DF, Woodward M. Body mass index and cardiovascular disease in the Asia-Pacific Region: an overview of 33 cohorts involving 310 000 participants. International Journal of Epidemiology. 2004;**33**:751–8.

170. Vague J. The degree of masculine differentiation of obesities: a factor determining predisposition to diabetes, atherosclerosis, gout, and uric calculous disease. American Journal of Clinical Nutrition 1956;**4**(1):20–34.

171. Shadid S, Koutsari C, Jensen MD. Direct free fatty acid uptake into human adipocytes in vivo: relation to body fat distribution. Diabetes. 2007;56(5):1369–75.

172. Chau YY, Bandiera R, Serrels A, Martínez-Estrada OM, Qing W, Lee M, et al. Visceral and subcutaneous fat have different origins and evidence supports a mesothelial source. Nature Cell Biology. 2014;16(4):367–75.

173. Bakker L, Boon M, van der Linden R, Arias-Bouda L, van Klinken J, Mit F, et al. Brown adipose tissue volume in healthy lean South Asian adults compared with white Caucasians: a prospective, case-controlled observational study. Lancet Diabetes & Endocrinology. 2013;2(3):210–17.

174. Admiraal WM. The Various Colours of Type 2 Diabetes–Pathogenesis and Epidemiology in Different Ethnic Groups [Doctorate]. Amsterdam: University of Amsterdam; 2013.

175. Veilleux A, Caron-Jobin M, Noel S, Laberge PY, Tchernof A. Visceral adipocyte hypertrophy is associated with dyslipidemia independent of body composition and fat distribution in women. Diabetes. 2011;60(5):1504–11.

176. Hunma S, Ramuth H, Miles-Chan JL, Schutz Y, Montani JP, Joonas N, et al. Body composition-derived BMI cut-offs for overweight and obesity in Indians and Creoles of Mauritius: comparison with Caucasians. International Journal of Obesity. 2016;40:1906–14.

177. Chandalia M, Lin P, Seenivasan T, Livingston EH, Snell PG, Grundy SM, et al. Insulin resistance and body fat distribution in South Asian men compared to Caucasian men. PLoS ONE. 2007;2(8):e812.

178. Stanfield KM, Wells JC, Fewtrell MS, Frost C, Leon DA. Differences in body composition between infants of South Asian and European ancestry: the London Mother and Baby Study. International Journal of Epidemiology. 2012;41(5):1409–18.

179. Nightingale CM, Rudnicka AR, Owen CG, Cook DG, Whincup PH. Patterns of body size and adiposity among UK children of South Asian, black African–Caribbean and white European origin: Child Heart And health Study in England (CHASE Study). International Journal of Epidemiology. 2011;40(1):33–44.

180. Biswas T, Islam A, Islam MS, Pervin S, Rawal LB. Overweight and obesity among children and adolescents in Bangladesh: a systematic review and meta-analysis. Public Health. 2017;142:94–101.

181. van Steijn L, Karamali NS, Kanhai HH, Ariens GA, Fall CH, Yajnik CS, et al. Neonatal anthropometry: thin-fat phenotype in fourth to fifth generation South Asian neonates in Surinam. International Journal of Obesity (London). 2009;33(11):1326–9.

182. D'Angelo S, Yajnik CS, Kumaran K, Joglekar C, Lubree H, Crozier SR, et al. Body size and body composition: a comparison of children in India and the UK through infancy and early childhood. Journal of Epidemiology & Community Health. 2015;69(12):1147–53.

183. Snijder MB, van Dam RM, Visser M, Seidell JC. What aspects of body fat are particularly hazardous and how do we measure them? International Journal of Epidemiology. 2006;35(1):83–92.

184. Snijder MB, Visser M, Dekker JM, Goodpaster BH, Harris TB, Kritchevsky SB, et al. Low subcutaneous thigh fat is a risk factor for unfavourable glucose and lipid levels, independently of high abdominal fat. The Health ABC Study. Diabetologia. 2005;48(2):301–8.

185. Snijder MB, Dekker JM, Visser M, Bouter LM, Stehouwer CDA, Yudkin JS, et al. Trunk fat and leg fat have independent and opposite associations with fasting and postload glucose levels. Diabetes Care. 2004;**27**(2):372–7.

186. Misra A, Vikram NK. Clinical and pathophysiological consequences of abdominal adiposity and abdominal adipose tissue depots. Nutrition. 2003;**19**:457–66.

187. Nazare JA, Smith JD, Borel AL, Haffner SM, Balkau B, Ross R, et al. Ethnic influences on the relations between abdominal subcutaneous and visceral adiposity, liver fat, and cardiometabolic risk profile: the International Study of Prediction of Intra-Abdominal Adiposity and Its Relationship With Cardiometabolic Risk/Intra-Abdominal Adiposity. American Journal of Clinical Nutrition. 2012;**96**(4):714–26.

188. Wells JC. Ecogeographical associations between climate and human body composition: analyses based on anthropometry and skinfolds. American Journal of Physical Anthropology. 2012;**147**(2):169–86.

189. Rush EC, Freitas I, Plank LD. Body size, body composition and fat distribution: comparative analysis of European, Maori, Pacific Island and Asian Indian adults. British Journal of Nutrition. 2009;**102**(4):632–41.

190. Ali AT, Ferris WF, Naran NH, Crowther NJ. Insulin resistance in the control of body fat distribution: a new hypothesis. Hormone and Metabolic Research. 2011;**43**(2):77–80.

191. Yajnik CS, Lubree HG, Rege SS, Naik SS, Deshpande JA, Deshpande SS, et al. Adiposity and hyperinsulinemia in Indians are present at birth. Journal of Endocrinolgy and Metabolism. 2002;**87**(12):5575–80.

192. Yajnik CS, Fall CHD, Coyaji KJ, Hirve SS, Rao S, Barker DJP, et al. Neonatal anthropometry: the thin-fat Indian baby. The Pune Maternal Nutrition Study. International Journal of Obesity and Related Metabolic Disorders. 2003;**27**(2):173–80.

193. Sletner L, Nakstad B, Yajnik CS, Morkrid K, Vangen S, Vardal MH, et al. Ethnic differences in neonatal body composition in a multi-ethnic population and the impact of parental factors: a population-based cohort study. PLoS One. 2013;**8**(8):e73058.

194. Modi N, Thomas EL, Uthaya SN, Umranikar S, Bell JD, Yajnik C. Whole body magnetic resonance imaging of healthy newborn infants demonstrates increased central adiposity in Asian Indians. Pediatric Research. 2009;**65**(5):584–7.

195. Uthaya S, Thomas EL, Hamilton G, Dore CJ, Bell J, Modi N. Altered adiposity after extremely preterm birth. Pediatric Research. 2005;**57**(2):211–15.

196. Harrington TA, Thomas EL, Frost G, Modi N, Bell JD. Distribution of adipose tissue in the newborn. Pediatric Research. 2004;**55**(3):437–41.

197. McKeigue PM, Pierpoint T, Ferrie JE, Marmot MG. Relationship of glucose intolerance and hyperinsulinaemia to body fat pattern in South Asians and Europeans. Diabetologia. 1992;**35**:785–91.

198. Rush E, Plank L, Chandu V, Laulu M, Simmons D, Swinburn B, et al. Body size, body composition, and fat distribution: a comparison of young New Zealand men of European, Pacific Island, and Asian Indian ethnicities. New Zealand Medical Journal. 2004;**117**(1207):U1203.

199. Kohli S, Sniderman AD, Tchernof A, Lear SA. Ethnic-specific differences in abdominal subcutaneous adipose tissue compartments. Obesity. 2010;**18**(11):2177–83.

200. **Sandhu JS, Esht V, Shenoy S.** Cardiovascular risk factors in middle age obese Indians: a cross-sectional study on association of per cent body fat and intra-abdominal fat mass. Heart Asia. 2012;**4**(1):1–5.

201. **Wang J, Thornton JC, Russell M, Burastero S, Heymsfield S, Pierson RN.** Asians have lower body mass index (BMI) but higher percent body fat than do whites: comparisons of anthropometric measurements. American Journal of Clinical Nutrition. 1994;**60**(1):23–8.

202. **Okosun IS, Liao Y, Rotimi CN, Dever GE, Cooper RS.** Impact of birth weight on ethnic variations in subcutaneous and central adiposity in American children aged 5–11 years. A study from the Third National Health and Nutrition Examination Survey. International Journal of Obesity. 2000;**24**(4):479–84.

203. **Horvath TL, Stachenfeld NS, Diano S.** A temperature hypothesis of hypothalamus-driven obesity. Yale Journal of Biology and Medicine. 2014;**87**(2):149–58.

204. **Lear SA, Kohli S, Bondy GP, Tchernof A, Sniderman AD.** Ethnic variation in fat and lean body mass and the association with insulin resistance. Journal of Clinical Endocrinology Metabolism. 2009;**94**(12):4696–702.

205. **Wells JCK.** Body composition and susceptibility to type 2 diabetes: an evolutionary perspective. European Journal of Clinical Nutrion. 2017;**71**(7):881–9.

206. **Wells JCK, Nesse RM, Sear R, Johnstone RA, Stearns SC.** Evolutionary public health: introducing the concept. Lancet. 2017;**390**(10093):500–9.

207. **Wells JCK.** Ethnic variability in adiposity and cardiovascular risk: the variable disease selection hypothesis. International Journal of Epidemiology. 2009;**38**(1):63–71.

208. **Chambers JC, Eda S, Bassett P, Karim Y, Thompson SG, Gallimore JR, et al.** C-reactive protein, insulin resistance, central obesity, and coronary heart disease risk in Indian Asians from the United Kingdom compared with European whites. Circulation. 2001;**104**:145–6.

209. **Heitmann BL, Lissner L.** Hip Hip Hurrah! Hip size inversely related to heart disease and total mortality. Obesity Reviews. 2011;**12**(6):478–81.

210. **Heitmann BL, Frederiksen P.** Thigh circumference and risk of heart disease and premature death: prospective cohort study. BMJ. 2009;**339**:b3292.

211. **Sachdev HS, Fall CH, Osmond C, Lakshmy R, Dey Biswas SK, Leary SD, et al.** Anthropometric indicators of body composition in young adults: relation to size at birth and serial measurements of body mass index in childhood in the New Delhi birth cohort. American Journal of Clinical Nutrition. 2005;**82**(2):456–66.

212. **Hall LML, Moran CN, Milne GR, Wilson J, MacFarlane NG, Forouhi NG, et al.** Fat oxidation, fitness and skeletal muscle expression of oxidative/lipid metabolism genes in South Asians: Implications for insulin resistance? PLoS ONE. 2010;**5**(12):e14197.

213. **Ehtisham S, Crabtree N, Clark P, Shaw N, Barrett T.** Ethnic differences in insulin resistance and body composition in United Kingdom adolescents. Journal of Clinical Endocrinology & Metabolism. 2005;**90**(7):3963–9.

214. **Chahal NS, Lim TK, Jain P, Chambers JC, Kooner JS, Senior R.** The increased prevalence of left ventricular hypertrophy and concentric remodeling in UK Indian Asians compared with European whites. Journal of Human Hypertension. 2013;**27**(5):288–93.

215. **Dulloo AG.** Collateral fattening: When a deficit in lean body mass drives overeating. Obesity (Silver Spring). 2017;**25**(2):277–9.

216. **Sinha S, Misra A, Rathi M, Kumar V, Pandey RM, Luthra K**, et al. Proton magnetic resonance spectroscopy and biochemical investigation of type 2 diabetes mellitus in Asian Indians: observation of high muscle lipids and C-reactive protein levels. Magnetic Resonance Imaging. 2009;**27**(1):94–100.

217. **Misra A, Nigam P, Hills AP, Chadha DS, Sharma V, Deepak KK**, et al. Consensus physical activity guidelines for Asian Indians. Diabetes Technology & Therapeutics. 2012;**14**(1):83–98.

218. **Misra A, Alappan NK, Vikram NK, Goel K, Gupta N, Mittal K**, et al. Effect of supervised progressive resistance-exercise training protocol on insulin sensitivity, glycemia, lipids, and body composition in Asian Indians with type 2 diabetes. Diabetes Care. 2008;**31**(7):1282–7.

219. **Paajanen TA, Oksala NKJ, Kuukasjärvi P, Karhunen PJ**. Short stature is associated with coronary heart disease: a systematic review of the literature and a meta-analysis. European Heart Journal. 2010;**31**(14):1802–9.

220. **Poh BK, Wong JE, Norimah AK, Deurenberg P**. Differences in body build in children of different ethnic groups and their impact on the prevalence of stunting, thinness, overweight, and obesity. Food and Nutrition Bulletin. 2016;**37**(1):3–13.

221. **McKeigue PM, Shah B, Marmot MG**. Relation of central obesity and insulin resistance with high diabetes prevalence and cardiovascular risk in South Asians. Lancet. 1991;**337**(8738):382–6.

222. **Belsare PV, Watve MG, Ghaskadbi SS, Bhat DS, Yajnik CS, Jog M**. Metabolic syndrome: aggression control mechanisms gone out of control. Medical Hypotheses. 2010;**74**(3):578–89.

223. **Bhatnagar P, Townsend N, Shaw A, Foster C**. The physical activity profiles of South Asian ethnic groups in England. Journal of Epidemiology and Community Health. 2016;**70**(6):602–8.

224. **Nightingale CM, Rudnicka AR, Kerry-Barnard SR, Donin AS, Brage S, Westgate KL**, et al. The contribution of physical fitness to individual and ethnic differences in risk markers for type 2 diabetes in children: The Child Heart and Health Study in England (CHASE). Pediatric Diabetes. 2018;**19**(4):603–10.

225. **Kuhn TS**. The Structure of Scientific Revolutions. Third edition. Chicago: The University of Chicago Press; 1996.

226. **Barker DJP**. Fetal and Infant Origins of Adult Disease. London: BMJ; 1992.

227. **Subbiah MT, Deitemeyer D, Yunker RL**. Decreased atherogenic response to dietary cholesterol in pigeons after stimulation of cholesterol catabolism in early life. Journal of Clinical Investigation. 1983;**71**(5):1509–13.

228. **Barker DJP**. Mothers, Babies and Disease in Later Life. London: BMJ Publishing Group; 1994.

229. **Barker DJP, Osmond C**. Infant mortality, childhood nutrition, and ischaemic heart disease in England and Wales. Lancet. 1986;(I):1077–81.

230. **Arnesen E, Forsdahl A**. The Tromso heart study: coronary risk factors and their association with living conditions during childhood. Journal of Epidemiology and Community Health. 1985;**39**(3):210–14.

231. **Bradley PJ**. Re: 'Decline in incidence of epidemic glucose intolerance in Nauruans: implications for the 'thrifty genotype'. American Journal of Epidemiology. 1992;**136**(4):499–500.

232. **Bradley PJ.** Obesity and risk of coronary heart disease in women. New England Journal of Medicine. 1990;**323**(16):1143–6.

233. **Bradley PJ.** Is obesity an advantageous adaptation? International Journal of Obesity. 1982;**6**(1):43–52.

234. **Krishnaveni GV, Yajnik CS.** Developmental origins of diabetes an Indian perspective. European Journal of Clinical Nutrion. 2017;**71**(7):865–9.

235. **Lawlor DA.** The developmental origins of health and disease: where do we go from here? Epidemiology. 2008;**19**(2):206–8.

236. **Hillier TA, Pedula KL, Schmidt MM, Mullen JA, Charles MA, Pettitt DJ.** Childhood obesity and metabolic imprinting: The ongoing effects of maternal hyperglycemia. Diabetes Care. 2007;**30**(9):2287–92.

237. **Gluckman PD, Hanson MA, Bateson P, Beedle AS, Law CM, Bhutta ZA, et al.** Towards a new developmental synthesis: adaptive developmental plasticity and human disease. Lancet. 2009;**373**(9675):1654–7.

238. **Saben Jessica L, Boudoures Anna L, Asghar Z, Thompson A, Drury A, Zhang W, et al.** Maternal metabolic syndrome programs mitochondrial dysfunction via germline changes across three generations. Cell Reports. **16**(1):1–8.

239. **Hardikar AA, Satoor SN, Karandikar MS, Joglekar MV, Puranik AS, Wong W, et al.** Multigenerational undernutrition increases susceptibility to obesity and diabetes that is not reversed after dietary recuperation. Cell Metabolism. 2015;**22**(2):312–19.

240. **Seaton SE, Yadav KD, Field DJ, Khunti K, Manktelow BN.** Birthweight centile charts for South Asian infants born in the UK. Neonatology. 2011;**100**(4):398–403.

241. **Villar J, Cheikh IL, Victora CG, Ohuma EO, Bertino E, Altman DG, et al.** International standards for newborn weight, length, and head circumference by gestational age and sex: the Newborn Cross-Sectional Study of the INTERGROWTH-21st Project. Lancet. 2014;**384**(9946):857–68.

242. **Yajnik CS, Fall CHD, Vaidya U, Pandit AN, Bavdekar A, Bhat DS, et al.** Fetal growth and glucose and insulin metabolism in four-year-old Indian children. Diabetic Medicine. 1995;**12**(4):330–6.

243. **Wells JC, DeSilva JM, Stock JT.** The obstetric dilemma: an ancient game of Russian roulette, or a variable dilemma sensitive to ecology? American Journal of Physical Anthropology. 2012;**149** Suppl 55:40–71.

244. **Ekstrom EC, Lindstrom E, Raqib R, El Arifeen S, Basu S, Brismar K, et al.** Effects of prenatal micronutrient and early food supplementation on metabolic status of the offspring at 4.5 years of age. The MINIMat randomized trial in rural Bangladesh. International Journal of Epidemiology. 2016;**45**(5):1656–67.

245. **Kulkarni B, Kuper H, Radhakrishna KV, Hills AP, Byrne NM, Taylor A, et al.** The association of early life supplemental nutrition with lean body mass and grip strength in adulthood: evidence from APCAPS. American Journal of Epidemiology. 2014;**179**(6):700–9.

246. **Potdar RD, Sahariah SA, Gandhi M, Kehoe SH, Brown N, Sane H, et al.** Improving women's diet quality preconceptionally and during gestation: effects on birth weight and prevalence of low birth weight–a randomized controlled efficacy trial in India (Mumbai Maternal Nutrition Project). American Journal of Clinical Nutrition. 2014;**100**(5):1257–68.

247. **Viegas OA, Scott PH, Cole TJ, Mansfield HN, Wharton P, Wharton BA.** Dietary protein energy supplementation of pregnant Asian mothers at Sorrento, Birmingham. I: Unselective during second and third trimesters. British Medical Journal. 1982;**285**:589–95.

248. **Bakeo, AC.** Trends in live births by mother's country of birth and other factors affecting low birthweight in England and Wales, 1983–2001. Health Statistics Quarterly 2004;**23** (Autumn):25–33.

249. **Harding S, Rosato MG, Cruickshank JK.** Lack of change in birthweights of infants by generational status among Indian, Pakistani, Bangladeshi, Black Caribbean, and Black African mothers in a British cohort study. International Journal of Epidemiology. 2004;**33**(6):1279–85.

250. **Kinra S, Rameshwar Sarma KV, Ghafoorunissa, Mendu VV, Ravikumar R, Mohan V,** et al. Effect of integration of supplemental nutrition with public health programmes in pregnancy and early childhood on cardiovascular risk in rural Indian adolescents: long term follow-up of Hyderabad nutrition trial. BMJ. 2008;**337**:a605.

251. **McFadyen IR, Campbell-Brown M, Abraham R, North WR, Haines AP.** Factors affecting birthweights in Hindus, Moslems and Europeans. British Journal of Obstetrics and Gynaecology. 1984;**91**(10):968–72.

252. **Dhawan S.** Birth weights of infants of first generation Asian women in Britain compared with second generation Asian women. BMJ. 1995;**311**:86–8.

253. **Bansal N, Chalmers JWT, Fischbacher CM, Steiner MFC, Bhopal RS.** Ethnicity and first birth: age, smoking, delivery, gestation, weight and feeding: Scottish health and ethnicity linkage study. European Journal of Public Health. 2014;**24**:910–15.

254. **West J, Lawlor DA, Fairley L, Bhopal R, Cameron N, McKinney PA,** et al. UK-born Pakistani-origin infants are relatively more adipose than White British infants: findings from 8704 mother-offspring pairs in the Born-in-Bradford prospective birth cohort. Journal of Epidemiology and Community Health. 2013;**67**:544–51.

255. **Simmons D.** Differences in umbilical cord insulin and birth weight in non-diabetic pregnancies of women from different ethnic groups in New Zealand. Diabetologia. 1994;**37**:930–6.

256. **Bryant M, Santorelli G, Lawlor DA, Farrar D, Tuffnell D, Bhopal R,** et al. A comparison of South Asian specific and established BMI thresholds for determining obesity prevalence in pregnancy and predicting pregnancy complications: findings from the Born in Bradford cohort. International Journal of Obesity (London). 2013;**38**(3):444–50.

257. **Farrar D, Fairley L, Santorelli G, Tuffnell D, Sheldon TA, Wright J,** et al. Association between hyperglycaemia and adverse perinatal outcomes in south Asian and white British women: analysis of data from the Born in Bradford cohort. Lancet Diabetes & Endocrinology. 2015;**3**(10):795–804.

258. **Patel RR, Steer P, Doyle P, Little MP, Elliott P.** Does gestation vary by ethnic group? A London-based study of over 122,000 pregnancies with spontaneous onset of labour. International Journal of Epidemiology. 2004;**33**(1):107–13.

259. **Zipursky AR, Park AL, Urquia ML, Creatore MI, Ray JG.** Influence of paternal and maternal ethnicity and ethnic enclaves on newborn weight. Journal of Epidemiology and Community Health. 2014;**68**(10):942–9.

260. **Schreider E.** Ecological rules, body-heat regulation, and human evolution. Evolution. 1964;**18**:1–9.

261. **Wells JC, Cole TJ.** Birth weight and environmental heat load: a between-population analysis. American Journal of Physical Anthropology. 2002;**119**(3):276–82.

262. **Wells JC.** Thermal environment and human birth weight. Journal of Theoretical Biology. 2002;**214**(3):413–25.

263. **Wells JC.** Environmental temperature and human growth in early life. Journal of Theoretical Biology. 2000;**204**(2):299–305.

264. **Wurtz P, Wang Q, Niironen M, Tynkkynen T, Tiainen M, Drenos F,** et al. Metabolic signatures of birthweight in 18,288 adolescents and adults. International Journal of Epidemiology. 2016;**45**(5):1539–50.

265. **Freathy RM, Bennett AJ, Ring SM, Shields B, Groves CJ, Timpson NJ,** et al. Type 2 diabetes risk alleles are associated with reduced size at birth. Diabetes. 2009;**58**(6):1428–33.

266. **Meier JJ.** Linking the genetics of type 2 diabetes with low birth weight: a role for prenatal islet maldevelopment? Diabetes. 2009;**58**(6):1255–6.

267. **West J, Wright J, Fairley L, Sattar N, Whincup P, Lawlor DA.** Do ethnic differences in cord blood leptin levels differ by birthweight category? Findings from the Born in Bradford cohort study. International Journal of Epidemiology. 2013;**43**(1):249–54.

268. **Norris T, Tuffnell D, Wright J, Cameron N.** Modelling foetal growth in a bi-ethnic sample: results from the Born in Bradford (BiB) birth cohort. Annals of Human Biology. 2014;**41**(6):481–7.

269. **Yajnik CS.** The insulin resistance epidemic in India: small at birth, big as adult? International Diabetes Federation Bulletin. 1998;**43**:23–8.

270. **Horikoshi M, Beaumont RN, Day FR, Warrington NM, Kooijman MN, Fernandez-Tajes J,** et al. Genome-wide associations for birth weight and correlations with adult disease. Nature. 2016;**538**(7624):248–52.

271. **Wells JC, Yao P, Williams JE, Gayner R.** Maternal investment, life-history strategy of the offspring and adult chronic disease risk in South Asian women in the UK. Evolution, Medicine and Public Health. 2016;**2016**(1):133–45.

272. **Kuzawa CW, Sweet E.** Epigenetics and the embodiment of race: developmental origins of US racial disparities in cardiovascular health. American Journal of Human Biology. 2009;**21**(1):2–15.

273. **Bijker R, Agyemang C.** The influence of early-life conditions on cardiovascular disease later in life among ethnic minority populations: a systematic review. Internal and Emergency Medicine. 2015;**11**(3):341–53.

274. **Kramer MS, Zhang X, Dahhou M, Yang S, Martin RM, Oken E,** et al. Does fetal growth restriction cause later obesity? pitfalls in analyzing causal mediators as confounders. American Journal of Epidemiology. 2017;**185**(7):585–90.

275. **Krishnaveni GV, Veena SR, Hill JC, Karat SC, Fall CH.** Cohort profile: Mysore parthenon birth cohort. International Journal of Epidemiology. 2015;**44**(1):28–36.

276. **Stein CE, Fall CH, Kumaran K, Osmond C, Cox V, Barker DJ.** Fetal growth and coronary heart disease in South India. Lancet. 1996;**348**(9037):1269–73.

277. Hanna LC, Hunt SM, Bhopal RS. Using the Rose Angina Questionnaire cross-culturally: the importance of consulting lay people when translating epidemiological questionnaires. Ethnicity & Health. 2011;**17**(3):241–51.

278. Kumaran K, Fall CHD, Martyn CN, Vijayakamar M, Stein C, Shier R. Blood pressure, arterial compliance, and left ventricular mass: no relation to small size at birth in South Indian adults. Heart. 2000;**83**:272–7.

279. Bhargava SK, Sachdev HS, Fall CH, Osmond C, Lakshmy R, Barker DJ, et al. Relation of serial changes in childhood body-mass index to impaired glucose tolerance in young adulthood. New England Journal of Medicine. 2004;**350**(9):865–75.

280. Fall CH, Sachdev HS, Osmond C, Lakshmy R, Biswas SD, Prabhakaran D, et al. Adult metabolic syndrome and impaired glucose tolerance are associated with different patterns of BMI gain during infancy: Data from the New Delhi Birth Cohort. Diabetes Care. 2008;**31**(12):2349–56.

281. Lakshmy R, Fall CH, Sachdev HS, Osmond C, Prabhakaran D, Biswas SD, et al. Childhood body mass index and adult pro-inflammatory and pro-thrombotic risk factors: data from the New Delhi birth cohort. International Journal of Epidemiology. 2011;**40**(1):102–11.

282. Raghupathy P, Antonisamy B, Geethanjali FS, Saperia J, Leary SD, Priya G, et al. Glucose tolerance, insulin resistance and insulin secretion in young south Indian adults: Relationships to parental size, neonatal size and childhood body mass index. Diabetes Research and Clinical Practice. 2010;**87**(2):283–92.

283. Kumar R, Bandyopadhyay S, Aggarwal AK, Khullar M. Relation between birthweight and blood pressure among 7–8 year old rural children in India. International Journal of Epidemiology. 2004;**33**(1):87–91.

284. Bavdekar A, Yajnik CS, Fall CH, Bapat S, Pandit AN, Deshpande V, et al. Insulin resistance syndrome in 8-year-old Indian children: small at birth, big at 8 years, or both? Diabetes. 1999;**48**(12):2422–9.

285. Yajnik CS, Katre PA, Joshi SM, Kumaran K, Bhat DS, Lubree HG, et al. Higher glucose, insulin and insulin resistance (HOMA-IR) in childhood predict adverse cardiovascular risk in early adulthood: the Pune Children's Study. Diabetologia. 2015;**58**(7):1626–36.

286. Yajnik CS, Deshmukh US. Maternal nutrition, intrauterine programming and consequential risks in the offspring. Reviews in Endocrine and Metabolic Disorders. 2008;**9**(3):203–11.

287. Yajnik CS, Deshpande SS, Jackson AA, Refsum H, Rao S, Fisher DJ, et al. Vitamin B12 and folate concentrations during pregnancy and insulin resistance in the offspring: the Pune Maternal Nutrition Study. Diabetologia. 2008;**51**(1):29–38.

288. Rao S, Kanade AN, Yajnik CS, Fall CH. Seasonality in maternal intake and activity influence offspring's birth size among rural Indian mothers–Pune Maternal Nutrition Study. International Journal of Epidemiology. 2009;**38**(4):1094–103.

289. Winder NR, Krishnaveni GV, Hill JC, Karat CL, Fall CH, Veena SR, et al. Placental programming of blood pressure in Indian children. Acta Paediatrica. 2011;**100**(5):653–60.

290. Nightingale CM, Rudnicka AR, Owen CG, Newton SL, Bales JL, Donin AS, et al. Birthweight and risk markers for type 2 diabetes and cardiovascular disease in

childhood: the Child Heart and Health Study in England (CHASE). Diabetologia. 2015;**58**(3):474–84.

291. **Whincup PH, Nightingale CM, Owen CG, Rudnicka AR, Gibb I, McKay CM,** et al. Early emergence of ethnic differences in type 2 diabetes precursors in the UK: The Child Heart and Health Study in England (CHASE Study). PLoS Med. 2010;**7**(4):e1000263.

292. **Harding S, Whitrow M, Lenguerrand E, Maynard M, Teyhan A, Cruickshank JK,** et al. Emergence of ethnic differences in blood pressure in adolescence: the determinants of adolescent social well-being and health study. Hypertension. 2010;**55**(4):1063–9.

293. **Cruickshank JK, Silva MJ, Molaodi OR, Enayat ZE, Cassidy A, Karamanos A,** et al. Ethnic differences in and childhood influences on early adult pulse wave velocity: the Determinants of Adolescent, now Young Adult, Social Wellbeing, and Health longitudinal study. Hypertension. 2016;**67**(6):1133–41.

294. **Alvear J, Brooke OG.** Fetal growth in different racial groups. Archives of Diseases of Childhood. 1978;**53**(1):27–32.

295. **Brooke OG, Wood C.** Growth in British Asians: longitudinal data in the first year. Journal of Human Nutrition. 1980;**34**(5):355–9.

296. **Wright J, Small N, Raynor P, Tuffnell D, Bhopal R, Cameron N,** et al. Cohort profile: The Born in Bradford multi-ethnic family cohort study. International Journal of Epidemiology. 2013;**42**(4):978–91.

297. **Lawlor DA, West J, Fairley L, Nelson SM, Bhopal RS, Tuffnell D,** et al. Pregnancy glycaemia and cord-blood levels of insulin and leptin in Pakistani and white British mother-offspring pairs: findings from a prospective pregnancy cohort. Diabetologia. 2014;**57**(12):2492–500.

298. **Anand SS, Gupta MK, Schulze KM, Desai D, Abdalla N, Wahi G,** et al. What accounts for ethnic differences in newborn skinfold thickness comparing South Asians and White Caucasians? Findings from the START and FAMILY Birth Cohorts. International Journal of Obesity. 2016;**40**(2):239–44.

299. **Fairley L, Santorelli G, Lawlor D, Bryant M, Bhopal R, Petherick E,** et al. The relationship between early life modifiable risk factors for childhood obesity, ethnicity and body mass index at age 3 years: findings from the Born in Bradford birth cohort study. BMC Obesity. 2015;**2**:9.

300. **Cezard G, Smith L, Petherick E, Cameron N, West J, Lawlor D,** et al. 1.11-P19 Ethnic differences in early life adiposity trajectories between White British and Pakistani children: results from the Born in Bradford cohort study in the UK. European Journal of Public Health. 2018;**28**(suppl_1):cky048.3–cky.3.

301. **Bansal N, Ayoola OO, Gemmell I, Vyas A, Koudsi A, Oldroyd J,** et al. Effects of early growth on blood pressure of infants of British European and South Asian origin at one year of age: the Manchester children's growth and vascular health study. Journal of Hypertension. 2008;**26**(3):412–18.

302. **Yajnik CS.** The insulin resistance epidemic in India: fetal origins, later lifestyle, or both? Nutr Rev; 2001; **59**(1 Pt 1):1–9.

303. **Yu ZB, Han SP, Zhu GZ, Zhu C, Wang XJ, Cao XG,** et al. Birth weight and subsequent risk of obesity: a systematic review and meta-analysis. Obesity Reviews. 2011;**12**(7):525–42.

304. Stocks T, Renders CM, Bulk-Bunschoten AM, Hirasing RA, van BS, Seidell JC. Body size and growth in 0- to 4-year-old children and the relation to body size in primary school age. Obesity Reviews. 2011;**12**(8):637–52.

305. Vasan SK, Roy A, Samuel VT, Antonisamy B, Bhargava SK, Alex AG, et al. IndEcho study: cohort study investigating birth size, childhood growth and young adult cardiovascular risk factors as predictors of midlife myocardial structure and function in South Asians. BMJ Open. 2018;**8**(4):e019675.

306. Fleming TP, Watkins AJ, Velazquez MA, Mathers JC, Prentice AM, Stephenson J, et al. Origins of lifetime health around the time of conception: causes and consequences. Lancet. 2018;**391**(10132):1842–52.

307. Katre PYC. Pune Experience: Influence of early life environment on risk of non-communicable diseases (NCDs) in Indians. Sight and Life. 2015;**29**(1):91–7.

308. Yajnik CS, Katre PA, Joshi SM, Kumaran K, Bhat DS, Lubree HG, et al. Higher glucose, insulin and insulin resistance (HOMA-IR) in childhood predict adverse cardiovascular risk in early adulthood: the Pune Children's Study. Diabetologia. 2015;**58**(7):1626–36.

309. Rao S, Yajnik CS, Kanade A, Fall CH, Margetts BM, Jackson AA, et al. Intake of micronutrient-rich foods in rural Indian mothers is associated with the size of their babies at birth: Pune Maternal Nutrition Study. Journal of Nutrition. 2001;**131**(4):1217–24.

310. Bhate V, Deshpande S, Bhat D, Joshi N, Ladkat R, Watve S, et al. Vitamin B12 status of pregnant Indian women and cognitive function in their 9-year-old children. Food and Nutrition Bulletin. 2008;**29**(4):249–54.

311. Kanade AN, Rao S, Kelkar RS, Gupte S. Maternal nutrition and birth size among urban affluent and rural women in India. Journal of the American College of Nutrition. 2008;**27**(1):137–45.

312. Hill JC, Krishnaveni GV, Annamma I, Leary SD, Fall CH. Glucose tolerance in pregnancy in South India: relationships to neonatal anthropometry. Acta Obstetricia et Gynecologica Scandinavica. 2005;**84**(2):159–65.

313. Raichlen DA, Pontzer H, Harris JA, Mabulla AZP, Marlowe FW, Josh Snodgrass J, et al. Physical activity patterns and biomarkers of cardiovascular disease risk in hunter-gatherers. American Journal of Human Biology. 2016;**29**(2):1–13.

314. O'Dea K. Marked improvement in carbohydrate and lipid metabolism in diabetic Australian aborigines after temporary reversion to traditional lifestyle. Diabetes. 1984;**33**(6):596–603.

315. Tuan Abdul Aziz TA, Teh LK, Md Idris MH, Bannur Z, Ashari LS, Ismail AI, et al. Increased risks of cardiovascular diseases and insulin resistance among the Orang Asli in Peninsular Malaysia. BMC Public Health. 2016;**16**(1):284.

316. Kaplan H, Thompson RC, Trumble BC, Wann LS, Allam AH, Beheim B, et al. Coronary atherosclerosis in indigenous South American Tsimane: a cross-sectional cohort study. Lancet. 2017;**389**(10080):1730–9.

317. Lawson RA, Murphy RH, Williamson CR. The relationship between income, economic freedom, and BMI. Public Health. 2016;**134**:18–25.

318. Gruer L, Cezard G, Clark E, Douglas A, Steiner M, Millard A, et al. Life expectancy of different ethnic groups using death records linked to population census data for 4.62 million people in Scotland. Journal of Epidemiology and Community Health. 2016;**70**:1251–4.

319. Wohland P, Rees P, Nazroo J, Jagger C. Inequalities in healthy life expectancy between ethnic groups in England and Wales in 2001. Ethnicity and Health. 2015;**20**(4):341–53.

320. Ebrahim S, Kinra S, Bowen L, Andersen E, Ben-Shlomo Y, Lyngdoh T, et al. The effect of rural-to-urban migration on obesity and diabetes in India: A cross-sectional study. PLoS Med. 2010;**7**(4):e1000268.

321. Siddiqui ST, Kandala NB, Stranges S. Urbanisation and geographic variation of overweight and obesity in India: a cross-sectional analysis of the Indian Demographic Health Survey 2005–2006. International Journal of Public Health. 2015;**60**(6):717–26.

322. Vidale S, Campana C. Ambient air pollution and cardiovascular diseases: From bench to bedside. European Journal of Preventive Cardiology. 2018;**25**(8):818–25.

323. Teo K, Chow CK, Vaz M, Rangarajan S, Yusuf S. The Prospective Urban Rural Epidemiology (PURE) study: examining the impact of societal influences on chronic noncommunicable diseases in low-, middle-, and high-income countries. American Heart Journal. 2009;**158**(1):1–7.

324. Ranasinghe P, Mathangasinghe Y, Jayawardena R, Hills AP, Misra A. Prevalence and trends of metabolic syndrome among adults in the Asia-Pacific region: a systematic review. BMC Public Health. 2017;**17**(1):101.

325. Katikireddi SV, Morling JR, Bhopal R. Is there a divergence in time trends in the prevalence of impaired glucose tolerance and diabetes? A systematic review in South Asian populations. International Journal of Epidemiology. 2011;**40**(6):1542–53.

326. Mohan V, Deepa M, Deepa R, Shanthirani CS, Farooq S, Ganesan A, et al. Secular trends in the prevalence of diabetes and impaired glucose tolerance in urban South India—the Chennai Urban Rural Epidemiology Study (CURES-17). Diabetologia 2006;**49**(6):1175–8.

327. Gupta R, Guptha S, Gupta V, Agrawal A, Gaur K, Deedwania PC. Twenty-year trends in cardiovascular risk factors in India and influence of educational status. European Journal of Preventive Cardiology. 2012;**19**(6):1258–71.

328. Gupta R, Joshi P, Mohan V, Reddy KS, Yusuf S. Epidemiology and causation of coronary heart disease and stroke in India. Heart. 2008;**94**(1):16–26.

329. Beasley AW. A story of heartache: the understanding of angina pectoris in the pre-surgical period. Journal of the Royal College of Physicians Edinburgh. 2011;**41**(4):361–5.

330. Dawber T, Kannel W, Lyell L. An approach to longitudinal studies in a community: the Framingham study. Annals New York Academy of Sciences. 1963;**107**:539–56.

331. Janssens S, Werf FVd. Acute coronary syndromes: Virchow's triad revisited. Lancet. 1996;**348**(supplI):sII2.

332. Levy D, Thom TJ. Death rates from coronary disease—progress and a puzzling paradox. New England Journal of Medicine. 1998;**339**(13):915–17.

333. Harding S, Rosato M, Teyhan A. Trends for coronary heart disease and stroke mortality among migrants in England and Wales, 1979-2003: slow declines notable for some groups. Heart. 2008;**94**(4):463–70.

334. Sekikawa A, Miyamoto Y, Miura K, Nishimura K, Willcox BJ, Masaki KH, et al. Continuous decline in mortality from coronary heart disease in Japan despite a

continuous and marked rise in total cholesterol: Japanese experience after the Seven Countries Study. International Journal of Epidemiology. 2015;44(5):1614–24.

335. **Müller-Nordhorn J, Binting S, Roll S, Willich SN.** An update on regional variation in cardiovascular mortality within Europe. European Heart Journal. 2008;29(10):1316–26.

336. **Marmot M, Elliott P.** Coronary Heart Disease Epidemiology: From aetiology to public health. Second edition. New York, United States: Oxford University Press; 2005. 932 p.

337. **Rodgers A, Woodward A, Swinburn B, Dietz WH.** Prevalence trends tell us what did not precipitate the US obesity epidemic. Lancet Public Health. 2018;3(4):e162–3.

338. **Jayawardena R, Ranasinghe P, Byrne NM, Soares MJ, Katulanda P, Hills AP.** Prevalence and trends of the diabetes epidemic in South Asia: a systematic review and meta-analysis. BMC Public Health. 2012;12:380.

339. **Roth GA, Huffman MD, Moran AE, Feigin V, Mensah GA, Naghavi M,** et al. Global and regional patterns in cardiovascular mortality from 1990 to 2013. Circulation. 2015;132(17):1667–78.

340. **Adab P, Pallan MJ, Lancashire ER, Hemming K, Frew E, Barrett T,** et al. Effectiveness of a childhood obesity prevention programme delivered through schools, targeting 6 and 7 year olds: cluster randomised controlled trial (WAVES study). BMJ. 2018;360:K211.

341. **Reddy KS, Prabhakaran D, Jeemon P, Thankappan KR, Joshi P, Chaturvedi V,** et al. Educational status and cardiovascular risk profile in Indians. Proceedings of the National Academy of Sciences. 2007;104(41):16263–8.

342. **Allen L, Williams J, Townsend N, Mikkelsen B, Roberts N, Foster C,** et al. Socioeconomic status and non-communicable disease behavioural risk factors in low-income and lower-middle-income countries: a systematic review. Lancet Global Health. 2017;5(3):e277–e89.

343. **Genne-Bacon EA.** Thinking evolutionarily about obesity. Yale Journal of Biology Medicine. 2014;87(2):99–112.

344. **Kinra S, Andersen E, Ben-Shlomo Y, Bowen L, Lyngdoh T, Prabhakaran D,** et al. Association between urban life-years and cardiometabolic risk. American Journal of Epidemiology. 2011;174(2):154–64.

345. **Lofink HE.** 'The worst of the Bangladeshi and the worst of the British': exploring eating patterns and practices among British Bangladeshi adolescents in East London. Ethnicity & Health. 2012;17(4):385–401.

346. **Bowen L, Ebrahim S, De Stavola B, Ness A, Kinra S, Bharathi AV,** et al. Dietary intake and rural-urban migration in India: a cross-sectional study. PLoS One. 2011;6(6):e14822.

347. **Hernandez AV, Pasupuleti V, Deshpande A, Bernabe-Ortiz A, Miranda JJ.** Effect of rural-to-urban within-country migration on cardiovascular risk factors in low- and middle-income countries: a systematic review. Heart. 2012;98(3):185–94.

348. **Hemingway H, Marmot M.** Psychosocial factors in the aetiology and prognosis of coronary heart disease: systematic review of prospective cohort studies. British Medical Journal. 1999;318:1460–7.

349. **Rosengren A, Hawken S, Ounpuu S, Sliwa K, Zubaid M, Almahmeed WA,** et al. Association of psychosocial risk factors with risk of acute myocardial infarction in

11119 cases and 13648 controls from 52 countries (the INTERHEART study): case-control study. Lancet. 2004;**364**(9438):953–62.

350. **Williams ED, Steptoe A, Chambers JC, Kooner JS.** Psychosocial risk factors for coronary heart disease in UK South Asian men and women. Journal of Epidemiology and Community Health. 2009;**63**(12):986–91.

351. **Sara JD, Prasad M, Eleid MF, Zhang M, Widmer RJ, Lerman A.** Association between work-related stress and coronary heart disease: a review of prospective studies through the job strain, effort-reward balance, and organizational justice models. Journal of the American Heart Association. 2018;**7**(9): pii: e008073.

352. **James GD.** Human evolution and chronic diseases: genes, allostasis, and cut-points. Anthropology. 2014;**2**(3):1000e122.

353. **Tawakol A, Ishai A, Takx RAP, Figueroa AL, Ali A, Kaiser Y,** et al. Relation between resting amygdalar activity and cardiovascular events: a longitudinal and cohort study. Lancet. 2017;**389**(10071):834–45.

354. **Chu P, Gotink RA, Yeh GY, Goldie SJ, Hunink MM.** The effectiveness of yoga in modifying risk factors for cardiovascular disease and metabolic syndrome: A systematic review and meta-analysis of randomized controlled trials. European Journal of Preventive Cardiology. 2014;**23**(3):291–307.

355. **Levine GN, Lange RA, Bairey-Merz CN, Davidson RJ, Jamerson K, Mehta PK,** et al. Meditation and cardiovascular risk reduction. Journal of the American Heart Association. 2017;**6**(10):e002218.

356. **Patel C, Marmot MG, Terry DJ, Carruthers M, Hunt B, Patel M.** Trial of relaxation in reducing coronary risk: four year follow up. British Medical Journal (Clinical research edition). 1985;**290**(6475):1103–6.

357. **Bathula R, Hughes AD, Panerai R, Potter J, Thom SA, Francis DP,** et al. Indian Asians have poorer cardiovascular autonomic function than Europeans: this is due to greater hyperglycaemia and may contribute to their greater risk of heart disease. Diabetologia. 2010;**53**(10):2120–8.

358. **Chaturvedi N, Bathula R, Shore AC, Panerai R, Potter J, Kooner J,** et al. South Asians have elevated postexercise blood pressure and myocardial oxygen consumption compared to europeans despite equivalent resting pressure. Journal of the American Heart Association. 2012;**1**(5).

359. **Hemingway H, Whitty CJM, Shipley MJ, Stansfeld S, Bruner E, Fuhrer R,** et al. Psychosocial risk factors for coronary disease in white, South Asian and Afro-Caribbean civil servants: the Whitehall II Study. Ethnicity and Health. 2006;**11**(3):391–400.

360. **Fischbacher CM, White M, Bhopal RS, Unwin NC.** Self-reported work strain is lower in south asian than european people: cross-sectional survey. Ethnicity & Health. 2005;**10**:279–92.

361. **Williams R, Bhopal R, Hunt K.** Coronary risk in a British Punjabi population: Comparative profile of non-biochemical factors. International Journal of Epidemiology. 1994;**23**(1):28–37.

362. **Pollard TM, Carlin, LE, Bhopal R, Unwin N, White M, Fischbacher C.** Social networks and coronary heart disease risk factors in South Asians and Europeans in the United Kingdom. Ethnicity & Health. 2003;**8**:263–75.

363. **Williams ED, Steptoe A, Chambers JC, Kooner JS.** Ethnic and gender differences in the relationship between hostility and metabolic and autonomic risk factors for coronary heart disease. Psychosomatic Medicine. 2011;**73**(1):53–8.

364. **Williams ED, Nazroo JY, Kooner JS, Steptoe A.** Subgroup differences in psychosocial factors relating to coronary heart disease in the UK South Asian population. Journal of Psychosom Research. 2010;**69**(4):379–87.

365. **Williams ED, Kooner I, Steptoe A, Kooner JS.** Psychosocial factors related to cardiovascular disease risk in UK South Asian men: a preliminary study. British Journal of Health Psychology. 2007;**12**(4):559–70.

366. **Modood T, Berthoud R, Lakey J, Nazroo J, Smith P, Virdee SB, S.** Ethnic Minorities in Britain: Diversity and Disadvantage. London: Policy Studies Institute; 1997.

367. **Bansal N, Bhopal RF, Netto GF, Lyons DF, Steiner MF, Sashidharan SP.** Disparate patterns of hospitalisation reflect unmet needs and persistent ethnic inequalities in mental health care: the Scottish health and ethnicity linkage study. Ethnicity and Health. 2014;**19**(2):217–39.

368. **Paradies Y.** A systematic review of empirical research on self-reported racism and health. International Journal of Epidemiology. 2006;**35**(4):888–901.

369. **Williams R, Hunt K.** Psychological distress among British South Asians: the contribution of stressful situations and subcultural differences in the West of Scotland Twenty-07 Study. Psychological Medicine. 1997;**27**:1173–81.

370. **Rankin J, Bhopal R.** Understanding of heart disease and diabetes in a South Asian community: cross-sectional study testing the 'snowball' sample method. Public Health. 2001;**115**:253–60.

371. **Darr A, Astin F, Atkin K.** Causal attributions, lifestyle change, and coronary heart disease: Illness beliefs of patients of South Asian and European origin living in the United Kingdom. Heart & Lung: Journal of Acute and Critical Care. 2008;**37**(2):91–104.

372. **Poulter NR, Khaw KT, Hopwood BE, Mugambi M, Peart WS, Rose G, et al.** The Kenyan Luo migration study: observations on the initiation of a rise in blood pressure. BMJ. 1990;**300**(6730):967–72.

373. **Mathur KS, Patney NL, Kumar V.** Atherosclerosis in India. An autopsy study of the aorta and the coronary, cerebral, renal and pulmonary arteries. Circulation. 1961;**24**(1):68–75.

374. **Danaraj TJ, Acker MS, Danaraj W, Wong HO, Tan BY.** Ethnic group differences in coronary heart disease in Singapore: an analysis of necropsy records. American Heart Journal. 1959;**58**:516–26.

375. **Razum O.** Commentary: Of salmon and time travelers–musing on the mystery of migrant mortality. International Journal of Epidemiology. 2006;**35**(4):919–21.

376. **Judd PA, Kassam-Khamis T, Thomas JE.** The Composition and Nutrient Content of Foods Commonly Consumed by South Asians in the UK. London: The Aga Khan Health Board (AKHB), UK; 2000.

377. **Bhardwaj S, Passi SJ, Misra A, Pant KK, Anwar K, Pandey RM, et al.** Effect of heating/reheating of fats/oils, as used by Asian Indians, on trans fatty acid formation. Food Chemistry. 2016;**212**:663–70.

378. Ramachandran A, Sathyamurthy I, Snelhalatha C, Satyavani K, Sivasankari S, Misra J, et al. Risk variables for coronary artery disease in Asian Indians. American Journal of Cardiology. 2001;87:267–71.

379. Teo KK, Ounpuu S, Hawken S, Pandey MR, Valentin V, Hunt D, et al. Tobacco use and risk of myocardial infarction in 52 countries in the INTERHEART study: a case-control study. Lancet. 2006;368(9536):647–58.

380. Kakde S, Bhopal RS, Jones CM. A systematic review on the social context of smokeless tobacco use in the South Asian population: Implications for public health. Public Health. 2012;126:635–45.

381. Rabanal KS, Meyer HE, Tell GS, Igland J, Pylypchuk R, Mehta S, et al. Can traditional risk factors explain the higher risk of cardiovascular disease in South Asians compared to Europeans in Norway and New Zealand? Two cohort studies. BMJ Open. 2017;7(12):e016819.

382. Rose G. Sick individuals and sick populations. International Journal of Epidemiology. 1985;14:32–8.

383. Eastwood SV, Tillin T, Chaturvedi N, Hughes AD. ethnic differences in associations between blood pressure and stroke in South Asian and European men. Hypertension. 2015;66(3):481–8.

384. Lawes CM, Bennett DA, Feigin VL, Rodgers A. Blood pressure and stroke: an overview of published reviews. Stroke. 2004;35(3):776–85.

385. Whelton PK, Carey RM, Aronow WS, Casey DE, Collins KJ, Dennison Himmelfarb C, et al. 2017 ACC/AHA/AAPA/ABC/ACPM/AGS/APhA/ASH/ASPC/NMA/PCNA Guideline for the prevention, detection, evaluation, and management of high blood pressure in adults. A report of the American College of Cardiology/American Heart Association Task Force on Clinical Practice Guidelines. Journal of the American College of Cardiology. 2018;71(19):e127–e248.

386. O'Donnell MJ, Xavier D, Liu L, Zhang H, Chin SL, Rao-Melacini P, et al. Risk factors for ischaemic and intracerebral haemorrhagic stroke in 22 countries (the INTERSTROKE study): a case-control study. Lancet. 2010;376(9735):112–23.

387. Lopez AD, Mathers CD, Ezzati M, Jamison DT, Murray CJ. Global and regional burden of disease and risk factors, 2001: systematic analysis of population health data. Lancet. 2006;367(9524):1747–57.

388. Wild S, McKeigue P. Cross sectional analysis of mortality by country of birth in England and Wales, 1970–92. BMJ. 1997;314(7082):705–10.

389. Modesti PA, Reboldi G, Cappuccio FP, Agyemang C, Remuzzi G, Rapi S, et al. Panethnic differences in blood pressure in Europe: a systematic review and meta-analysis. PLoS One. 2016;11(1):e0147601.

390. Agyemang C, Bhopal R, Bruijnzeels M. Do variations in blood pressure of South Asians, African descent and Chinese children reflect those of the adult populations in the UK? A review of cross-sectional data. Ethnicity & Health. 2005;9:S68–S9.

391. Agyemang C, Bhopal R. Is the blood pressure of people from African origin adults in the UK higher or lower than that in European origin white people? A review of cross-sectional data. Journal of Human Hypertension. 2003;17(8):523–34.

392. Agyemang C, Bhopal RS. Is the blood pressure of South Asian adults in the UK higher or lower than that in European white adults? A review of cross-sectional data. Journal of Human Hypertension. 2002;16(11):739–51.

393. Agyemang C, Bhopal R, Bruijnzeels M. Do variations in blood pressure of South Asians, African descent and Chinese children reflect those of the adult population in the UK? A review of cross-sectional data. Journal of Human Hypertension. 2003;18(4):229–37.

394. Agyemang C, Humphry RW, Bhopal R. Divergence with age in blood pressure in African-Caribbean and White populations in England: implications for screening for hypertension. American Journal of Hypertension. 2012;25(1):89–96.

395. Young JH, Chang YP, Kim JD, Chretien JP, Klag MJ, Levine MA, et al. Differential susceptibility to hypertension is due to selection during the out-of-Africa expansion. PLoS Genet. 2005;1(6):e82.

396. Bhopal R, Rahemtulla T, Sheikh A. Persistent high stroke mortality in Bangladeshi populations. BMJ. 2005;331:1096–7.

397. Bathula R, Hughes AD, Panerai RB, Potter JF, McG Thom SA, Tillin T, et al. South Asians have adverse cerebrovascular haemodynamics, despite equivalent blood pressure, compared with Europeans. This is due to their greater hyperglycaemia. International Journal of Epidemiology. 2011;40(6):1490–8.

398. Brar I, Robertson AD, Hughson RL. Increased central arterial stiffness and altered cerebrovascular haemodynamic properties in South Asian older adults. Journal of Human Hypertension. 2016;30(5):309–14.

399. Faconti L, Nanino E, Mills CE, Cruickshank KJ. Do arterial stiffness and wave reflection underlie cardiovascular risk in ethnic minorities? JRSM Cardiovascular Disease. 2016;5:1–9.

400. Sluyter JD, Hughes AD, Thom SAM, Lowe A, Camargo Jr CA, Hametner B, et al. Arterial waveform parameters in a large, population-based sample of adults: relationships with ethnicity and lifestyle factors. Journal of Human Hypertension. 2017;31(5):305–12.

401. Philips JC, Marchand M, Scheen AJ. Squatting amplifies pulse pressure increase with disease duration in patients with type 1 diabetes. Diabetes Care. 2008;31(2):322–4.

402. Culic V. Triggering of cardiovascular incidents by micturition and defecation. International Journal of Cardiology. 2005;20:1–3.

403. Chakrabarti SD, Ganguly R, Chatterjee SK, Chakravarty A.. Is squatting a triggering factor for stroke in Indians? Acta Neurologica Scandinavica. 2002;105:124–7.

404. Murakami T. Squatting: the hemodynamic change is induced by enhanced aortic wave reflection. American Journal of Hypertension. 2002;15(11):986–8.

405. Hanson P, Slane PR, Rueckert PA, Clark SV. Squatting revisited: comparison of haemodynamic responses in normal individuals and heart transplantation recipients. British Heart Journal. 1995;74(2):154–8.

406. Martin Eastwood WDM, A.N. Smith. Straining, sitting, and squatting at stool. Lancet. 1975;306(7923):18–19.

407. Sacks FM, Lichtenstein AH, Wu JHY, Appel LJ, Creager MA, Kris-Etherton PM, et al. Dietary fats and cardiovascular disease: A presidential advisory from the American Heart Association. Circulation. 2017;136(3):e1–e23.

408. Mente A, Dehghan M, Rangarajan S, McQueen M, Dagenais G, Wielgosz A, et al. Association of dietary nutrients with blood lipids and blood pressure in 18 countries: a cross-sectional analysis from the PURE study. Lancet Diabetes & Endocrinology. 2017;5(10):774–87.

409. Jensen MK, Aroner SA, Mukamal KJ, Furtado JD, Post WS, Tsai MY, et al. High-density lipoprotein subspecies defined by presence of apolipoprotein C-III and incident coronary heart disease in four cohorts. Circulation. 2018;137(13):1364–73.

410. Steinberg D, Parthasarathy S, Carew TE, Khoo JC, Witztum JL. Beyond cholesterol. Modifications of low-density lipoprotein that increase its atherogenicity. New England Journal of Medicine. 1989;320(14):915–24.

411. Voight BF, Peloso GM, Orho-Melander M, Frikke-Schmidt R, Barbalic M, Jensen MK, et al. Plasma HDL cholesterol and risk of myocardial infarction: a Mendelian randomisation study. Lancet. 2012;380(9841):572–80.

412. Kulkarni KR, Markovitz JH, Nanda NC, Segrest JP. Increased prevalence of smaller and denser LDL particles in Asian Indians. Arteriosclerosis, Thrombosis and Vascular Biology. 1999;19:2749–55.

413. Halcox J, Misra A. Type 2 diabetes mellitus, metabolic syndrome, and mixed dyslipidemia: How similar, how different, and how to treat? Metabolic Syndrome and Related Disorders. 2014;13(1):1–21.

414. Donin AS, Nightingale CM, Owen CG, Rudnicka AR, McNamara MC, Prynne CJ, et al. Ethnic differences in blood lipids and dietary intake between UK children of black African, black Caribbean, South Asian, and white European origin: the Child Heart and Health Study in England (CHASE). American Journal of Clinical Nutrition. 2010;92(4):776–83.

415. Misra A, Shrivastava U. Obesity and dyslipidemia in South Asians. Nutrients. 2013;5(7):2708–33.

416. Shaper AG, Jones KW. Serum-cholesterol, diet and coronary heart-disease in African and Asians in Uganda. Lancet. 1959;10:534–7.

417. Karthikeyan G, Teo KK, Islam S, McQueen MJ, Pais P, Wang X, et al. Lipid profile, plasma apolipoproteins, and risk of a first myocardial infarction among Asians: an analysis from the INTERHEART Study. Journal of the American College of Cardiology. 2009;53(3):244–53.

418. Enas EA, Dharmarajan TS, Varkey B. Consensus statement on the management of dyslipidemia in Indian subjects: A different perspective. Indian Heart Journal. 2015;62(2).

419. Enas EA, Chacko V, Senthilkumar A, Puthumana N, Mohan V. Elevated lipoprotein(a)–a genetic risk factor for premature vascular disease in people with and without standard risk factors: a review. Disease-a-Month. 2006;52(1):5–50.

420. Anand SS, Enas EA, Pogue J, Haffner S, Pearson T, Yusuf S. Elevated lipoprotein(a) levels in South Asians in North America. Metabolism: Clinical & Experimental. 1998;47:182–4.

421. Misra A, Khurana L. The metabolic syndrome in South Asians: epidemiology, determinants, and prevention. Metabolic Syndrome and Related Disorders. 2009;7(6):497–514.

422. Alberty R, Albertyová D. Lipoprotein(a) in Children of Asian Indian Descendants and their Caucasian neighbors: The Slovak Lipid Community Study. Indian Journal of Clinical Biochemistry. 2012;27(3):231–8.

423. Tavridou A, Unwin N, Bhopal R, Laker M. Predictors of lipoprotein (a) levels in a European and South Asian population in the Newcastle Heart Project. European Journal of Clinical Investigation. 2003;33:686–92..

424. **Nordestgaard BG, Chapman MJ, Ray K, Borén J, Andreotti F, Watts GF,** et al. Lipoprotein(a) as a cardiovascular risk factor: current status. European Heart Journal. 2010;**31**(23):2844–53.

425. **Stefanadis C, Antoniou CK, Tsiachris D, Pietri P.** Coronary atherosclerotic vulnerable plaque: current perspectives. Journal of the American Heart Association. 2017;**6**(3):e005543.

426. **Karthikeyan G, Teo KK, Islam S, McQueen MJ, Pais P, Wang X,** et al. Lipid profile, plasma apolipoproteins, and risk of a first myocardial infarction Among Asians: an analysis from the INTERHEART Study. Journal of the American College of Cardiology. 2009;**53**(3):244–53.

427. **de Souza RJ, Mente A, Maroleanu A, Cozma AI, Ha V, Kishibe T,** et al. Intake of saturated and trans unsaturated fatty acids and risk of all cause mortality, cardiovascular disease, and type 2 diabetes: systematic review and meta-analysis of observational studies. BMJ. 2015;**351**:h3978.

428. **Chowdhury R, Warnakula S, Kunutsor S, Crowe F, Ward HA, Johnson L,** et al. Association of dietary, circulating, and supplement fatty acids with coronary risk: a systematic review and meta-analysis. Annals of Internal Medicine. 2014;**160**(9):658.

429. **Ascherio A, Katan MB, Zock PL, Stampfer MJ, Willett WC.** Trans fatty acids and coronary heart disease. New England Journal of Medicine. 1999;**340**(25):1994–8.

430. **Byers T.** hardened fats, hardened arteries? New England Journal of Medicine. 1997;**337**(21):1544–5.

431. **Radtke T, Schmid A, Trepp A, Dahler F, Coslovsky M, Eser P,** et al. Short-term effects of trans fatty acids from ruminant and industrial sources on surrogate markers of cardiovascular risk in healthy men and women: A randomized, controlled, double-blind trial. European Journal of Preventive Cardiology. 2016;**24**(5):534–43.

432. **Stender S, Astrup A, Dyerberg J.** Tracing artificial trans fat in popular foods in Europe: a market basket investigation. BMJ Open. 2014;**4**(5):e005218.

433. **Gulati S, Misra A, Sharma M.** Dietary fats and oils in India. Current Diabetes Reviews. 2017;**13**(5):438–43.

434. **Downs SM, Marie Thow A, Ghosh-Jerath S, Leeder SR.** Aligning food-processing policies to promote healthier fat consumption in India. Health Promotion International. 2015;**30**(3):595–605.

435. **Waziry R, Jawad M, Ballout RA, Al Akel M, Akl EA.** The effects of waterpipe tobacco smoking on health outcomes: an updated systematic review and meta-analysis. International Journal of Epidemiology. 2017;**46**(1):32–43.

436. **Gupta PC, Pednekar MS, Parkin DM, Sankaranarayanan R.** Tobacco associated mortality in Mumbai (Bombay) India. Results of the Bombay Cohort Study. International Journal of Epidemiology. 2005;**34**:1395–402.

437. **Hackshaw A, Morris JK, Boniface S, Tang JL, Milenkovic D.** Low cigarette consumption and risk of coronary heart disease and stroke: meta-analysis of 141 cohort studies in 55 study reports. BMJ. 2018;**360**:j5855.

438. **West R, McNeill A, Raw M.** Smokeless tobacco cessation guidelines for health professionals in England. British Dental Journal. 2004;**196**(10):611–18.

439. **Qasim H, Karim ZA, Rivera JO, Khasawneh FT, Alshbool FZ.** Impact of electronic cigarettes on the cardiovascular system. Journal of the American Heart Association. 2017;**6**(9):pii: e006353.

440. **Benowitz NL.** The role of nicotine in smoking-related cardiovascular disease. Preventative Medicine. 1997;**26**(4):412–17.

441. **Mohan I, Gupta R, Misra A, Sharma KK, Agrawal A, Vikram NK, et al.** Disparities in prevalence of cardiometablic risk factors in rural, urban-poor, and urban-middle class women in India. PLoS One. 2016;**11**(2):e0149437.

442. **Nierkens V.** Smoking in a multicultural society:Implications for prevention: Academic Medical Center, University of Amsterdam; 2006.

443. **Agyemang C, Stronks K, Tromp N, Bhopal R, Zaninotto P, Unwin N, et al.** A cross-national comparative study of smoking prevalence and cessation between English and Dutch South Asian and African origin populations: the role of national context. Nicotine & Tobacco Research. 2010;**12**(6):557–66.

444. **Bradby H, Williams R.** Is religion or culture the key feature in changes in substance use after leaving school? Young Punjabis and a comparison group in Glasgow. Ethnicity and Health. 2006;**11**(3):307–24.

445. **Karlsen S, Millward D, Sandford A.** Investigating ethnic differences in current cigarette smoking over time using the health surveys for England. European Journal of Public Health. 2012;**22**(2):254–6.

446. **Karlsen S, Nazroo JY.** Religious and ethnic differences in health: evidence from the Health Surveys for England 1999 and 2004. Ethnicity & Health. 2010;**15**(6):549–68.

447. **Bradby H.** Watch out for the Aunties! Young British Asians' accounts of identity and substance use. Sociology of Health and Illness. 2007;**29**(5):656–72.

448. **Balarajan R, Bulusu L, Adelstein AM, Shukla V.** Patterns of mortality among migrants to England and Wales from the Indian subcontinent. BMJ. 1984;**289**(6453):1185–7.

449. **Longman JM, Pritchard C, McNeill A, Csikar J, Croucher RE.** Accessibility of chewing tobacco products in England. Journal of Public Health. 2010;**32**(3):372–8.

450. **Nunez-de la Mora A, Jesmin F, Bentley G.** Betel nut use among first and second generation Bangladeshi Women in London, UK. Journal of Immigrant and Minority Health. 2007;**9**(4):299–306.

451. **Kassim S, Al-Haboubi M, Croucher R.** Short-term smoking cessation in English resident adults of Bangladeshi origin: a service review. Nicotine and Tobacco Research. 2015;**18**(4):410–15.

452. **Srinath RK, Shah B, Varghese C, Ramadoss A.** Responding to the threat of chronic diseases in India. Lancet. 2005;**366**(9498):1744–9.

453. **Willi C, Bodenmann P, Ghali WA, Faris PD, Cornuz J.** Active smoking and the risk of type 2 diabetes: a systematic review and meta-analysis. JAMA. 2007;**298**(22):2654–64.

454. **Pan A, Wang Y, Talaei M, Hu FB, Wu T.** Relation of active, passive, and quitting smoking with incident type 2 diabetes: a systematic review and meta-analysis. Lancet Diabetes & Endocrinology. 2015;**3**(12):958–67.

455. **Bush H, Williams R, Bradby H, Anderson A, Lean M.** Family hospitality and ethnic tradition among South Asian, Italian and general population women in the West of Scotland. Sociology of Health & Illness. 1998;**20**(3):351–80.

456. **Misra A, Khurana L, Isharwal S, Bhardwaj S.** South Asian diets and insulin resistance. British Journal of Nutrition. 2009;**1012**(4):465–73.

457. **Azar KM, Chen E, Holland A, Palaniappan L.** Festival foods in the immigrant diet. Journal of Immigrant and Minority Health. **15**(5):953–60.

458. Lawton J, Ahmad N, Hanna L, Douglas M, Bains H, Hallowell N. 'We should change ourselves, but we can't': accounts of food and eating practices amongst British Pakistanis and Indians with type 2 diabetes. Ethnicity & Health. 2008;**13**(4):305–19.

459. Sarfraz J. Food and eating practices in multigenerational, Pakistani, Muslim families living in Edinburgh; a qualitative study [PhD thesis]. Edinburgh: University of Edinburgh; 2015.

460. Harcombe Z, Baker JS, DiNicolantonio JJ, Grace F, Davies B. Evidence from randomised controlled trials does not support current dietary fat guidelines: a systematic review and meta-analysis. Open Heart. 2016;**3**(2):e000409.

461. Bakker LE, van Schinkel LD, Guigas B, Streefland TC, Jonker JT, van Klinken JB, et al. A 5-day high-fat, high-calorie diet impairs insulin sensitivity in healthy, young South asian men but not in caucasian men. Diabetes. 2014;**63**(1):248–58.

462. Gulati S, Misra A. Abdominal obesity and type 2 diabetes in Asian Indians: dietary strategies including edible oils, cooking practices and sugar intake. European Journal of Clinical Nutrition. 2017;**71**(7):850–7.

463. Mozaffarian D. Dietary and policy priorities for cardiovascular disease, diabetes, and obesity: a comprehensive review. Circulation. 2016;**133**(2):187–225.

464. Lovegrove JA, Givens DI. Dairy food products: good or bad for cardiometabolic disease? Nutrition Research Reviews. 2016;**29**(2):249–67E.

465. Vos MB, Kaar JL, Welsh JA, Van Horn LV, Feig DI, Anderson CAM, et al. Added sugars and cardiovascular disease risk in children: a scientific statement from the American Heart Association. Circulation. 2017;**135**(19):e1017–e34.

466. Mohan V, Gayathri R, Jaacks LM, Lakshmipriya N, Anjana RM, Spiegelman D, et al. Cashew nut consumption increases hdl cholesterol and reduces systolic blood pressure in Asian Indians with type 2 diabetes: a 12-week randomized controlled trial. Journal of Nutrition. 2018;**148**(1):63–9.

467. Loveman E, Colquitt J, Rees K. Cochrane corner: does increasing intake of dietary fibre help prevent cardiovascular disease? Heart. 2016;**102**(20):1607–9.

468. Gulati S, Misra A, Pandey RM. Effects of 3 g of soluble fiber from oats on lipid levels of Asian Indians – a randomized controlled, parallel arm study. Lipids in Health and Disease. 2017;**16**(1):71.

469. Miller V, Mente A, Dehghan M, Rangarajan S, Zhang X, Swaminathan S, et al. Fruit, vegetable, and legume intake, and cardiovascular disease and deaths in 18 countries (PURE): a prospective cohort study. Lancet. 2017;**390**(10107):2037–49.

470. Shridhar K, Dhillon PK, Bowen L, Kinra S, Bharathi AV, Prabhakaran D, et al. The association between a vegetarian diet and cardiovascular disease (CVD) risk factors in India: the Indian Migration Study. PLoS One. 2014;**9**(10):e110586.

471. Esposito K, Kastorini CM, Panagiotakos DB, Giugliano D. Prevention of type 2 diabetes by dietary patterns: a systematic review of prospective studies and meta-analysis. Metabolic Syndrome and Related Disorders. 2010;**8**(6):471–6.

472. Thorning TK, Raben A, Tholstrup T, Soedamah-Muthu SS, Givens I, Astrup A. Milk and dairy products: good or bad for human health? An assessment of the totality of scientific evidence. Food and Nutrition Research. 2016;**60**:32527.

473. Etemadi A, Sinha R, Ward MH, Graubard BI, Inoue-Choi M, Dawsey SM, et al. Mortality from different causes associated with meat, heme iron, nitrates, and nitrites

in the NIH-AARP Diet and Health Study: population based cohort study. BMJ. 2017;**357**:j1957.

474. **Micha R, Wallace SK, Mozaffarian D.** Red and processed meat consumption and risk of incident coronary heart disease, stroke, and diabetes mellitus: a systematic review and meta-analysis. Circulation. 2010;**121**(21):2271–83.

475. **Sayon-Orea C, Carlos S, Martinez-Gonzalez MA.** Does cooking with vegetable oils increase the risk of chronic diseases?: a systematic review. British Journal of Nutrition. 2015;**113**(S2):S36–S48.

476. **Martinez-Gonzalez MA, Fuente-Arrillaga C, Nunez-Cordoba JM, Basterra-Gortari FJ, Beunza JJ, Vazquez Z,** et al. Adherence to Mediterranean diet and risk of developing diabetes: prospective cohort study. BMJ. 2008;**336**(7657).

477. **Joint Working Party of the Royal College of Physicians of London and the British Cardiac Society, Royal College of Physicians of London and British Cardiac Society.** Prevention of coronary heart disease–Report of the Joint Working Party of the Royal College of Physicians of London and the British Cardiac Society. Journal of the Royal College of Physicians London. 1976;**10**(3):213–75.

478. **Anand SS, Islam S, Rosengren A, Franzosi MG, Steyn K, Yusufali AH,** et al. Risk factors for myocardial infarction in women and men: insights from the INTERHEART study. European Heart Journal. 2008;**29**(7):932–40.

479. **Leong DP, Smyth A, Teo KK, McKee M, Rangarajan S, Pais P,** et al. Patterns of alcohol consumption and myocardial infarction risk: observations from 52 countries in the INTERHEART case–control study. Circulation. 2014;**130**(5):390–8.

480. **Gepner Y, Golan R, Harman-Boehm I, Henkin Y, Schwarzfuchs D, Shelef I,** et al. Effects of initiating moderate alcohol intake on cardiometabolic risk in adults with type 2 diabetes. A 2-year randomized, controlled trial. Annals of Internal Medicine. 2015;**163**(8):569–79.

481. **Haseeb S, Alexander B, Baranchuk A.** Wine and cardiovascular health. A comprehensive review. Circulation. 2017;**136**(15):1434–48.

482. **Mozaffarian D, Fahimi S, Singh GM, Micha R, Khatibzadeh S, Engell RE,** et al. Global sodium consumption and death from cardiovascular causes. New England Journal of Medicine. 2014;**371**(7):624–34.

483. **Liu G, Zong G, Hu FB, Willett WC, Eisenberg DM, Sun Q.** Cooking methods for red meats and risk of type 2 diabetes: a prospective study of U.S. women. Diabetes Care. 2017;**40**(8):1041–9.

484. **Gibney MJ, Forde CG, Mullally D, Gibney ER.** Ultra-processed foods in human health: a critical appraisal. American Journal of Clinical Nutrition. 2017;**106**(3):717–24.

485. **Poti JM, Braga B, Qin B.** Ultra-processed food intake and obesity: what really matters for health—processing or nutrient content? Current Obesity Reports. 2017;**6**(4):420–31.

486. **Gadiraju TV, Patel Y, Gaziano JM, Djousse L.** Fried food consumption and cardiovascular health: a review of current evidence. Nutrients. 2015;**7**(10):8424–30.

487. **Nigam P, Bhatt S, Misra A, Chadha DS, Vaidya M, Dasgupta J,** et al. Effect of a 6-month intervention with cooking oils containing a high concentration of monounsaturated fatty acids (olive and canola oils) compared with control oil in

male Asian Indians with nonalcoholic fatty liver disease. Diabetes Technology & Therapeutics. 2014;**16**(4):255–61.

488. **Vlassara H, Cai W, Crandall J, Goldberg T, Oberstein R, Dardaine V,** et al. Inflammatory mediators are induced by dietary glycotoxins, a major risk factor for diabetic angiopathy. Proceedings of the National Academy of Sciences. 2002;**99**(24):15596–601.

489. **Tessier FJ, Birlouez-Aragon I.** Health effects of dietary Maillard reaction products: the results of ICARE and other studies. Amino Acids. 2012;**42**(4):1119–31.

490. **Birlouez-Aragon I, Saavedra G, Tessier FJ, Galinier A, it-Ameur L, Lacoste F,** et al. A diet based on high-heat-treated foods promotes risk factors for diabetes mellitus and cardiovascular diseases. American Journal of Clinical Nutrition. 2010;**91**(5):1220–6.

491. **Liu G, Zong G, Wu K, Hu Y, Li Y, Willett WC,** et al. Meat cooking methods and risk of type 2 diabetes: results from three prospective cohort studies. Diabetes Care. 2018;**41**:1049–60.

492. **Sartorius K, Sartorius B, Madiba TE, Stefan C.** Does high-carbohydrate intake lead to increased risk of obesity? A systematic review and meta-analysis. BMJ Open. 2018;**8**(2):e018449.

493. **Parackal S.** Dietary transition in the South Asian diaspora: implications for diabetes prevention strategies. Current Diabetes Reviews. 2016;**12**.

494. **Hall KD.** A review of the carbohydrate-insulin model of obesity. European Journal of Clinical Nutrition. 2017;**71**(3):323–6.

495. **Hall LML, Sattar N, Gill JS.** Risk of metabolic and vascular disease in South Asians: potential mechanisms for increased insulin resistance. Future Lipidology. 2008;**3**(4):411–24.

496. **Joshi MS, Lamb R.** New foods for old? The diet of South Asians in the UK. Psychology & Developing Societies. 2000;**12**(1):83–103.

497. **Misra A, Singhal N, Khurana L.** Obesity, the metabolic syndrome, and type 2 diabetes in developing countries: role of dietary fats and oils. Journal of the American College of Nutrition. 2010;**29**(3 Suppl):289S–301S.

498. **Martha P, McMurry MS, Cerqueira MT, Sonja L, Connor MSea.** Changes in lipid and lipoprotein levels and body weight in Tarahumara Indians after consumption of an affluent diet. New England Journal of Medicine. 1991;**325**:1704–8.

499. **Yadav K, Krishnan A.** Changing patterns of diet, physical activity and obesity among urban, rural and slum populations in north India. Obesity Reviews. 2008;**9**(5):400–8.

500. **Kumar BN, Meyer HE, Wandel M, Dalen I, Holmboe-Ottesen G.** Ethnic differences in obesity among immigrants from developing countries, in Oslo, Norway. International Journal of Obesity (London). 2006;**30**(4):684–90.

501. **Kumar BN.** Ethnic Differences in Obesity and Related Risk Factors for Cardiovascular Diseases among Immigrants in Oslo, Norway: A cross sectional study of ethnic differences in obesity and selected risk factors and their associations among adolescents and adults in Oslo [PhD thesis]. Oslo: University of Oslo; 2006.

502. **Raheja BS.** Ghee, cholesterol, and heart disease. Lancet. 1987; **2**(8568):1144–5.

503. **Department of Health.** Health Survey for England 1999: the health of minority ethnic groups. Vol 1 and Vol 2. London: The Stationery Office; 2001.

504. **Miller GJ, Kotecha S, Wilkinson WH, Wilkes H, Stirling Y, Sanders TA,** et al. Dietary and other characteristics relevant for coronary heart disease in men of Indian, West Indian and European descent in London. Atherosclerosis. 1988;**70**(1–2):63–72.

505. **Misra A, Khurana L.** Obesity and the metabolic syndrome in developing countries. Journal of Clinical Endocrinology Metabolism. 2008;**93**(11_Supplement_1):s9–30.

506. **Iqbal R, Anand S, Ounpuu S, Islam S, Zhang X, Rangarajan S,** et al. Dietary patterns and the risk of acute myocardial infarction in 52 Countries. Circulation. 2008;**118**(19):1929–37.

507. **Emadian A, England CY, Thompson JL.** Dietary intake and factors influencing eating behaviours in overweight and obese South Asian men living in the UK: mixed method study. BMJ Open. 2017;**7**(7):e016919.

508. **Garduno-Diaz SD, Khokhar S.** South Asian dietary patterns and their association with risk factors for the metabolic syndrome. Journal of Human Nutrition and Dietetics. 2013;**26**(2):145–55.

509. **Leung G, Stanner S.** Diets of minority ethnic groups in the UK: influence on chronic disease risk and implications for prevention. Nutrition Bulletin. 2011;**36**(2):161–98.

510. **Gerstein HC, Islam S, Anand S, Almahmeed W, Damasceno A, Dans A,** et al. Dysglycaemia and the risk of acute myocardial infarction in multiple ethnic groups: an analysis of 15,780 patients from the INTERHEART study. Diabetologia. 2010;**53**(12):2509–17.

511. **Pradeepa R, Nazir A, Mohan V.** Type 2 diabetes and cardiovascular diseases: do they share a common soil? The Asian Indian experience. Heart Asia. 2012;**4**(1):69–76.

512. **Bellary S, O'Hare JP, Raymond NT, Mughal S, Hanif WM, Jones A,** et al. Premature cardiovascular events and mortality in south Asians with type 2 diabetes in the United Kingdom Asian Diabetes Study–effect of ethnicity on risk. Current Medical Research & Opinion. 2010;**26**(8):1873–9.

513. **Ma S, Cutter J, Tan CE, Chew SK, Tai ES.** Assocations of diabetes mellitus and ethnicity with mortality in a mulitethnic Asian population: data from the 1992 Singapore National Health Survey. American Journal of Epidemiology. 2003;**158**:543–52.

514. **WHO.** Definition, diagnosis and classification of diabetes mellitus and its complications. Report of a WHO consultation. Part 1: diagnosis and classification of diabetes mellitus. Geneva: Department of Noncommunicable Disease Surveillance; 1999.

515. **WHO.** Definition and diagnosis of diabetes mellitus and intermediate hyperglycaemia. Report of a WHO/IDF consultation. Geneva; 2006.

516. **Raymond NT, Varadhan L, Reynold DR, Bush K, Sankaranarayanan S, Bellary S,** et al. Higher prevalence of retinopathy in diabetic patients of South Asian ethnicity compared with white Europeans in the community: a cross-sectional study. Diabetes Care. 2009;**32**(3):410–15.

517. **Bellary S, O'Hare JP, Raymond NT, Gumber A, Mughal S, Szczepura A,** et al. Enhanced diabetes care to patients of south Asian ethnic origin (the United Kingdom Asian Diabetes Study): a cluster randomised controlled trial. Lancet. 2008;**371**(9626):1769–76.

518. **Anjana RM, Shanthi Rani CS, Deepa M, Pradeepa R, Sudha V, Divya NH,** et al. Incidence of diabetes and prediabetes and predictors of progression among Asian

Indians: 10-year follow-up of the Chennai Urban Rural Epidemiology Study (CURES). Diabetes Care. 2015;38(8):1441–8.

519. **Vistisen D, Witte DR, Brunner EJ, Kivimaki M, Tabak A, Jorgensen ME, et al.** Risk of cardiovascular disease and death in individuals with prediabetes defined by different criteria: The Whitehall II Study. Diabetes Care. 2018; 41(4):899–906.

520. **Dilley J, Ganesan A, Deepa R, Deepa M, Sharada G, Williams OD, et al.** Association of A1C with cardiovascular disease and metabolic syndrome in Asian Indians with normal glucose tolerance. Diabetes Care. 2007;30:1527–32.

521. **Likhari T, Gama R.** Ethnic differences in glycated haemoglobin between white subjects and those of South Asian origin with normal glucose tolerance. Journal of Clinical Pathology. 2010;63(3):278–80.

522. **Thomas C, Nightingale C, Rudnicka A, Owen C, Sattar N, Cook D, et al.** Ethnic differences in type 2 diabetes risk markers in children in the UK are not explained by socio-economic status: Child Heart and Health Study in England. Journal of Epidemiology and Community Health. 2010;64(Suppl 1):A7–A8.

523. **Stern M.** Glycemia and Cardiovascular Risk. Diabetes Care. 1997;20:501–2.

524. **Huang Y, Cai X, Mai W, Li M, Hu Y.** Association between prediabetes and risk of cardiovascular disease and all cause mortality: systematic review and meta-analysis. BMJ. 2016;355:i5953.

525. **Gale EA.** Glucose control in the UKPDS: what did we learn? Diabetic Medicine. 2008;25 Suppl 2:9–12.

526. **Hopper I, Billah B, Skiba M, Krum H.** Prevention of diabetes and reduction in major cardiovascular events in studies of subjects with prediabetes: meta-analysis of randomised controlled clinical trials. European Journal of Cardiovascular Prevention and Rehabilitation. 2011;18(6):813–23.

527. **Li G, Zhang P, Wang J, An Y, Gong Q, Gregg EW, et al.** Cardiovascular mortality, all-cause mortality, and diabetes incidence after lifestyle intervention for people with impaired glucose tolerance in the Da Qing Diabetes Prevention Study: a 23-year follow-up study. Lancet Diabetes Endocrinol. 2014;2(6):474–80.

528. **Venn BJ, Williams SM, Mann JI.** Comparison of postprandial glycaemia in Asians and Caucasians. Diabetic Medicine. 2010;27:1205–8.

529. **Group IDMAP.** A proposed India-specific algorithm for management of type 2 diabetes. Diabetes Technology & Therapeutics. 2016;18(6):346–50.

530. **Misra A, Vikram NK, Arya S, Pandey RM, Dhingra V, Chatterjee A, et al.** High prevalence of insulin resistance in postpubertal Asian Indian children is associated with adverse truncal body fat patterning, abdominal adiposity and excess body fat. International Journal of Obesity 2004;28:1217–26.

531. **Yajnik CS.** Early life origins of insulin resistance and type 2 diabetes in India and other Asian countries. Journal of Nutrition. 2004;134(1):205–10.

532. **Ikehara S, Tabak AG, Akbaraly TN, Hulman A, Kivimaki M, Forouhi NG, et al.** Age trajectories of glycaemic traits in non-diabetic South Asian and white individuals: the Whitehall II cohort study. Diabetologia. 2015;58(3):534–42.

533. **Rattarasarn C.** Dysregulated lipid storage and its relationship with insulin resistance and cardiovascular risk factors in non-obese Asian patients with type 2 diabetes. Adipocyte. 2018;6(4):1–10.

534. **Bellisari A.** Evolutionary origins of obesity. Obesity Reviews. 2008;9(2):165–80.

535. **Deurenberg P, Deurenberg-Yap M, Guricci S.** Asians are different from Caucasians and from each other in their body mass index/body fat per cent relationship. Obesity Reviews. 2002;3:141–6.

536. **Deurenberg P.** Relationships between indices of obesity and its co-morbidities in multi-ethnic Singapore. International Journal of Obesity. 2001;25(10):1554–62.

537. **Deurenberg P, Yap M, van Staveren WA.** Body mass index and percent body fat: a meta analysis among different ethnic groups. International Journal of Obesity. 1998;22:1164–71.

538. **Dudeja V, Misra A, Pandey RM, Devina G, Kumar G, Vikram NK.** BMI does not accurately predict overweight in Asian Indians in northern India. British Journal of Nutrition. 2001;86:105–12.

539. **Razak F, Anand SS, Shannon H, Vuksan V, Davis B, Jacobs R, et al.** Defining obesity cut points in a multiethnic population. Circulation. 2007;115(16):2111–18.

540. **Gray LJ, Yates T, Davies MJ, Brady E, Webb DR, Sattar N, et al.** Defining obesity cut-off points for migrant South Asians. PLoS ONE. 2011;6(10):e26464.

541. **Ntuk UE, Gill JM, Mackay DF, Sattar N, Pell JP.** Ethnic-specific obesity cutoffs for diabetes risk: cross-sectional study of 490,288 UK biobank participants. Diabetes Care. 2014;37(9):2500–7.

542. **Hayes L, White M, McNally RJQ, Unwin N, Tran A, Bhopal R.** Do cardiometabolic, behavioural and socioeconomic factors explain the 'healthy migrant effect' in the UK? Linked mortality follow-up of South Asians compared with white Europeans in the Newcastle Heart Project. Journal of Epidemiology and Community Health. 2017;71:863–9.

543. **Kim SH, Despres JP, Koh KK.** Obesity and cardiovascular disease: friend or foe? European Heart Journal. 2015;37(48):3560–8.

544. **Kelishadi R.** Childhood overweight, obesity, and the metabolic syndrome in developing countries. Epidemiologic Reviews. 2007;29;62–76.

545. **Satija A, Hu FB, Bowen L, Bharathi AV, Vaz M, Prabhakaran D, et al.** Dietary patterns in India and their association with obesity and central obesity. Public Health Nutrition. 2015;18(16):3031–41.

546. **Gepner Y, Shelef I, Schwarzfuchs D, Zelicha H, Tene L, Yaskolka Meir A, et al.** Effect of distinct lifestyle interventions on mobilization of fat storage pools: CENTRAL magnetic resonance imaging randomized controlled trial. Circulation. 2018;137(11):1143–57.

547. **Smith J, Al-Amri M, Dorairaj P, Sniderman A.** The adipocyte life cycle hypothesis. Clinical Science. 2006;110(1):1–9.

548. **Misra A, Khurana L.** Obesity-related non-communicable diseases: South Asians vs White Caucasians. Interational Journal of Obesity. 2011;35(2):167–87.

549. **Johannsen DL, Tchoukalova Y, Tam CS, Covington JD, Xie W, Schwarz JM, et al.** Effect of 8 weeks of overfeeding on ectopic fat deposition and insulin sensitivity: testing the 'adipose tissue expandability' hypothesis. Diabetes Care. 2014;37(10):2789–97.

550. **Ahn SG, Lim HS, Joe DY, Kang SJ, Choi BJ, Choi SY, et al.** Relationship of epicardial adipose tissue by echocardiography to coronary artery disease. Heart. 2007;94:e7.

551. **Kiefer FW, Cohen P, Plutzky J.** Fifty shades of brown. Circulation. 2012;126(9):1012–15.

552. **Danaei G, Robins JM, Young JG, Hu FB, Manson JE, Hern+ín MA.** Weight loss and coronary heart disease: sensitivity analysis for unmeasured confounding by undiagnosed disease. Epidemiology. 2016;**27**(2):302–10.

553. **Garg SK, Lin F, Kandula N, Ding J, Carr J, Allison M, et al.** Ectopic fat depots and coronary artery calcium in South Asians compared with other racial/ethnic groups. Journal of the American Heart Association. 2016;**5**(11):e004257.

554. **Viner RM, Cole TJ, Fry T, Gupta S, Kinra S, McCarthy D, et al.** Insufficient evidence to support separate BMI definitions for obesity in children and adolescents from south Asian ethnic groups in the UK. International Journal of Obesity (London). 2010;**34**(4):656–8.

555. **Patel S, Unwin N, Bhopal R, White M, Harland J, Ayis SA, et al.** A comparison of proxy measures of abdominal obesity in Chinese, European and South Asian adults. Diabetic Medicine. 1999;**16**:853–60.

556. **Unwin N, Bhopal R, Hayes L, White M, Patel S, Ragoobirsingh D, et al.** A comparison of the new International Diabetes Federation definition of metabolic syndrome to WHO and NCEP definitions in Chinese, European and South Asian origin adults. Ethnicity & Disease. 2007;**17**(3):522–8.

557. **Krishnaveni GV, Hill JC, Veena SR, Leary SD, Saperia J, Chachyamma KJ, et al.** Truncal adiposity is present at birth and in early childhood in South Indian children. Indian Pediatrics. 2005;**42**(6):527–38.

558. **Power C, Thomas C.** Changes in BMI, duration of overweight and obesity, and glucose metabolism: 45 years of follow-up of a birth cohort. Diabetes Care. 2011;**34**(9):1986–91.

559. **Zheng H, Dirlam J.** The body mass index-mortality link across the life course: two selection biases and their effects. PLoS One. 2016;**11**(2):e0148178.

560. **Vazquez G, Duval S, Jacobs DR, Jr., Silventoinen K.** Comparison of body mass index, waist circumference, and waist/hip ratio in predicting incident diabetes: a meta-analysis. Epidemiologic Reviews. 2007;**29**(1):115–28.

561. **Diemer FS, Brewster LM, Haan YC, Oehlers GP, van Montfrans GA, Nahar-van Venrooij LMW.** Body composition measures and cardiovascular risk in high-risk ethnic groups. Clinical Nutrition. 2017:1–7.

562. **Sattar N, Gill JM.** Type 2 diabetes as a disease of ectopic fat? BMC Medicine. 2014;**12**:123.

563. **Cheng FW, Gao X, Jensen GL.** Weight change and all-cause mortality in older adults: a meta-analysis. Journal of Nutrition in Gerontology and Geriatrics. 2015;**34**(4):343–68.

564. **Willett WC.** Weight changes and health in Cuba. BMJ. 2013;**346**:f1777.

565. **Whincup PH, Gilg JA, Papacosta O, Seymour C, Miller GJ, Alberti KG, et al.** Early evidence of ethnic differences in cardiovascular risk: cross sectional comparison of British South Asian and white children. BMJ. 2002;**324**(7338):635–8.

566. **Whincup PH, Gilg JA, Owen CG, Odoki K, Alberti KG, Cook DG.** British South Asians aged 13–16 years have higher fasting glucose and insulin levels than Europeans. Diabetic Medicine. 2005;**22**(9):1275–7.

567. **Reddy KS, Prabhakaran D, Shah P, Shah B.** Differences in body mass index and waist: hip ratios in North Indian rural and urban populations. Obesity Reviews. 2002;**3**(3):197–202.

568. Abdullah A, Wolfe R, Stoelwinder JU, de Courten M, Stevenson C, Walls HL, et al. The number of years lived with obesity and the risk of all-cause and cause-specific mortality. International Journal of Epidemiology. 2011;40(4):985–96.

569. Song M, Hu FB, Wu K, Must A, Chan AT, Willett WC, et al. Trajectory of body shape in early and middle life and all cause and cause specific mortality: results from two prospective US cohort studies. BMJ. 2016;353:i2195.

570. Bruijnzeels M, Kumar BN, Agyemang C, Stronks K. Diabetes mellitus type II and cardiovascular risk profile in immigrant groups in three North Western European countries: Norway, Netherlands and UK. In: Tellnes G, editor. Urbanisation and Health–New Challenges in Health Promotion and Prevention. Oslo: Oslo Academic Press; 2007. p. 268–84.

571. de Mutsert R, Sun Q, Willett WC, Hu FB, van Dam RM. Overweight in early adulthood, adult weight change, and risk of type 2 diabetes, cardiovascular diseases, and certain cancers in men: a cohort study. American Journal of Epidemiology. 2014;179(11):1353–65.

572. Zheng W, McLerran DF, Rolland B, Zhang X, Inoue M, Matsuo K, et al. Association between body-mass index and risk of death in more than 1 million Asians. New England Journal of Medicine. 2011;364(8):719–29.

573. Cordain L, Gotshall RW, Eaton SB, Eaton SB, 3rd. Physical activity, energy expenditure and fitness: an evolutionary perspective. International Journal of Sports Medicine 1998;19(5):328–35.

574. Tremblay A, Therrien F. Physical activity and body functionality: implications for obesity prevention and treatment. Canadian Journal of Physiology and Pharmacology 2006;84(2):149–56.

575. Ranasinghe CD, Ranasinghe P, Jayawardena R, Misra A. Physical activity patterns among South-Asian adults: a systematic review. International Journal of Behavioral Nutrition and Physical Activity 2013;10(1):116.

576. Fischbacher CM, Hunt S, Alexander L. How physically active are South Asians in the United Kingdom? A literature review. Journal of Public Health (Oxford). 2004;26(3):250–8.

577. Sumner J, Uijtdewilligen L, Chu AH, Ng SH, Barreira TV, Sloan RA, et al. Stepping volume and intensity patterns in a multi-ethnic urban Asian population. BMC Public Health. 2018;18(1):539.

578. Rawlins E, Baker G, Maynard M, Harding S. Perceptions of healthy eating and physical activity in an ethnically diverse sample of young children and their parents: the DEAL prevention of obesity study. Journal of Human Nutrition and Dietetics. 2013;26(2):132–44.

579. Horne M, Skelton DA, Speed S, Todd C. Attitudes and beliefs to the uptake and maintenance of physical activity among community-dwelling South Asians aged 60–70 years: A qualitative study. Public Health. 2012;126(5):417–23.

580. Morrison Z, Douglas A, Bhopal R, Sheikh A. Understanding experiences of participating in a weight loss lifestyle intervention trial: a qualitative evaluation of South Asians at high risk of diabetes. BMJ Open. 2014;4(6):e004736.

581. Horne M, Skelton DA, Speed S, Todd C. Perceived barriers to initiating and maintaining physical activity among South Asian and White British adults in

their 60s living in the United Kingdom: a qualitative study. Ethnicity and Health. 2013;**18**(6):626–45.

582. **Sriskantharajah J, Kai J.** Promoting physical activity among South Asian women with coronary heart disease and diabetes: what might help? Family Practice. 2007;**24**(1):71–6.

583. **Lawton J, Ahmad N, Hanna L, Douglas M, Hallowell N.** 'I can't do any serious exercise': barriers to physical activity amongst people of Pakistani and Indian origin with Type 2 diabetes. Health Education Research. 2006;**21**(1):43–54.

584. **Samitz G, Egger M, Zwahlen M.** Domains of physical activity and all-cause mortality: systematic review and dose-response meta-analysis of cohort studies. International Journal of Epidemiology. 2011;**40**(5):1382–400.

585. **Gill JM, Celis-Morales CA, Ghouri N.** Physical activity, ethnicity and cardio-metabolic health: does one size fit all? Atherosclerosis. 2014;**232**(2):319–33.

586. **Aguiar EJ, Morgan PJ, Collins CE, Plotnikoff RC, Callister R.** Efficacy of interventions that include diet, aerobic and resistance training components for type 2 diabetes prevention: a systematic review with meta-analysis. International Journal of Behavioral Nutrition and Physical Activity. 2014;**11**:2.

587. **Murtagh EM, Nichols L, Mohammed MA, Holder R, Nevill AM, Murphy MH.** The effect of walking on risk factors for cardiovascular disease: An updated systematic review and meta-analysis of randomised control trials. Preventive Medicine. 2015;**72**(1):34–43.

588. **Schwingshackl L, Dias S, Hoffmann G.** Impact of long-term lifestyle programmes on weight loss and cardiovascular risk factors in overweight/obese participants: a systematic review and network meta-analysis. Systematic Reviews. 2014;**3**(1):130.

589. **Davey GJG, Roberts JD, Patel S, Pierpoint IF, Godsland IF, Davies B,** et al. Effects of exercise on insulin resistance in South Asians and Europeans. Journal of Exercise Physiology [Internet]. 2000; 3.

590. **Owen CG, Nightingale CM, Rudnicka AR, Cook DG, Ekelund U, Whincup PH.** Ethnic and gender differences in physical activity levels among 9-10-year-old children of white European, South Asian and African-Caribbean origin: the Child Heart Health Study in England (CHASE Study). International Journal of Epidemiology. 2009;**38**(4):1082–93.

591. **Hayes L, White M, Unwin N, Bhopal R, Fischbacher C, Harland J, Alberti KG,** et al. Patterns of physical activity and relationship with risk markers for cardiovascular disease and diabetes in Indian, Pakistani, Bangladeshi and European adults in a UK population. Journal of Public Health Medicine. 2002;**24**:170–8.

592. **Bhatnagar P, Shaw A, Foster C.** Generational differences in the physical activity of UK South Asians: a systematic review. International Journal of Behavioral Nutrition and Physical Activity. 2015;**12**(1):96.

593. **Nightingale CM, Donin AS, Kerry SR, Owen CG, Rudnicka AR, Brage S,** et al. Cross-sectional study of ethnic differences in physical fitness among children of South Asian, black African–Caribbean and white European origin: the Child Heart and Health Study in England (CHASE). BMJ Open. 2016;**6**:e011131.

594. **Konopka AR, Asante A, Lanza IR, Robinson MM, Johnson ML, Dalla MC,** et al. Defects in mitochondrial efficiency and H_2O_2 emissions in obese women are restored to a lean phenotype with aerobic exercise training. Diabetes. 2015;**64**(6):2104–15.

595. Osei-Kwasi HA, Nicolaou M, Powell K, Terragni L, Maes L, Stronks K, et al. Systematic mapping review of the factors influencing dietary behaviour in ethnic minority groups living in Europe: a DEDIPAC study. International Journal of Behavioral Nutrition and Physical Activity. 2016;13:85.

596. Koshoedo S, Paul-Ebhohimhen V, Jepson R, Watson M. Understanding the complex interplay of barriers to physical activity amongst black and minority ethnic groups in the United Kingdom: a qualitative synthesis using meta-ethnography. BMC Public Health. 2015;15(1):643.

597. Jepson R, Harris FM, Bowes A, Robertson R, Avan G, Sheikh A. Physical activity in South asians: an in-depth qualitative study to explore motivations and facilitators. PLoS One. 2012;7(10):e45333.

598. Hendriks AM, Gubbels JS, Jansen MW, Kremers SP. Health beliefs regarding dietary behavior and physical activity of Surinamese immigrants of Indian descent in The Netherlands: a qualitative study. ISRN Obesity. 2012;2012:903868.

599. Cross-Bardell L, George T, Bhoday M, Tuomainen H, Qureshi N, Kai J. Perspectives on enhancing physical activity and diet for health promotion among at-risk urban UK South Asian communities: a qualitative study. BMJ Open. 2015;5(2):e007317.

600. Grace C, Begum R, Subhani S, Kopelman P, Greenhalgh T. Prevention of type 2 diabetes in British Bangladeshis: qualitative study of community, religious, and professional perspectives. BMJ. 2008;337:a1931.

601. Hajek P, Myers K, Dhanji AR, West O, McRobbie H. Weight change during and after Ramadan fasting. Journal of Public Health. 2012;34(3):377–81.

602. Johnson C, Mohan S, Rogers K, Shivashankar R, Thout SR, Gupta P, et al. Mean dietary salt intake in urban and rural areas in India: a population survey of 1395 persons. Journal of the American Heart Association. 2017;6(1): e004547.

603. Dhanjal TS, Lal M, Haynes R, Lip G. A comparison of cardiovascular risk factors among Indo-Asian and caucasian patients admitted with acute myocardial infarction in Kuala Lumpur, Malaysia and Birmingham, England. International Journal of Clinical Practice. 2001;55(10):665–8.

604. Parackal S, Stewart J, Ho E. Exploring reasons for ethnic disparities in diet- and lifestyle-related chronic disease for Asian sub-groups in New Zealand: a scoping exercise. Ethnicity & Health. 2017;22(4):333–47.

605. Sattar N, McConnachie A, Shaper AG, Blauw GJ, Buckley BM, de Craen AJ, et al. Can metabolic syndrome usefully predict cardiovascular disease and diabetes? Outcome data from two prospective studies. Lancet. 2008;371(9628):1927–35.

606. Tzoulaki I, Ebbels TMD, Valdes A, Elliott P, Ioannidis JPA. Design and analysis of metabolomics studies in epidemiologic research: a primer on -omic technologies. American Journal of Epidemiology. 2014;180(2):129–39.

607. Danesh J, Erqou S, Walker M, Thompson SG, Tipping R, Ford C, et al. The Emerging Risk Factors Collaboration: analysis of individual data on lipid, inflammatory and other markers in over 1.1 million participants in 104 prospective studies of cardiovascular diseases. European Journal of Epidemiology. 2007;22(12):839–69.

608. Ahmed E, El-Menyar A. South Asian ethnicity and cardiovascular risk: the known, the unknown, and the paradox. Angiology. 2014;66(5):405–15.

609. Holick MF, Binkley NC, Bischoff-Ferrari HA, Gordon CM, Hanley DA, Heaney RP, et al. Evaluation, treatment, and prevention of vitamin d deficiency: an Endocrine

Society Clinical Practice Guideline. Journal of Clinical Endocrinology & Metabolism. 2011;**96**(12):3908.

610. **Norman AW, Bouillon R.** Vitamin D nutritional policy needs a vision for the future. Experimental Biology and Medicine. 2010;**235**(9):1034–45.

611. **Grandi NC, Breitling LP, Brenner H.** Vitamin D and cardiovascular disease: Systematic review and meta-analysis of prospective studies. Preventative Medicine. 2010;**51**(3-4):228–33.

612. **Mousa A, Naderpoor N, de Courten MP, Teede H, Kellow N, Walker K,** et al. Vitamin D supplementation has no effect on insulin sensitivity or secretion in vitamin D–deficient, overweight or obese adults: a randomized placebo-controlled trial. American Journal of Clinical Nutrition. 2017;**105**(6):1372–81.

613. **Sluyter JD, Camargo Jr CA, Stewart AW, Waayer D, Lawes CMM, Toop L,** et al. Effect of monthly, high-dose, long-term vitamin D supplementation on central blood pressure parameters: a randomized controlled trial substudy. Journal of American Heart Association. 2017; **6**(10). pii: e006802.

614. **Sluyter JD, Camargo CA, Stewart AW, Waayer D, Lawes CMM, Toop L,** et al. Effect of monthly, high-dose, long-term vitamin d supplementation on central blood pressure parameters: a randomized controlled trial substudy. Journal of the American Heart Association. 2017;**6**(10):e006802.

615. **Scragg R, Wishart J, Stewart A, Ofanoa M, Kerse N, Dyall L,** et al. No effect of ultraviolet radiation on blood pressure and other cardiovascular risk factors. Journal of Hypertension. 2011;**29**(9):1749–56.

616. **Ginde AA, Scragg R, Schwartz RS, Camargo CA, Jr.** Prospective study of serum 25-hydroxyvitamin D level, cardiovascular disease mortality, and all-cause mortality in older U.S. adults. Journal of the American Geriatrics Society. 2009;**57**(9):1595–603.

617. **Witham MD, Dove FJ, Dryburgh M, Sugden JA, Morris AD, Struthers AD.** The effect of different doses of vitamin D(3) on markers of vascular health in patients with type 2 diabetes: a randomised controlled trial. Diabetologia. 2010;**53**(10):2112–19.

618. **Autier P, Mullie P, Macacu A, Dragomir M, Boniol M, Coppens K,** et al. Effect of vitamin D supplementation on non-skeletal disorders: a systematic review of meta-analyses and randomised trials. Lancet Diabetes & Endocrinology. 2017;**5**(12):986–1004.

619. **Smith M.** Seasonal, ethnic and gender variations in serum vitamin D3 levels in the local population of Peterborough. Bioscience Horizons. 2010;**3**(2):124–31.

620. **Krishnaveni GV, Veena SR, Winder NR, Hill JC, Noonan K, Boucher BJ,** et al. Maternal vitamin D status during pregnancy and body composition and cardiovascular risk markers in Indian children: the Mysore Parthenon Study. American Journal of Clinical Nutrition. 2011;**93**(3):628–35.

621. **Shaunak S, Colston K, Ang L, Patel SP, Maxwell JD.** Vitamin D deficiency in adult British Hindu Asians: a family disorder. BMJ. 1985;**291**:1166–8.

622. **Ford JA, Colhoun EM, McIntosh WB, Dunnigan MG.** Rickets and osteomalacia in the Glasgow Pakistani community, 1961-1971. BMJ. 1972;**2**:677–80.

623. **Pittas AG, Chung M, Trikalinos T, Mitri J, Brendel M, Patel K,** et al. Systematic review: vitamin d and cardiometabolic outcomes. Annals of Internal Medicine. 2010;**152**(5):307–14.

624. Jablonski NG, Chaplin G. Human skin pigmentation as an adaptation to UV radiation. Proceedings of the National Academy of Sciences. 2010;**107**(Supplement 2):8962–8.

625. **Dunnigan MG, McIntosh WB, Sutherland GR, Gardee R, al e.** Policy for prevention of Asian rickets in Britain: a preliminary assessment of the Glasgow Rickets Campaign. British Medical Journal. 1981;**288**:357–60.

626. **Nagpal J, Pande JN, Bhartia A.** A double-blind, randomized, placebo-controlled trial of the short-term effect of vitamin D3 supplementation on insulin sensitivity in apparently healthy, middle-aged, centrally obese men. Diabetic Medicine. 2009;**26**(1):19–27.

627. **Madar AA, Knutsen KV, Stene LC, Brekke M, Meyer HE, Lagerlov P.** Effect of vitamin D3 supplementation on glycated hemoglobin (HbA1c), fructosamine, serum lipids, and body mass index: a randomized, double-blinded, placebo-controlled trial among healthy immigrants living in Norway. BMJ Open Diabetes Research and Care 2014;**2**(1):e000026.

628. **von Hurst PR, Stonehouse W, Coad J.** Vitamin D supplementation reduces insulin resistance in South Asian women living in New Zealand who are insulin resistant and vitamin D deficient–a randomised, placebo-controlled trial. British Journal of Nutrition. 2009;**103**(4):549–55.

629. **McCully KS.** Homocysteine, folate, vitamin b6, and cardiovascular disease. Journal of the American Medical Association. 1998;**279**:392–3.

630. **Rush EC, Katre P, Yajnik CS.** Vitamin B12: one carbon metabolism, fetal growth and programming for chronic disease. Europeran Journal of Clinical Nutrition. 2014;**68**(1):2–7.

631. **Misra A, Vikram NK, Pandey RM, Dwivedi M, Ahmad FU, Luthra K,** et al. Hyperhomocysteinemia and low intake of folic acid and vitamin B12 in urban North India. European Journal of Nutrition. 2002;**41**:68–77.

632. **Chakraborty S, Chopra M, Mani K, Giri AK, Banerjee P, Sahni NS,** et al. Prevalence of vitamin B12 deficiency in healthy Indian school-going adolescents from rural and urban localities and its relationship with various anthropometric indices: a cross-sectional study. Journal of Human Nutrition and Dietetics. 2018;**31**:12541.

633. **Mahalle N, Kulkarni MV, Garg MK, Naik SS.** Vitamin B12 deficiency and hyperhomocysteinemia as correlates of cardiovascular risk factors in Indian subjects with coronary artery disease. Journal of Cardiology. 2013;**61**(4):289–94.

634. **Khokhar S, Oyelade OJ, Marletta L, Shahar D, Ireland J, de HS.** Vitamin composition of ethnic foods commonly consumed in Europe. Food and Nutrition Research. 2012;**56**;5639.

635. **Refsum H, Yajnik CS, Gadkari M, Schneede J, Vollset SE, Orning L,** et al. Hyperhomocysteinemia and elevated methylmalonic acid indicate a high prevalence of cobalamin deficiency in Asian Indians. American Journal of Clinical Nutrition 2001;**74**(2):233–41.

636. **Homocysteine Lowering Trialists' Collaboration.** Lowering blood homocysteine with folic acid based supplements: meta-analysis of randomised trials. British Medical Journal. 1998;**316**:894–8.

637. **Panwar RB, Gupta R, Gupta BK, Raja S, Vaishnav J, Khatri M,** et al. Atherothrombotic risk factors & premature coronary heart disease in India: a case-control study. Indian Journal of Medical Research. 2011;**134**(1):26–32.

638. Iqbal MP, Ishaq M, Kazmi KA, Yousuf FA, Mehboobali N, Ali SA, et al. Role of vitamins B6, B12 and folic acid on hyperhomocysteinemia in a Pakistani population of patients with acute myocardial infarction. Nutrition Metabolism and Cardiovascular Diseases 2005;**15**(2):100–8.

639. Bond TA, Joglekar CV, Marley-Zagar E, Lubree HG, Kumaran K, Yajnik CS, et al. Maternal vitamin B12 and folate status during pregnancy and insulin resistance and body composition in the offspring at 12 years in a rural Indian birth cohort: data from the Pune Maternal Nutrition Study. Proceedings of the Nutrition Society. 2013;**72**(OCE4).

640. Deshmukh U, Katre P, Yajnik CS. Influence of maternal vitamin B12 and folate on growth and insulin resistance in the offspring. Nestle Nutrition Institute Workshop Series. 2013;**74**:145–54.

641. Krishnaveni GV, Hill JC, Veena SR, Bhat DS, Wills AK, Karat CL, et al. Low plasma vitamin B12 in pregnancy is associated with gestational 'diabesity' and later diabetes. Diabetologia. 2009;**52**(11):2350–8.

642. Miller MA, Cappuccio FP. Ethnicity and inflammatory pathways–implications for vascular disease, vascular risk and therapeutic intervention. Current Medicinal Chemistry 2007;**14**(13):1409–25.

643. Stefler D, Bhopal R, Fischbacher CM. Might infection explain the higher risk of coronary heart disease in South Asians? Systematic review comparing prevalence rates with white populations in developed countries. Public Health. 2012;**126**(5):397–409.

644. Fischbacher CM, Blackwell CC, Bhopal R, Ingram R, Unwin NC, White M. Serological evidence of *Helicobacter pylori* infection in UK South Asian and European populations: implications for gastric cancer and coronary heart disease. Journal of Infection. 2004;**48**:168–74.

645. Fischbacher CM, Bhopal R, Blackwell CC, Ingram R, Unwin NC, et al. IgG is higher in South Asians than Europeans: Does infection contribute to ethnic variation in cardiovascular disease? Arteriosclerosis, Thrombosis and Vascular Biology. 2003;**23**:703–4.

646. Mehta JL, Saldeen TG, Rand K. Interactive role of infection, inflammation and traditional risk factors in atherosclerosis and coronary artery disease. Journal of the American College of Cardiology. 1998;**31**(6):1217–25.

647. Jacobson MS. Cholesterol oxides in Indian ghee: possible cause of unexplained high risk of atherosclerosis in Indian immigrant populations. Lancet. 1987;**2**:656–8.

648. Chatha K, Anderson NR, Gama R. Ethnic variation in C-reactive protein: UK resident Indo-Asians compared with Caucasians. Journal of Cardiovascular Risk. 2002;**9**:139–41.

649. Forouhi NG, Sattar N, McKeigue PM. Relation of C-reactive protein to body fat distribution and features of the metabolic syndrome in Europeans and South Asians. International Journal of Obesity. 2001;**25**:1327–31.

650. Miller MA, Cappuccio FP. Cellular adhesion molecules and their relationship with measures of obesity and metabolic syndrome in a multiethnic population. International Journal of Obesity (London). 2006;**30**(8):1176–82.

651. Miller MA, McTernan PG, Harte AL, Silva NF, Strazzullo P, Alberti KG, et al. Ethnic and sex differences in circulating endotoxin levels: A novel marker of atherosclerotic

and cardiovascular risk in a British multi-ethnic population. Atherosclerosis 2008;**203**(2):494–502.

652. Miller MA, McTernan PG, Harte AL, Silva NF, Strazzullo P, Alberti KG, et al. Ethnic and sex differences in circulating endotoxin levels: A novel marker of atherosclerotic and cardiovascular risk in a British multi-ethnic population. Atherosclerosis. 2009;**203**(2):494–502.

653. Miller MA, Sagnella GA, Kerry SM, Strazzullo P, Cook DG, Cappuccio FP. Ethnic differences in circulating soluble adhesion molecules. The Wandsworth Heart and Stroke Study. Clinical Science 1993;**104**(6):591–8.

654. Becker E, Boreham R, Chaudhary M, Craig R, Deverill C, Doyle M, et al. Health Survey for England: Methodology and documentation. Leeds: The Information Centre; 2006.

655. Elliott P, Chambers JC, Zhang W, Clarke R, Hopewell JC, Peden JF, et al. Genetic loci associated with c-reactive protein levels and risk of coronary heart disease. JAMA. 2009;**302**(1):37–48.

656. Danesh J, Collins R, Appleby P, Peto R. Association of fibrinogen, C-reactive protein, albumin, or leukocyte count with coronary heart disease: meta-analyses of prospective studies. JAMA. 1998;**279**:1477–82.

657. Keavney B, Danesh J, Parish S, Palmer A, Clark S, Youngman L, et al. Fibrinogen and coronary heart disease: test of causality by 'Mendelian randomization'. International Journal of Epidemiology. 2006;**35**(4):935–43.

658. Kain K, Catto AJ, Young J, Bamford J, Bavington J, Grant PJ. Increased fibrinogen, von Willebrand factor and tissue plasminogen activator levels in insulin resistant South Asian patients with ischaemic stroke. Atherosclerosis. 2002;**163**(2):371–6.

659. Kain K, Catto AJ, Grant PJ. Associations between insulin resistance and thrombotic risk factors in high-risk South Asian subjects. Diabetic Medicine. 2003;**20**(8):651–5.

660. Hunt BJ, Jurd KM. Endothelial cell activation. A central pathophysiological process. British Medical Journal. 1998;**316**:1328–9.

661. Mendall MA. Inflammatory responses and coronary heart disease. The 'dirty chicken' hypothesis of cardiovascular risk factors. British Medical Journal. 1998;**316**:953–4.

662. Bergh C, Fall K, Udumyan R, Sjöqvist H, Fröbert O, Montgomery S. Severe infections and subsequent delayed cardiovascular disease. European Journal of Preventive Cardiology. 2017;**24**(18):1958–66.

663. Danesh J, Appleby P. Persistent infection and vascular disease: a systematic review. Expert Opinion on Investigational Drugs. 1998;**7**:691–713.

664. Mendis S, Arseculeratne YM, Withana N, Samitha S. *Chlamydia pneumoniae* infection and its association with coronary heart disease and cardiovascular risk factors in a sample South Asian population. International Journal of Cardiology. 2001;**79**:191–6.

665. Cook DG, Davies PD, Wise R, Honeybourne D. *Chlamydia pneumoniae* infection and ethnic origin. ethnicity and health. 1998;**3**(4):237–46.

666. Heianza Y, Ma W, Manson JE, Rexrode KM, Qi L. Gut microbiota metabolites and risk of major adverse cardiovascular disease events and death: a systematic review and meta-analysis of prospective studies. Journal of the American Heart Association. 2017;**6**(7):e004947.

667. Musso G, Gambino R, Cassader M. Obesity, diabetes, and gut microbiota: the hygiene hypothesis expanded? Diabetes Care. 2010;**33**(10):2277–84.

668. Misra A, Tandon N, Ebrahim S, Sattar N, Alam D, Shrivastava U, et al. Diabetes, cardiovascular disease, and chronic kidney disease in South Asia: current status and future directions. BMJ. 2017;**357**:j1420.

669. Burden AC, McNally PG, Feehally J, Walls J. Increased incidence of end-stage renal failure secondary to diabetes mellitus in Asian ethnic groups in the United Kingdom. Diabetic Medicine. 1992;**9**(7):641–5.

670. Roderick PJ, Jones I, Raleigh VS, McGeown M, Mallick N. Population need for renal replacement therapy in Thames regions: ethnic dimension. British Medical Journal. 1994;**309**:1111–14.

671. Roderick PJ, Jeffrey RF, Yuen HM, Godfrey KM, West J, Wright J. Smaller kidney size at birth in South Asians: findings from the Born in Bradford birth cohort study. Nephrology, Dialysis, Transplantation. 2016;**31**(3):455–65.

672. Tillin T, Forouhi N, McKeigue P, Chaturvedi N. Microalbuminuria and coronary heart disease risk in an ethnically diverse UK population: a prospective cohort study. Journal of the American Society of Nephrology. 2005;**16**(12):3702–10.

673. Agyemang C, van V, I, van den Born BJ, Stronks K. Prevalence of microalbuminuria and its association with pulse pressure in a multi-ethnic population in Amsterdam, The Netherlands. The SUNSET Study. Kidney & Blood Pressure Research. 2008;**31**(1):38–46.

674. Fischbacher C, Bhopal R, Ruttert MK, Unwin N, Marshall SM, White M, et al. Microalbuminuria is more frequent in South Asian than in European origin populations: a comparative study in Newcastle, UK. Diabetic Medicine. 2003;**20**(1):31–6.

675. McKeigue PM, Adelstein AM, Shipley MJ, Riemersma RA, Marmot MG, Hunt SP, et al. Diet and risk factors for coronary heart disease in Asians in northwest London. Lancet. 1985;**326**(8464):1086–90.

676. Fowler PBS. Diet and risk factors for coronary heart disease in Asians in North West London. Lancet. 1985;**2**(8464):1363–4.

677. Rodondi N, den Elzen WP, Bauer DC, Cappola AR, Razvi S, Walsh JP, et al. Subclinical hypothyroidism and the risk of coronary heart disease and mortality. JAMA. 2010;**304**(12):1365–74.

678. Matthews SB, Waud JP, Roberts AG, Campbell AK. Systemic lactose intolerance: a new perspective on an old problem. Postgrad Medical Journal. 2005;**81**:167–73.

679. Gaskin DJ, Ilich JZ. Lactose maldigestion revisited: diagnosis, prevalence in ethnic minorities, and dietary recommendations to overcome it. American Journal of Lifestyle Medicine. 2009;**3**(3):212–18.

680. Holmboe-Ottesen G, Wandel M. Changes in dietary habits after migration and consequences for health: a focus on South Asians in Europe. Food & Nutrion Research. 2012;**56**.

681. Oliver MF. Serum cholesterol-the knave of hearts and the joker. Lancet. 1981;**318**(8255):1090–5.

682. Iqbal TH, Wood GM, Lewis KO, Leek JP, Cooper BT. Prevalence of primary lactase deficiency in adult residents of west Birmingham. BMJ. 1993;**306**(6888):1303.

683. Tandon RK, Joshi YK, Singh DS, Narendranathan M, Balakrishnan V, Lal K. Lactose intolerance in North and South Indians. American Journal of Clinical Nutrition. 1981;**34**:943–6.

684. **Segall JJ.** Cardiovascular disease in South Asians. Lancet. 2000;356(9244):1853.

685. **Gilbert PA, Khokhar S.** Changing dietary habits of ethnic groups in Europe and implications for health. Nutrition Reviews. 2008;66(4):203–15.

686. **Park CM, March K, Ghosh AK, Jones S, Coady E, Tuson C,** et al. Left-ventricular structure in the Southall And Brent REvisited (SABRE) study: Explaining ethnic differences. Hypertension. 2013;61(5):1014–20.

687. **Zindrou D, Taylor KM, Bagger JP.** Coronary artery size and disease in UK South Asian and Caucasian men. European Journal of Cardio-Thoracic Surgery 2006;29(4):492–5.

688. **Hasan RK, Ginwala NT, Shah RY, Kumbhani DJ, Wilensky RL, Mehta NN.** Quantitative angiography in South Asians reveals differences in vessel size and coronary artery disease severity compared to Caucasians. American Journal of Cardiovascular Disease 2011;1(1):31–7.

689. **Lip GY, Rathore VS, Katira R, Watson RD, Singh SP.** Do Indo-Asians have smaller coronary arteries? Postgrad Medical Journal. 1999;75(886):463–6.

690. **Tillin T, Dhutia H, Chambers J, Malik I, Coady E, Mayet J,** et al. South Asian men have different patterns of coronary artery disease when compared with European men. Int J Cardiol. 2008;129(3):406–13.

691. **Bennett PC, Gill PS, Silverman S, Blann AD, Lip GYH.** Ethnic differences in common carotid intima–media thickness, and the relationship to cardiovascular risk factors and peripheral arterial disease: the Ethnic-Echocardiographic Heart of England Screening Study. QJM. 2011;104(3):245–54.

692. **Chahal NS, Lim TK, Jain P, Chambers JC, Kooner JS, Senior R.** Does subclinical atherosclerosis burden identify the increased risk of cardiovascular disease mortality among United Kingdom Indian Asians? A population study. American Heart Journal. 2011;162(3):460–6.

693. **Anand SS, Yusuf S, Vuksan V, Devanesen S, Teo KK, Montague PA,** et al. Differences in risk factors, atherosclerosis, and cardiovascular disease between ethnic groups in Canada: the Study of Health Assessment and Risk in Ethnic Groups (SHARE). Lancet. 2000;356:279–84.

694. **Anand SS, Yusuf S, Jacobs R, Davis AD, Yi Q, Gerstein H.** Risk factors, atherosclerosis, and cardiovascular disease among Aboriginal people in Canada: the study of health assessment and risk evaluation in Aboriginal people (SHARE-AP). Lancet. 2001;358:1147–52.

695. **Feder G, Crook AM, Magee P, Banerjee S, Timmis AD, Hemingway H.** Ethnic differences in invasive management of coronary disease: prospective cohort study of patients undergoing angiography. BMJ. 2002;324(7336):511–16.

696. **Weir-McCall JR, Cassidy DB, Belch JJF, Gandy SJ, Houston JG, Lambert MA,** et al. Whole-body cardiovascular MRI for the comparison of atherosclerotic burden and cardiac remodelling in healthy South Asian and European adults. British Journal of Radiology. 2016;89(1065):20160342.

697. **Chaturvedi N, Coady E, Mayet J, Wright AR, Shore AC, Byrd S,** et al. Indian Asian men have less peripheral arterial disease than European men for equivalent levels of coronary disease. Atherosclerosis. 2007;193(1):204–12.

698. **Koulaouzidis G, Jenkins PJ, McArthur T.** Comparison of coronary calcification among South Asians and Caucasians in the UK. International Journal of Cardiology. 2013;168(2):1647–8.

699. **Villadsen PR, Petersen SE, Dey D, Patel S, Naderi H, Davies LC**, et al. Impact of South Asian ethnicity on total plaque volume, calcified plaque volume and non-calcified plaque volume in the coronary arteries: a coronary CT angiography study in East London (UK). European Heart Journal 2013;**34**(supp 1):4683-P.

700. **Snijder MB, Stronks K, Agyemang C, Busschers WB, Peters RJ, van den Born BJ.** Ethnic differences in arterial stiffness the Helius study. International Journal of Cardiology. 2015;**191**:28–33.

701. **Webb DR, Khunti K, Lacy P, Gray LJ, Mostafa S, Talbot D**, et al. Conduit vessel stiffness in British South Asians of Indian descent relates to 25-hydroxyvitamin D status. Jouranl of Hypertension. 2012;**30**(8):1588–96.

702. **Kasliwal RR, Mahansaria K, Bansal M.** Central aortic blood pressure and pulse wave velocity as additional markers in patients with hypertension. Hypertension Journal. 2015;**1**(2):73–82.

703. **Eeftinck Schattenkerk DW, van Gorp J, Snijder MB, Zwinderman AH, Agyemang CO, Peters RJ**, et al. Ethnic differences in arterial wave reflection are mostly explained by differences in body height–cross-sectional analysis of the HELIUS Study. PLoS One. 2016;**11**(7):e0160243.

704. **Fischbacher C, Bhopal R, Patel S, White M, Unwin N, Alberti KG.** Anaemia in Chinese, South Asian, and European populations in Newcastle upon Tyne: cross-sectional study. BMJ. 2001;**322**:958–9.

705. **Naotunna NP, Dayarathna M, Maheshi H, Amarasinghe GS, Kithmini VS, Rathnayaka M**, et al. Nutritional status among primary school children in rural Sri Lanka; a public health challenge for a country with high child health standards. BMC Public Health. 2017;**17**(1):57.

706. **Adaikalakoteswari A, Balasubramanyam M, Mohan V.** Telomere shortening occurs in Asian Indian Type 2 diabetic patients. Diabetic Medicine. 2005;**22**(9):1151–6.

707. **Fossel M.** Telomerase and the Aging Cell. Implications for human health. Journal of the American Medical Association. 1998;**279**:1732–5.

708. **St-Onge MP, Grandner MA, Brown D, Conroy MB, Jean-Louis G, Coons M**, et al. Sleep duration and quality: impact on lifestyle behaviors and cardiometabolic health: a scientific statement From the American Heart Association. Circulation. 2016;**134**(18):e367–e86.

709. **Kohinor MJ, Stronks K, Nicolaou M, Haafkens JA.** Considerations affecting dietary behaviour of immigrants with type 2 diabetes: a qualitative study among Surinamese in the Netherlands. Ethnicity & Health. 2011;**16**(3):245–58.

710. **Martin RM, Gunnell D, Smith GD.** Breastfeeding in infancy and blood pressure in later life: systematic review and meta-analysis. American Jounral of Epidemiology. 2005;**161**(1):15–26.

711. **Leeson CP, Kattenhorn M, Deanfield JE, Lucas A.** Duration of breast feeding and arterial distensibility in early adult life: population based study. BMJ. 2001;**322**(7287):643–7.

712. **Reynolds RM, Fischbacher C, Bhopal R, Byrne CD, White M, Unwin N**, et al. Differences in cortisol concentrations in South Asian and European men living in the United Kingdom. Clinical Endocrinology. 2006;**64**(5):530–4.

713. **Ward AMV, Fall CHD, Stein CE, Kumaran K, Veena SR, Wood PJ**, et al. Cortisol and the metabolic syndrome in South Asians. Clinical Endocrinology. 2003;**58**:500–5.

714. Krishna M, Kalyanaraman K, Veena SR, Krishanveni GV, Karat SC, Cox V, et al. Cohort profile: The 1934–66 Mysore Birth Records Cohort in South India. International Journal of Epidemiology. 2015;**44**(6):1833–41.

715. Naimi TS, Brown DW, Brewer RD, Giles WH, Mensah G, Serdula MK, et al. Cardiovascular risk factors and confounders among non-drinking and moderate-drinking US adults. American Journal of Preventive Medicine. 2005;**28**(4):369–73.

716. Cochrane R, Sukhwant B. The drinking habits of Sikh, Hindu, Muslim and White men in the West Midlands: a community survey. British Journal of Addiction. 1990;**85**:759–69.

717. Kiechl S, Willeit J. Complex association between alcohol consumption and myocardial infarction: always good for a new paradox. Circulation. 2014;**130**(5):383–6.

718. Rudan I, Smolej-Narancic N, Campbell H, Carothers A, Wright A, Janicijevic B, et al. Inbreeding and the genetic complexity of human hypertension. Genetics. 2003;**163**(3):1011–21.

719. Bittles AH, Black ML. Consanguinity, human evolution, and complex diseases. Proceedings of the National Academy of Sciences. 2010;**107**(suppl 1):1779–86.

720. Bittles AH. Consanguinity in Context. New York: Cambridge University Press; 2012.

721. Bhopal RS, Petherick ES, Wright J, Small N. Potential social, economic and general health benefits of consanguineous marriage: results from the Born in Bradford cohort study. European Journal of Public Health. 2014;**24**(5):862–9.

722. Campbell H, Rudan I, Bittles AH, Wright AF. Human population structure, genome autozygosity and human health. Genome Medicine. 2009;**1**(9):91.

723. Campbell H, Carothers AD, Rudan I, Hayward C, Biloglav Z, Barac L, et al. Effects of genome-wide heterozygosity on a range of biomedically relevant human quantitative traits. Human Molecular Genetics 2007;**16**(2):233–41.

724. Ismail J, Jafar TH, Jafary FH, White F, Faruqui AM, Chaturvedi N. Risk factors for non-fatal myocardial infarction in young South Asian adults. Heart. 2004;**90**(3):259–63.

725. GBD 2016 Causes of Death Collaborators. Global, regional, and national age-sex specific mortality for 264 causes of death, 1980–2016: a systematic analysis for the Global Burden of Disease Study 2016. Lancet. 2017;**390**(10100):1151–210.

726. Lozano R, Naghavi M, Foreman K, Lim S, Shibuya K, Aboyans V, et al. Global and regional mortality from 235 causes of death for 20 age groups in 1990 and 2010: a systematic analysis for the Global Burden of Disease Study 2010. Lancet. 2012;**380**(9859):2095–128.

727. Shrivastava U, Misra A, Gupta R, Viswanathan V. Socioeconomic factors relating to diabetes and its management in India. Journal of Diabetes. 2016;**8**(1):12–23.

728. Battu HS, Bhopal R, Agyemang C. Heterogeneity in blood pressure in UK Bangladeshi, Indian and Pakistani, compared to White, populations: divergence of adults and children. Journal of Human Hypertension. 2018 Sep 4. doi: 10.1038/s41371-018-0095-5. [Epub ahead of print]

729. Anjana RM, Pradeepa R, Deepa M, Datta M, Sudha V, Unnikrishnan R, et al. Prevalence of diabetes and prediabetes (impaired fasting glucose and/or impaired glucose tolerance) in urban and rural India: phase I results of the Indian Council of Medical Research-INdia DIABetes (ICMR-INDIAB) study. Diabetologia. 2011;**54**(12):3022–7.

730. **Zargar AH, Khan AK, Masoodi SR, Laway BA, Wani AI, Bashir MI**, et al. Prevalence of Type 2 diabetes mellitus and impaired glucose tolerance in the Kashmir Valley of the Indian subcontinent. Diabetes Research and Clinical Practice. 2000;**47**(2):135–46..

731. **Reichenbach DD.** Autopsy incidence of diseases among Southwestern American Indians. Archives of Pathology. 1967;**84**(1):81–6.

732. **Padmavati S, Sandhu I.** Incidence of coronary artery disease in Delhi from medicolegal autopies. Indian Journal of Medical Research. 1969;**57**:465–76.

733. **Reddy CR, Jagabandhu N.** Thromboembolic complications seen at autopsy in South India. Archives of Pathology. 1967;**83**(4):399–402.

734. **Koska J, Saremi A, Howell S, Bahn G, De Courten B, Ginsberg H**, et al. Advanced glycation end products, oxidation products, and incident cardiovascular events in patients with type 2 diabetes. Diabetes Care. 2018;**41**(3):570–6.

735. **Saremi A, Howell S, Schwenke DC, Bahn G, Beisswenger PJ, Reaven PD.** Advanced glycation end products, oxidation products, and the extent of atherosclerosis during the va diabetes trial and follow-up study. Diabetes Care. 2017;**40**(4):591–8.

736. **Ahn CH, Min SH, Lee DW, Oh TJ, Kim KM, Moon JH**, et al. Hemoglobin glycation index is associated with cardiovascular diseases in people with impaired glucose metabolism. Journal of Clinical Endocrinology & Metabolism. 2017;**102**(8):2905–13.

737. **Aarabi M, Jackson PR.** Coronary risk in South Asians: role of ethnicity and blood sugar. European Journal of Cardiovascular Prevention and Rehabilitation 2004;**11**(5):389–93.

738. **Saulnier PJ, Wheelock KM, Howell S, Weil EJ, Tanamas SK, Knowler WC**, et al. Advanced glycation end products predict loss of renal function and correlate with lesions of diabetic kidney disease in American Indians with type 2 diabetes. Diabetes. 2016;**65**(12):3744–53.

739. **Vlassara H, Striker LJ, Teichberg S, Fuh H, Li YM, Steffes M.** Advanced glycation end products induce glomerular sclerosis and albuminuria in normal rats. Proceedings of the National Academy of Sciences 1994;**91**(24):11704–8.

740. **Yates T, Haffner SM, Schulte PJ, Thomas L, Huffman KM, Bales CW**, et al. Association between change in daily ambulatory activity and cardiovascular events in people with impaired glucose tolerance (NAVIGATOR trial): a cohort analysis. Lancet. 2014;**383**(9922):1059–66.

741. **Priya MM, Amutha A, Pramodkumar TA, Ranjani H, Jebarani S, Gokulakrishnan K**, et al. Beta-cell function and insulin sensitivity in normal glucose-tolerant subjects stratified by 1-hour plasma glucose values. Diabetes Technology & Therapeutics. 2016;**18**(1):29–33.

742. **Hulman A, Simmons RK, Brunner EJ, Witte DR, Færch K, Vistisen D**, et al. Trajectories of glycaemia, insulin sensitivity and insulin secretion in South Asian and white individuals before diagnosis of type 2 diabetes: a longitudinal analysis from the Whitehall II cohort study. Diabetologia. 2017;**60**(7):1252–60.

743. **Chowdhury R, Narayan KM, Zabetian A, Raj S, Tabassum R.** Genetic studies of type 2 diabetes in South asians: a systematic overview. Current Diabetes Reviews 2014;**10**(4):258–74.

744. **Narayan KMV.** Type 2 diabetes: Why we are winning the battle but losing the war? 2015 Kelly West Award Lecture. Diabetes Care. 2016;**39**(5):653–63.

745. **Misra A, Anoop S, Gulati S, Mani K, Bhatt SP, Pandey RM.** Body fat patterning, hepatic fat and pancreatic volume of non-obese Asian Indians with type 2 diabetes in North India: A case-control study. PLoS One. 2015;**10**(10):e0140447.

746. **Fridlyand LE, Philipson LH.** Cold climate genes and the prevalence of type 2 diabetes mellitus. Medical Hypotheses. 2006;**67**(5):1034–41.

747. **Bhopal R.** Causes in epidemiology: the jewels in the public health crown. Journal of Public Health. 2008;**30**(3):224–5.

748. **Segal UA, Elliott D, Mayadas NS.** Immigration Worldwide Policies, Practices, and Trends. Oxford: Oxford University Press; 2010.

749. **Biswas T, Pervin S, Tanim MIA, Niessen L, Islam A.** Bangladesh policy on prevention and control of non-communicable diseases: a policy analysis. BMC Public Health. 2017;**17**(1):582.

750. **Vaidya A.** Tackling cardiovascular health and disease in Nepal: epidemiology, strategies and implementation. Heart Asia. 2011;**3**(1):87–91.

751. **Zhong Y, Rosengren A, Fu M, Welin L, Welin C, Caidahl K,** et al. Secular changes in cardiovascular risk factors in Swedish 50-year-old men over a 50-year period: The study of men born in 1913, 1923, 1933, 1943, 1953 and 1963. European Journal of Preventive Cardiology. 2017;**24**(6):612–20.

752. **Yang Q, Cogswell M, Flanders WD, Hong Y, Zhang Z, Loustalot F,** et al. Trends in Cardiovascular Health Metrics and Associations With All-Cause and CVD Mortality Among US Adults. JAMA. 2012;**307**(12):1273–83.

753. **Hardoon SL, Whincup PH, Lennon LT, Wannamethee SG, Capewell S, Morris RW.** How much of the recent decline in the incidence of myocardial infarction in British men can be explained by changes in cardiovascular risk factors? Evidence from a prospective population-based study. Circulation. 2008;**117**(5):598–604.

754. **Bhatnagar P, Wickramasinghe K, Williams J, Rayner M, Townsend N.** The epidemiology of cardiovascular disease in the UK 2014. Heart. 2015;**101**(15):1182–9.

755. **Saaristo T, Moilanen L, Korpi-Hyovalti E, Vanhala M, Saltevo J, Niskanen L,** et al. Lifestyle intervention for prevention of type 2 diabetes in primary health care: one-year follow-up of the Finnish National Diabetes Prevention Program (FIN-D2D). Diabetes Care. 2010;**33**(10):2146–51.

756. **Davies MJ, Tringham JR, Troughton J, Khunti KK.** Prevention of type 2 diabetes mellitus. A review of the evidence and its application in a UK setting. Diabetic Medicine. 2004;**21**(5):403–14.

757. **Cardona-Morrell M, Rychetnik L, Morrell S, Espinel P, Bauman A.** Reduction of diabetes risk in routine clinical practice: are physical activity and nutrition interventions feasible and are the outcomes from reference trials replicable? A systematic review and meta-analysis. BMC Public Health. 2010;**10**(1):653.

758. **Weber MB, Ranjani H, Staimez LR, Anjana RM, Ali MK, Narayan KM,** et al. The stepwise approach to diabetes prevention: Results From the D-CLIP randomized controlled trial. Diabetes Care. 2016;**39**(10):dc161241.

759. **Ambady R, Snehalatha C, Samith Shetty A, Nanditha A.** Primary prevention of Type 2 diabetes in South Asians–challenges and the way forward. Diabetic Medicine. 2013;**30**(1):26–34.

760. **Brown T, Smith S, Bhopal R, Kasim A, Summerbell C.** Diet and Physical activity interventions to prevent or treat obesity in South Asian children and adults: A

systematic review and meta-analysis. International Journal of Environmental Research and Public Health. 2015;**12**(1):566–94.

761. **Bhopal RS, Douglas A, Wallia S, Forbes JF, Lean M, Gill JMR,** et al. Weight change over three-years in South Asians at high risk of diabetes: effects and cost in a cluster-randomised trial of a lifestyle intervention. Lancet Diabetes & Endocrinology. 2013;**2**(3):218–27.

762. **Ramachandran A, Snehalatha C, Ram J, Selvam S, Simon M, Nanditha A,** et al. Effectiveness of mobile phone messaging in prevention of type 2 diabetes by lifestyle modification in men in India: a prospective, parallel-group, randomised controlled trial. Lancet Diabetes & Endocrinology. 2013;**1**(3):191–8.

763. **Ramachandran A, Snehalatha C, Mary S, Mukesh B, Bhaskar AD, Vijay V.** The Indian Diabetes Prevention Programme shows that lifestyle modification and metformin prevent type 2 diabetes in Asian Indian subjects with impaired glucose tolerance (IDPP-1). Diabetologia. 2006;**49**(2):289–97.

764. **Bhopal RS, Douglas A, Wallia S, Forbes JF, Lean MEJ, Gill JMR,** et al. Effect of a lifestyle intervention on weight change in south Asian individuals in the UK at high risk of type 2 diabetes: a family-cluster randomised controlled trial. Lancet Diabetes & Endocrinology. 2014;**2**(3):218–27.

765. **Knowler WC, Barrett-Connor E, Fowler SE, Hamman RF, Lachin JM, Walker EA,** et al. Reduction in the incidence of type 2 diabetes with lifestyle intervention or metformin. New England Journal of Medicine. 2002;**346**(6):393–403.

766. **Tuomilehto J, Lindstrom J, Eriksson JG, Valle TT, Hamalainen H, Ilanne-Parikka P,** et al. Prevention of type 2 diabetes mellitus by changes in lifestyle among subjects with impaired glucose tolerance. New England Journal of Medicine. 2001;**344**(18):1343–50.

767. **Zaman MJ, Philipson P, Chen R, Farag A, Shipley M, Marmot MG,** et al. South Asians and coronary disease: is there discordance between effects on incidence and prognosis? Heart. 2013;**99**(10):729–36.

768. **Zaman MJ, Bhopal RS.** New answers to three questions on the epidemic of coronary mortality in south Asians: Incidence or case fatality? Biology or environment? Will the next generation be affected? Heart. 2013;**99**:154–8.

769. **Liew R, Sulfi S, Ranjadayalan K, Cooper J, Timmis AD.** Declining case fatality rates for acute myocardial infarction in South Asian and white patients in the past 15 years. Heart. 2006;**92**(8):1030–4.

770. **Gupta M, Doobay AV, Singh N, Anand SS, Raja F, Mawji F,** et al. Risk factors, hospital management and outcomes after acute myocardial infarction in South Asian Canadians and matched control subjects. CMAJ. 2002;**166**:717–22.

771. **de Carvalho LP, Gao F, Chen Q, Hartman M, Sim LL, Koh TH,** et al. Differences in late cardiovascular mortality following acute myocardial infarction in three major Asian ethnic groups. European Heart Journal: Acute Cardiovascular Care. 2014;**3**(4):354–62.

772. **Prabhakaran D, Yusuf S, Mehta S, Pogue J, Avezum A, Budaj A,** et al. Two-year outcomes in patients admitted with non-ST elevation acute coronary syndrome: results of the OASIS registry 1 and 2. Indian Heart J. 2005;**57**(3):217–25.

773. **Gholap NN, Mehta RL, Khunti K, Davies MJ, Squire IB.** Survival following acute myocardial infarction in patients of South Asian and White European ethnicity in the UK. Heart. 2011;**97**(Suppl 1):A6–A.

774. Bhurji N, Javer J, Gasevic D, Khan NA. Improving management of type 2 diabetes in South Asian patients: a systematic review of intervention studies. BMJ Open. 2016;**6**(4):e008986.

775. Soljak MA, Majeed A, Eliahoo J, Dornhorst A. Ethnic inequalities in the treatment and outcome of diabetes in three English Primary Care Trusts. International Journal for Equity in Health 2007;**6**(1):8.

776. McElduff P, Edwards R, Burns JA, Young RJ, Heller R, Long B, et al. Comparison of processes and intermediate outcomes between South Asian and European patients with diabetes in Blackburn, north-west England. Diabetic Medicine. 2005;**22**(9):1226–33.

777. Wright AK, Kontopantelis E, Emsley R, Buchan I, Sattar N, Rutter MK, et al. Life expectancy and cause-specific mortality in type 2 diabetes: A population-based cohort study quantifying relationships in ethnic subgroups. Diabetes Care. 2017;**40**(3):338–45.

778. Ahmad N, Thomas GN, Chan C, Gill P. Ethnic differences in lower limb revascularisation and amputation rates. Implications for the aetiopathology of atherosclerosis? Atherosclerosis. 2014;**233**(2):503–7.

779. Chaturvedi N, Abbott CA, Whalley A, Widdows P, Leggetter SY, Boulton AJM. Risk of diabetes-related amputation in South Asians vs. Europeans in the UK. Diabetic Medicine. 2002;**19**(2):99–104.

780. Eastwood SV, Tillin T, Sattar N, Forouhi NG, Hughes AD, Chaturvedi N. Associations between prediabetes, by three different diagnostic criteria, and incident CVD differ in South Asians and Europeans. Diabetes Care. 2015;**38**(12):2325–32.

781. Gupta R, Misra A. Epidemiology of microvascular complications of diabetes in South Asians and comparison with other ethnicities. Journal of diabetes. 2016;**8**(4).

782. Misra A, Chowbey P, Makkar BM, Vikram NK, Wasir JS, Chadha D, et al. Consensus statement for diagnosis of obesity, abdominal obesity and the metabolic syndrome for Asian Indians and recommendations for physical activity, medical and surgical management. Journal of the Association of Physicians India. 2009;**57**:163–70.

783. Nishtar S. Prevention of coronary heart disease in south Asia. Lancet. 2002;**360**(9338):1015–18.

784. De Backer G, Ambrosioni E, Borch-Johnsen K, Brotons C, Cifkova R, Dallongeville J, et al. European guidelines on cardiovascular disease prevention in clinical practice: Third Joint Taskforce of European and other Societies on Cardiovascular Disease Prevention in Clinical Practice. European Heart Journal. 2003;**24**:1601–10.

785. JSB3. Joint British Societies' consensus recommendations for the prevention of cardiovascular disease (JBS3). Heart. 2014;**100**(ii):ii1–ii67.

786. Goff DC, Jr., Lloyd-Jones DM, Bennett G, Coady S, D'Agostino RB, Gibbons R, et al. 2013 ACC/AHA guideline on the assessment of cardiovascular risk: a report of the American College of Cardiology/American Heart Association Task Force on Practice Guidelines. Circulation. 2014;**129**(25 Suppl 2):S49–S73.

787. Martin CA, Gowda U, Smith BJ, Renzaho AMN. Systematic review of the effect of lifestyle interventions on the components of the metabolic syndrome in South Asian Migrants. J Immigr Minor Health. 2018;**20**(1):231–44.

788. Emadian A, Thompson J. A mixed-methods examination of physical activity and sedentary time in overweight and obese South Asian men living in the United Kingdom. International Journal of Environmental Research Public Health. 2017;**14**(4).

789. Kandula NR, Dave S, De Chavez PJ, Bharucha H, Patel Y, Seguil P, et al. Translating a heart disease lifestyle intervention into the community: the South Asian Heart Lifestyle Intervention (SAHELI) study; a randomized control trial. BMC Public Health 2015;**15**(1):1064.

790. Weber MB, Oza-Frank R, Staimez LR, Ali MK, Narayan KM. Type 2 diabetes in Asians: prevalence, risk factors, and effectiveness of behavioral intervention at individual and population levels. Annual Review of Nutrition. 2012;**32**:417–39.

791. Damen JA, Hooft L, Schuit E, Debray TP, Collins GS, Tzoulaki I, et al. Prediction models for cardiovascular disease risk in the general population: systematic review. BMJ. 2016;**353**:i2416.

792. Pylypchuk R, Wells S, Kerr A, Poppe K, Riddell T, Harwood M, et al. Cardiovascular disease risk prediction equations in 400000 primary care patients in New Zealand: a derivation and validation study. Lancet. 2018;**391**(10133):1897–907.

793. Ramachandran A, Snehalatha C, Samith Shetty A, Nanditha A. Predictive value of HbA1c for incident diabetes among subjects with impaired glucose tolerance–analysis of the Indian Diabetes Prevention Programmes. Diabetic Medicine. 2012;**29**(1):94–8.

794. Abdullah N, Abdul Murad NA, Mohd Haniff EA, Syafruddin SE, Attia J, Oldmeadow C, et al. Predicting type 2 diabetes using genetic and environmental risk factors in a multi-ethnic Malaysian cohort. Public Health. 2017;**149**:31–8.

795. Hippisley-Cox J, Coupland C, Robson J, Sheikh A, Brindle P. Predicting risk of type 2 diabetes in England and Wales: prospective derivation and validation of QDScore. BMJ. 2009;**338**:b880.

796. **Department of Health and Social Care.** National Service Framework for Coronary Heart Disease. Modern standards and service models London, Department of Health 2000.

797. Chou R, Dana T, Blazina I, Daeges M, Jeanne TL. Statins for prevention of cardiovascular disease in adults: Evidence report and systematic review for the US Preventive Services Task Force. JAMA. 2016;**316**(19):2008–24.

798. Tillin T, Hughes AD, Whincup P, Mayet J, Sattar N, McKeigue PM, et al. Ethnicity and prediction of cardiovascular disease: performance of QRISK2 and Framingham scores in a UK tri-ethnic prospective cohort study (SABRE–Southall And Brent REvisited). Heart. 2014;**100**(1):60–7.

799. Kandula NR, Kanaya AM, Liu K, Lee JY, Herrington D, Hulley SB, et al. Association of 10–year and lifetime predicted cardiovascular disease risk with subclinical atherosclerosis in South Asians: Findings From the Mediators of Atherosclerosis in South Asians Living in America (MASALA) Study. Journal of the American Heart Association. 2014;**3**(5): e001117.

800. Selvarajah S, Kaur G, Haniff J, Cheong KC, Hiong TG, van der Graaf Y, et al. Comparison of the Framingham Risk Score, SCORE and WHO/ISH cardiovascular risk prediction models in an Asian population. International Journal of Cardiology. 2014;**176**(1):211–18.

801. Kanjilal S, Rao VS, Mukherjee M, Natesha BK, Renuka KS, Sibi K, et al. Application of cardiovascular disease risk prediction models and the relevance of novel biomarkers to risk stratification in Asian Indians. Vascular Health and Risk Management 2008;**4**(1):199–211.

802. Bhopal R, Fischbacher C, Vartiainen E, Unwin N, White M, Alberti G. Predicted and observed cardiovascular disease in South Asians: application of FINRISK,

Framingham and SCORE models to Newcastle Heart Project data. Journal of Public Health (Oxford). 2005;27(1):93–100.

803. **Allan GM, Nouri F, Korownyk C, Kolber MR, Vandermeer B, McCormack J.** Agreement among cardiovascular disease risk calculators. Circulation. 2013;127(19):1948–56.

804. **Bhopal RS.** Statins: numbers needed to treat and personal decision making. BMJ. 2014;349:g4980.

805. **Keyes KM, Davey SG, Koenen KC, Galea S.** The mathematical limits of genetic prediction for complex chronic disease. Journal of Epidemiology & Community Health. 2015;69:574–9.

806. **Hippisley-Cox J, Coupland C, Brindle P.** Development and validation of QRISK3 risk prediction algorithms to estimate future risk of cardiovascular disease: prospective cohort study. BMJ. 2017;357:j2099.

807. **Gopal DP, Usher-Smith JA.** Cardiovascular risk models for South Asian populations: a systematic review. International Journal of Public Health. 2016;61(5):525–34.

808. **Bhopal RS.** Cardiovascular risk prediction and ethnicity: QRISK2 strengthens creaky foundations. Brit Med J [Internet]. 2008;336:[1475 p.].

809. **Hippisley-Cox J, Coupland C, Vinogradova Y, Robson J, Minhas R, Sheikh A**, et al. Predicting cardiovascular risk in England and Wales: prospective derivation and validation of QRISK2. BMJ. 2008;336(7659):1475–82.

810. **Yusuf S.** Why do people not take life-saving medications? The case of statins. Lancet. 2016;388(10048):943–5.

811. **Chapman J, Qureshi N, Kai J.** Effectiveness of physical activity and dietary interventions in South Asian populations: a systematic review. British Journal of General Practice. 2013;63(607):104–14.

812. **Leon B, Miller BV, III, Zalos G, Courville AB, Sumner AE, Powell-Wiley TM**, et al. Weight loss programs may have beneficial or adverse effects on fat mass and insulin sensitivity in overweight and obese Black women. Journal of Racial and Ethnic Health Disparities. 2014;1(3):140–7.

813. **Nicolaou M.** Diet and Overweight Perception–An explorative study among Turkish, Moroccan and Surinamese migrants living in the Netherlands. PhD Thesis. VU University Amsterdam; 2009.

814. **Pallan MJ, Hiam LC, Duda JL, Adab P.** Body image, body dissatisfaction and weight status in South Asian children: a cross-sectional study. BMC Public Health. 2011;11(1):21.

815. **Sommer C, Jenum AK, Waage CW, Morkrid K, Sletner L, Birkeland KI.** Ethnic differences in BMI, subcutaneous fat and serum leptin levels during and after pregnancy and risk of gestational diabetes. European Journal of Endocrinology. 2015;172(6).

816. **Bhopal R.** The inter-relationship of folk traditional and western medicine within an asian community in britain. Social Science & Medicine. 1986;22:99–105.

817. **Bhopal RS.** Bhye bhaddi: a food and health concept of Punjabi Asians. Social Science & Medicine. 1986;23:687–8.

818. **Misra A, Gulati S, Luthra A.** Ayurveda for diabetes in India; Authors' reply. Lancet Diabetes & Endocrinology. 2016;4(11):884–5.

819. **Healy MAM.** The Asian Community;Medicines and Traditions. Lancashire: Silver Link Publishing; 1990.

820. De Backer G. Epidemiology and prevention of cardiovascular disease: Quo vadis? European Journal of Preventive Cardiology. 2017;24(7):768–72.

821. Dowse GK, Gareeboo H, Alberti KG, Zimmet P, Tuomilehto J, Purran A, et al. Changes in population cholesterol concentrations and other cardiovascular risk factor levels after five years of the non-communicable disease intervention programme in Mauritius. Mauritius Non-communicable Disease Study Group. BMJ. 1995;311(7015):1255–9.

822. Zatonski WA, McMichael AJ, Powles JW. Ecological study of reasons for sharp decline in mortality from ischaemic heart disease in Poland since 1991. British Medical Journal. 1998;316:1047–51.

823. Subramanian SV, Corsi DJ, Subramanyam MA, Davey Smith G. Jumping the gun: the problematic discourse on socioeconomic status and cardiovascular health in India. International Journal of Epidemiology. 2013;42(5):1410–26.

824. Tunstall Pedoe H, Clayton D, Morris JN, Bridge W, McDonald L. Coronary heart-attack in East London. Lancet. 1975;ii:833–8.

825. Miller GJ, Beckles GL, Alexis SD, Byam NT, Price SG. Serum lipoproteins and susceptibility of men of Indian descent to coronary heart disease. The St James Survey, Trinidad. Lancet. 1982;2(8291):200–3.

826. Tuomilheto J, Zimmet P, Kankaapaa J, Wolf E, Hunt D, King H, et al. Prevalence of ishaemic ECG abnormalities according to the diabetes status in the population of Fiji and their assiciations with other risk factors. Diabetes Research & Clinical Practice. 1988;5(3):205–17.

827. Padmavati S, Gupta S, Pantulu GVA. Dietary fat, serum cholesterol levels and incidence of atherosclerosis in Delhi. Circulation. 1959;19:849–53.

828. Padmavati S. A five year survey of heart disease in Delhi. Indian Heart Journal. 1958;10:33.

829. Wig KL, Malhotra RP, Chitkara NL, Gupta SP. Prevalence of coronary atherosclerosis in Northern India. BMJ. 1962:510–13.

830. Malhotra RP, Pathania NS. Some aetiological aspects of coronary heart disease. BMJ. 1958:528–31.

831. Mathur KS, Sapru RP. Aetiology and incidence of heart disease: Changing pattern over the fifteen year period 1947 to 1961. Journal of the Association of Physicians of India. 1963;11:651.

832. Mathur KS, Patney NL, Kumar V. Prevalence of CHD in general population of Agra. Indian Journal Medical Research. 1961;69:605.

833. Malhotra SL. Geographical aspects of acute myocardial infarction in India with special reference to patterns of diet and eating. British Heart Journal. 1967;29(3):337–44.

834. Malhotra SL. Epidemiology of ischaemic heart disease in India with special reference to causation. British Heart Journal. 1967;29(6):895–905.

835. Gupta A, Gupta R, Sarna M, Rastogi S, Gupta VP, Kothari K, et al. Prevalence of diabetes, impaired fasting glucose and insulin resistance syndrome in an urban Indian population. Diabetes Research & Clinical Practice. 2003;61(1):69–76.

836. Gupta R, Kaul V, Bhagat N, Agrawal M, Gupta VP, Misra A, et al. Trends in prevalence of coronary risk factors in an urban Indian population: Jaipur Heart Watch-4. Indian Heart Journal 2007;59(4):346–53.

837. **Gupta R, Sharma KK, Gupta BK, Gupta A, Saboo B, Maheshwari A,** et al. Geographic epidemiology of cardiometabolic risk factors in middle class urban residents in India: cross-sectional study. Journal of Global Health. 2015;5(1):010411.

838. **Malhotra SL.** Serum lipids, dietary factors and ischemic heart disease. American Journal of Clinical Nutrition. 1967;20(5):462–74.

839. **Chadha SL, Ramachadran K, Shekhawat S, Tandon R, Gopinath N.** A 3-year follow-up study of coronary heart disease in Delhi. Bulletin of the World Health Organisation. 1993;71:67–72.

840. **Sehmi J, Salaheen D, Yeo Y, Zhang W, Das D, McCarthy MI,** et al. A genome-wide association study in Indian Asians identifies four susceptibility loci for type-2 diabetes. Heart. 2011;97(Suppl 1):A43–A.

841. **Admiraal WM, Vlaar EM, Nierkens V, Holleman F, Middelkoop BJC, Stronks K,** et al. Intensive lifestyle intervention in general practice to prevent type 2 diabetes among 18 to 60-year-old South Asians: 1-year effects on the weight status and metabolic profile of participants in a randomized controlled trial. PLoS ONE. 2013;8(7):e68605.

842. **Mathews G, Alexander J, Rahemtulla T, Bhopal R.** Impact of a cardiovascular risk control project for South Asians (Khush Dil) on motivation, behaviour, obesity, blood pressure and lipids. Journal of Public Health. 2007;29(4):388–97.

843. **Rush EC, Chandu V, Plank LD.** Reduction of abdominal fat and chronic disease factors by lifestyle change in migrant Asian Indians older than 50 years. Asia Pacific Journal of Clinical Nutrition 2007;16(4):671–6.

844. **Adab P, Barrett T, Bhopal R, Cade JE, Canaway A, Cheng KK,** et al. The West Midlands ActiVe lifestyle and healthy Eating in School children (WAVES) study: a cluster randomised controlled trial testing the clinical effectiveness and cost-effectiveness of a multifaceted obesity prevention intervention programme targeted at children aged 6-7 years. Health Technol Assessment. 2018;22(8):1–608.

845. **Sisti LG, Dajko M, Campanella P, Shkurti E, Ricciardi W, de Waure C.** The effect of multifactorial lifestyle interventions on cardiovascular risk factors: a systematic review and meta-analysis of trials conducted in the general population and high risk groups. Preventive Medicine. 2018;109:82–97.

846. **Doshmangir P, Jahangiry L, Farhangi MA, Doshmangir L, Faraji L.** The effectiveness of theory- and model-based lifestyle interventions on HbA1c among patients with type 2 diabetes: a systematic review and meta-analysis. Public Health. 2018;155:133–41.

847. **Cruickshank JK.** Challenging the orthodoxy of insulin resistance. Lancet. 1995;346:772–3.

848. **Lean MEJ, Leslie WS, Barnes AC, Brosnahan N, Thom G, McCombie L,** et al. Primary care-led weight management for remission of type 2 diabetes (DiRECT): an open-label, cluster-randomised trial. Lancet. 2017;391(10120):541–51.

849. **Hanson S, Jones A.** Is there evidence that walking groups have health benefits? A systematic review and meta-analysis. British Journal of Sports Medicine. 2015 49(11):710–15.

850. **Dehghan M, Mente A, Zhang X, Swaminathan S, Li W, Mohan V,** et al. Associations of fats and carbohydrate intake with cardiovascular disease and mortality in 18 countries from five continents (PURE): a prospective cohort study. Lancet. 2017;390(10107):2050–62.

851. Mack TM. The new pan-Asian paan problem. Lancet. 2001;**357**:1638–9.

852. Gupta Jain S, Puri S, Misra A, Gulati S, Mani K. Effect of oral cinnamon intervention on metabolic profile and body composition of Asian Indians with metabolic syndrome: a randomized double-blind control trial. Lipids in Health and Disease. 2017;**16**(1):113.

853. Gulati S, Misra A, Tiwari R, Sharma M, Pandey RM, Yadav CP. Effect of high-protein meal replacement on weight and cardiometabolic profile in overweight/obese Asian Indians in North India. British Journal of Nutrition. 2017;**117**(11):1531–40.

854. Mohan V, Anjana RM, Gayathri R, Ramya Bai M, Lakshmipriya N, Ruchi V, et al. Glycemic index of a novel high-fiber white rice variety developed in India–A randomized control trial study. Diabetes Technology & Therapeutics. 2016;**18**(3):164–70.

855. De Silva DA, Woon FP, Gan HY, Chen CP, Chang HM, Koh TH, et al. Arterial stiffness is associated with intracranial large artery disease among ethnic Chinese and South Asian ischemic stroke patients. Journal of Hypertension **27**(7):1453–1458. 2009;**27**(7):1453–8.

856. Ghouri N, Purves D, Deans KA, Logan G, McConnachie A, Wilson J, et al. An investigation of two-dimensional ultrasound carotid plaque presence and intima media thickness in middle-aged South Asian and European men living in the United Kingdom. PLoS One. 2015;**10**(4):e0123317.

857. Whincup PH, Nightingale CM, Owen CG, Rapala A, Bhowruth DJ, Prescott MH, et al. Ethnic differences in carotid intima-media thickness between UK Children of Black African-Caribbean and White European origin. Stroke. 2012;**43**:1747–54.

858. Stenmark KR, Davie N, Frid M, Gerasimovskaya E, Das M. Role of the adventitia in pulmonary vascular remodeling. Physiology (Bethesda). 2006;**21**:134–45.

859. World Health Organization. Diabetes mellitus: report of a study group. Geneva: 1985. Technical Report Series No. 727.

860. Petersen JL, McGuire DK,. Impaired glucose tolerance and impaired fasting glucose–a review of diagnosis, clinical implications and management. Diabetes & Vascular Disease Research. 2005;**2**(1):9–15.

861. de Courten B, de Courten MP, Soldatos G, Dougherty SL, Straznicky N, Schlaich M, et al. Diet low in advanced glycation end products increases insulin sensitivity in healthy overweight individuals: a double-blind, randomized, crossover trial. American Journal of Clinical Nutrition. 2016;**103**(6):1426–33.

862. Kellow NJ, Savige GS. Dietary advanced glycation end-product restriction for the attenuation of insulin resistance, oxidative stress and endothelial dysfunction: a systematic review. European Journal of Clinical Nutrition. 2013;**67**(3):239–48.

863. Xian H, Vasilopoulos T, Liu W, Hauger RL, Jacobson KC, Lyons MJ, et al. Steeper change in body mass across four decades predicts poorer cardiometabolic outcomes at midlife. Obesity (Silver Spring). 2017;**25**(4):773–80.

864. Finkelstein EA, Kruger E. Meta- and cost-effectiveness analysis of commercial weight loss strategies. Obesity(SilverSpring). 2014;**22**(9):1942–51.

865. Abraham C, Michie S. A taxonomy of behavior change techniques used in interventions. Health Psychology. 2008;**27**(3):379–87.

866. Carr S, Lhussier M, Forster N, Geddes L, Deane K, Pennington M, et al. An evidence synthesis of qualitative and quantitative research on component intervention

techniques, effectiveness, cost effectiveness, equity and acceptability of different versions of health-related lifestyle advisor role in improving health. Health Technology Assessment. 2011;15(9):iii–iv, 1–284.

867. Michie S, Jochelson K, Markham WA, Bridle C. Low-income groups and behaviour change interventions: a review of intervention content, effectiveness and theoretical frameworks. Journal of Epidemiology and Community Health. 2009;63(8):610–22.

868. Craig P, Dieppe P, Macintyre S, Michie S, Nazareth I, Petticrew M. Developing and evaluating complex interventions: the new Medical Research Council guidance. BMJ. 2008;337:a1655.

869. Davidson EM, Liu JJ, Bhopal RS, White M, Johnson MR, Netto G, et al. Behavior change interventions to improve the health of racial and ethnic minority populations: A tool kit of adaptation approaches. Milbank Quarterly 2013;91(4):811–51.

870. Wallia S, Douglas A, Bhopal R, Sharma A, Hutchison A, et al. Culturally adapting the prevention of diabetes and obesity in South Asians (PODOSA) trial. Health Promotion International. 2014;29(4):768–79.

871. Allender S, Owen B, Kuhlberg J, Lowe J, Nagorcka-Smith P, Whelan J, et al. A community based systems diagram of obesity causes. PLoS One 2015;10(7):e0129683.

872. Whelan J, Love P, Pettman T, Doyle J, Booth S, Smith E, et al. Cochrane update: Predicting sustainability of intervention effects in public health evidence: identifying key elements to provide guidance. Journal of Public Health. 2014;36(2):347–51.

873. Adams KF, Subramanian SV. Commentary: Is the concern regarding overweight/ obesity in India overstated? International Journal of Epidemiology. 2008;37(5):1005–7.

874. Garshick M, Wu F, Demmer R, Parvez F, Ahmed A, Eunus M, et al. The association between socioeconomic status and subclinical atherosclerosis in a rural Bangladesh population. Preventive Medicine. 2017;102:6–11.

875. Gupta R, Gupta VP, Ahluwalia NS. Educational status, coronary heart disease, and coronary risk factor prevalence in a rural population of India. British Medical Journal. 1994;309:1332–6.

876. Pais P, Pogue J, Gerstein H, Zachariah E, Savitha D, Nayak PR, et al. Risk factors for acute myocardial infarction in Indians: a case-control study. Lancet. 1996;348:358–63.

877. Gupta R, Misra A, Pais P, Rastogi P, Gupta VP. Correlation of regional cardiovascular disease mortality in India with lifestyle and nutritional factors. International Journal of Cardiology. 2006;108(3):291–300.

878. Enas EA, Singh V, Munjal YP, Bhandari S, Yadave RD, Manchanda SC. Reducing the burden of coronary artery disease in India: challenges and opportunities. Indian Heart Journal. 2008;60(2):161–75.

879. National Institute of Nutrition. Dietary Guidelines for Indians - A Manual. 2011. Available from: http://ninindia.org/DietaryGuidelinesforNINwebsite.pdf.

880. Enas EA, Kannan S. How to Beat the Heart Disease Epidemic Among South Asians: A Prevention and Management Guide for Asian Indians and Their Doctors. Chicago: Grace Printing; 2005.

881. Kooner JS. Coronary heart disease in UK Indian Asians: the potential for reducing mortality. Heart. 1997;78(6):530–2.

882. **Enas EA, Chacko V, Pazhoor SG, Chennikkara H, Devarapalli HP.** Dyslipidemia in South Asian patients. Current Atherosclerosis Reports 2007;**9**(5):367–74.

883. **Aarabi M, Jackson PR.** Predicting coronary risk in UK South Asians: an adjustment method for Framingham-based tools. European Journal of Cardiovascular Prevention and Rehabilitation 2005;**12**(1):46–51.

884. JBS 2: Joint British Societies' guidelines on prevention of cardiovascular disease in clinical practice. Heart. 2005;**91**(suppl 5):v1–v52.

885. Joint British recommendations on prevention of coronary heart disease in clinical practice. Heart. 1998;**80**(suppl 2):S1–S29.

886. **Kakde S, Bhopal RS, Bhardwaj S, Misra A.** Urbanized South Asians' susceptibility to coronary heart disease: The high-heat food preparation hypothesis. Nutrition. 2016;**33**:216–224.

887. **Malcolm G.** Cod liver oil and tuberculosis. BMJ. 2011;**343**:d7505.

888. **Battu HS, Bhopal R, Agyemang C.** Heterogeneity in blood pressure in UK Bangladeshi, Indian and Pakistani, compared to White, populations: divergence of adults and children. Journal of Human Hypertension. 2018 Sep 4. doi: 10.1038/s41371-018-0095-5. [Epub ahead of print]

Index

Tables, figures, and boxes are indicated by an italic *t*, *f*, and *b* following the page number.

plasminogen 181
plasticity 90
PODOSA trial 236
pollution 124, 192, 207
polymorphisms 40–1, 42–3
polyunsaturated fatty acids 11*t*
population case series (register) 28
population groups 27
population sciences 7, 12, 23
postprandial 10, 154, 159
poverty 16–17, 129, 132–3
predation release hypothesis 47*t*, 48–9, 54*b*
predicted risk 227, 230–1, 231*t*
pregnancy, post-partum weight loss 233
prevention 226–32
processed foods 126, 153, 154, 156
pro-coagulant state 180–1
programming 90
pro-inflammatory state 67, 179–80
prospective birth cohort studies 97, 98*t*, 106
prospective cohort study 28
psychosocial factors 19*t*, 122, 128–31, 134–6
publication bias 106
public health (policy) 224–5
Pune Maternal Nutrition Study 111–12, 120*b*, 272
PURE study 141, 170
pyridoxine 178

Q-risk model 231

racism 128, 129, 130, 131
Rafnsson, S.B. 55*b*
Raghupathy, P. 101*t*, 111
randomized, blinded and controlled trials 28–9
Rao, S. 104*t*, 112
Reaven, G.M. 10, 32*f*, 36*b*
recessive gene 43
reference populations 12–14
relative risk 30
renal function 184–5
research 224–5
retrospective cohort studies 97
rickets 176
risk scores 227, 230–1, 231*t*
rural populations 10, 124
rural-to-urban migration 124, 127–8, 144, 156

SABRE study 28, 236
Sachdev, H.S. 100*t*, 110
salt 154, 168
Sattar, N. 171*b*
saturated fats 152, 153
Scotland 3
Scragg, R. 248*t*, 266
selection bias 29

sex differences
    bodily dimensions 59
    obesity patterns 61, 63
sickle cell disease 43
single nucleotide polymorphisms (SNPs) 40–1, 43
skinfold thickness 114
sleep 191
smoking, *see* tobacco
Sniderman, A.D. 65*f*, 71*b*
socio-economic development 17, 122–38, 204*f*, 205, 207
    demographic and epidemiological transitions 122, 123–4
    lifestyle 122, 124
    poverty 132–3
    psychosocial factors 122, 128–31, 134–7
    wealth 133–4
soil toxins 192
soldier-to-diplomat hypothesis 75, 76, 77*f*, 78–9, 81, 82*b*
South Asia(ns), definitions 6–8
Speakman, J.R. 54*b*
Srivastava, U. 9, 10, 33*b*
Stein, C.E. 98*t*, 110
stress 128–31
stroke
    atherosclerosis 15, 125
    blood pressure 144
    haemorrhagic 15, 16–17, 125
    pathology 15–17
    socio-economics 125, 126
Stronks, K. 248*t*, 267
study design 27–9
subcutaneous/ cutaneous 55–66
superficial subcutaneous fat 62*t*, 65
syndrome X 83*b*, 193
systolic BP 144–5

telomeres 191
theory 30
thin-fat phenotype 64, 270
thresholds for action 238–9
thrifty genotype hypothesis 38–9, 41, 44–8, 51, 52*b*
thrifty phenotype hypothesis 93–6, 116*b*
thrombosis 180–1
thyroid dysfunction 185–6
Tillin, T. 171*b*
tobacco 11*t*, 18*t*, 20*t*, 126, 141, 149–52, 227, 228*t*, 240
toxins 192
traditional healing 234
trans fatty acids 19*t*, 137*b*, 138*b*, 148–9, 153, 156
trials 28–9
triglycerides 19*t*, 146
tropical diabetes 20
trunk 58